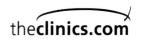

PEDIATRIC CLINICS
OF NORTH AMERICA

Scientific Foundations
of Clinical Practice, Part I

GUEST EDITORS
Ellis D. Avner, MD
Robert M. Kliegman, MD

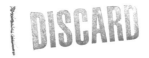

August 2006 • Volume 53 • Number 4

SAUNDERS

An Imprint of Elsevier, Inc.
PHILADELPHIA   LONDON   TORONTO   MONTREAL   SYDNEY   TOKYO

W.B. SAUNDERS COMPANY
A Division of Elsevier Inc.

1600 John F. Kennedy Boulevard • Suite 1800 • Philadelphia, Pennsylvania 19103

http://www.theclinics.com

THE PEDIATRIC CLINICS OF NORTH AMERICA	Volume 53, Number 4
August 2006	ISSN 0031-3955
Editor: Carla Holloway	ISBN 1-4160-3896-5

The ideas and opinions expressed in *The Pediatric Clinics of North America* do not necessarily reflect those o the Publisher. The Publisher does not assume any responsibility for any injury and/or damage to person or property arising out of or related to any use of the material contained in this periodical. The reader i advised to check the appropriate medical literature and the product information currently provided by the manufacturer of each drug to be administered to verify the dosage, the method and duration of adminis tration, or contraindications. It is the responsibility of the treating physician or other health care profes sional, relying on independent experience and knowledge of the patient, to determine drug dosages an the best treatment for the patient. Mention of any product in this issue should not be construed as endorse ment by the contributors, editors, or the Publisher of the product or manufacturers' claims.

The Pediatric Clinics of North America (ISSN 0031-3955) is published bi-monthly by W.B. Saunders, 360 Par Avenue South, New York, NY 10010-1710. Months of publication are February, April, June, August, Octo ber, and December. Business and Editorial Offices: 1600 John F. Kennedy Blvd., Suite 1800, Philadelphia PA 19103-2899. Accounting and Circulation Offices: 6277 Sea Harbor Drive, Orlando, FL 32887-4800 Periodicals postage paid at New York, NY and additional mailing offices. Subscription prices are $125.00 per year (US individuals), $260.00 per year (US institutions), $170.00 per year (Canadian indivi duals), $340.00 per year (Canadian institutions), $190.00 per year (international individuals), $340.00 pe year (international institutions), $65.00 per year (US students), $100.00 per year (Canadian students) and $100.00 per year (foreign students). To receive students/resident rare, orders must be accompanie by name of affiliated institution, date of term, and the signature of program/residency coordinator o institution letterhead. Orders will be billed at individual rate until proof of status is received. Foreig air speed delivery is included in all Clinics subscription prices. All prices are subject to change withou notice. POSTMASTER: Send address changes to *The Pediatric Clinics of North America*, Elsevier Periodical Customer Service, 6277 Sea Harbor Drive, Orlando, FL 32887-4800. **Customer Service: 1-800-654-245 (US). From outside of the US, call 1-407-345-4000.** E-mail: hhspcs@harcourt.com.

The Pediatric Clinics of North America is also published in Spanish by McGraw-Hill Inter-americana Editore S.A., Mexico City, Mexico; in Portuguese by Riechmann and Affonso Editores, Rua Comandante Coelh 1085, CEP 21250, Rio de Janeiro, Brazil; and in Greek by Althayia SA, Athens, Greece.

The Pediatric Clinics of North America is covered in *Index Medicus, Excerpta Medica, Current Contents, Curren Contents/Clinical Medicine, Science Citation Index, ASCA, ISI/BIOMED*, and *BIOSIS*.

Printed in the United States of America.

GUEST EDITORS

ELLIS D. AVNER, MD, Associate Dean for Research, Professor of Pediatrics, Medical College of Wisconsin; Director, Children's Research Institute, Children's Hospital and Health System of Wisconsin, Milwaukee, Wisconsin

ROBERT M. KLIEGMAN, MD, Muma Professor and Chair, Department of Pediatrics, Medical College of Wisconsin; Executive Vice President, Children's Research Institute, Children's Hospital and Health System of Wisconsin, Milwaukee, Wisconsin

CONTRIBUTORS

DEVENDRA K. AMRE, MBBS, PhD, Assistant Professor of Pediatrics, Department of Pediatrics, University of Montreal, Research Center, Saint-Justine Hospital, Montreal, Quebec, Canada

RAYMOND C. BARFIELD, MD, PHD, Assistant Member, Division of Stem Cell Transplantation, St. Jude Children's Research Hospital, Memphis, Tennessee

DAVID P. BICK, MD, Associate Professor, Division of Medical Genetics, Department of Pediatrics; Department of Obstetrics and Gynecology; and Human and Molecular Genetics Center, Medical College of Wisconsin, Milwaukee, Wisconsin

LAURE DEMATTIA, DO, Instructor of Family and Community Medicine, Medical College of Wisconsin, The NEW (Nutrition, Exercise, and Weight-management) Kids™ Program, Children's Hospital of Wisconsin, Milwaukee, Wisconsin

KENNETH W. GOW, MD, Assistant Professor, Department of Surgery, Division of Pediatric Surgery, Emory University School of Medicine, Atlanta, Georgia

WILLIAM J. GROSSMAN, MD, PhD, Assistant Professor, Division of Hematology/Oncology/Blood & Marrow Transplantation, Department of Pediatrics, Medical College of Wisconsin, Milwaukee, Wisconsin

MARTIN J. HESSNER, PhD, Associate Professor of Pediatrics, Section of Endocrinology, The Medical College of Wisconsin, Milwaukee, Wisconsin

RONALD N. HINES, PhD, Professor of Pediatrics and Pharmacology and Toxicology, Co-Chief, Section of Clinical Pharmacology, Pharmacogenetics and Teratology, Medical College of Wisconsin; Associate Director, Children's Research Institute, Children's Hospital and Health Systems, Milwaukee, Wisconsin

HOWARD J. JACOB, PhD, Warren P. Knowles Professor of Human and Molecular Genetics, Professor of Pediatrics (Genetics), and Professor of Physiology (Genetics), Medical College of Wisconsin and Children's Research Institute; and Director of Human and Molecular Genetics Center, Medical College of Wisconsin, Milwaukee, Wisconsin

CHANDY C. JOHN, MD, MS, Associate Professor, Department of Pediatrics and Medicine; Director, Global Pediatrics Program, University of Minnesota Medical School; University of Minnesota Children's Hospital, Minneapolis, Minnesota

ERIC KODISH, MD, F.J. O'Neill Professor and Chairman, Department of Bioethics, Cleveland Clinic Foundation, Lerner College of Medicine at Case, Cleveland, Ohio

SUBRA KUGATHASAN, MD, Associate Professor of Pediatrics, Department of Pediatrics, Medical College of Wisconsin, Milwaukee, Wisconsin

ANNE E. KWITEK, PhD, Associate Professor of Physiology, The Medical College of Wisconsin, Milwaukee, Wisconsin

EDUARDO C. LAU, PhD, Assistant Professor, Division of Medical Genetics, Department of Pediatrics and Human and Molecular Genetics Center, Medical College of Wisconsin, Milwaukee, Wisconsin

MINGYU LIANG, MB, PhD, Assistant Professor of Physiology, The Medical College of Wisconsin, Milwaukee, Wisconsin

JAMES V. LUSTIG, MD, Professor of Pediatrics (Allergy and Immunology), Medical College of Wisconsin and Children's Research Institute; and Director of Asthma and Allergy Center, Children's Hospital of Wisconsin, Milwaukee, Wisconsin

DAVID A. MARGOLIS, MD, Associate Professor of Pediatrics, Director of Blood and Marrow Transplantation, Division of Pediatric Hematology and Oncology, Medical College of Wisconsin, Milwaukee, Wisconsin

D. GAIL McCARVER, MD, Professor of Pediatrics and Pharmacology and Toxicology, Co-Chief, Section of Clinical Pharmacology, Pharmacogenetics and Teratology, Medical College of Wisconsin; Member, Children's Research Institute, Children's Hospital and Health Systems, Milwaukee, Wisconsin

JOHN R. MEURER, MD, MBA, Associate Professor of Pediatrics and Chief of General Pediatrics, Medical College of Wisconsin and Children's Research Institute; and Coalition Director and Principal Investigator, Fight Asthma Milwaukee Allies, Children's Hospital and Health System, Milwaukee, Wisconsin

LAWRENCE MILLER, PsyD, The NEW (Nutrition, Exercise, and Weight-management) Kids™ Program, Children's Hospital of Wisconsin, Milwaukee, Wisconsin

MICHAEL OLIVIER, PhD, Associate Professor of Physiology, Department of Physiology, Human and Molecular Genetics Center, Medical College of Wisconsin, Milwaukee, Wisconsin

FRANK PARK, PhD, Associate Professor, Department of Medicine, Kidney Disease Center; Department of Physiology, Medical College of Wisconsin, Milwaukee, Wisconsin

CONTRIBUTORS

LINDA M. REIS, MS, Certified Genetic Counselor, Children's Hospital of Wisconsin, Milwaukee, Wisconsin

MARK S. RUTTUM, MD, Professor of Ophthalmology, Director of Pediatric Ophthalmology, Medical College of Wisconsin, Milwaukee, Wisconsin

RUSSELL E. SCHEFFER, MD, Associate Professor of Psychiatry, Chucker Aring Professor of Psychiatry; Director, Child and Adolescent Psychiatry and Behavioral Medicine, Medical College of Wisconsin and Children's Hospital of Wisconsin, Milwaukee, Wisconsin

JOHN R. SCHREIBER, MD, Ruben-Bentson Chair in Pediatrics; Head, Department of Pediatrics, University of Minnesota Medical School; University of Minnesota Children's Hospital, Minneapolis, Minnesota

ELENA V. SEMINA, PhD, Associate Professor, Pediatric Genetics, Medical College of Wisconsin, Milwaukee, Wisconsin

JOSEPH A. SKELTON, MD, Assistant Professor of Pediatrics, Division of Pediatric Gastroenterology and Nutrition, Medical College of Wisconsin; The NEW (Nutrition, Exercise, and Weight-management) Kids™ Program, Children's Hospital of Wisconsin, Milwaukee, Wisconsin

JULIE-AN M. TALANO, MD, Assistant Professor of Pediatrics, Division of Pediatric Hematology and Oncology, Medical College of Wisconsin, Milwaukee, Wisconsin

JAMES W. VERBSKY, MD, PhD, Assistant Professor, Division of Rheumatology, Department of Pediatrics, Medical College of Wisconsin, Milwaukee, Wisconsin

CONTENTS

for adult- and pediatric-based therapies. This article provides a historical perspective, but most importantly, uses this background to illustrate important principles of the field. The application of pharmacogenomics to asthma therapy is presented as an example of the current status of pharmacogenomics as it is being applied to an important pediatric health problem. Finally, a discussion of future promises and challenges to the application of pharmacogenomics is presented, including economic and ethical issues.

Many pediatric diseases have now reached a therapeutic plateau using standard therapy. Gene therapy has emerged as an exciting new means to achieve specific therapeutic benefit. Although there have been important and promising breakthroughs in recent clinical trials, there have been some serious setbacks that have tempered this initial excitement. In this review, we discuss the important developments in the field of gene therapy as it applies to various pediatric diseases and relate the recent successes and failures to the future potential of gene therapy as a medical therapeutic application.

Many scientific advances in molecular medicine, such as those made in genomics, stem cell transplantation, and neurobiology, raise important ethical issues that are relevant to pediatrics. Although some of these novel issues appear to be nearly without precedent, others are illuminated by reflection on prior challenges. How do we approach such complex ethical questions in the context of pluralism? This article examines several important areas in molecular medicine exemplifying fundamental ethical questions that are broadly applicable.

Knowledge of the genetic mutations of primary immune deficiency syndromes has grown significantly over the last 30 years. In this article the authors present an overview of the clinical aspects, laboratory evaluation, and genetic defects of primary immunodeficiencies, with an emphasis on the pathophysiology of the known molecular defects. This article is designed to give the primary pediatrician a general knowledge of this rapidly expanding field.

FORTHCOMING ISSUES

RECENT ISSUES

PEDIATRIC CLINICS OF NORTH AMERICA AUGUST 2006

GOAL STATEMENT

The goal of *Pediatric Clinics of North America* is to keep practicing physicians and residents up to date with current clinical practice in pediatrics by providing timely articles reviewing the state-of-the-art in patient care.

ACCREDITATION

The *Pediatric Clinics of North America* is planned and implemented in accordance with the Essential Areas and Policies of the Accreditation Council for Continuing Medical Education (ACCME) through the joint sponsorship of the University of Virginia School of Medicine and Elsevier. The University of Virginia School of Medicine is accredited by the ACCME to provide continuing medical education for physicians.

The University of Virginia School of Medicine designates this educational activity for a maximum of 15 AMA PRA Category 1 Credits™. Physicians should only claim credit commensurate with the extent of their participation in the activity.

The American Medical Association has determined that physicians not licensed in the US who participate in this CME activity are eligible for 15 AMA PRA Category 1 Credits™.

Category 1 credit can be earned by reading the text material, taking the CME examination online at http://www.theclinics.com/home/cme, and completing the evaluation. After taking the test, you will be required to review any and all incorrect answers. Following completion of the test and evaluation, your credit will be awarded and you may print your certificate.

FACULTY DISCLOSURE/CONFLICT OF INTEREST

The University of Virginia School of Medicine, as an ACCME accredited provider, endorses and strives to comply with the Accreditation Council for Continuing Medical Education (ACCME) Standards of Commercial Support, Commonwealth of Virginia statutes, University of Virginia policies and procedures, and associated federal and private regulations and guidelines on the need for disclosure and monitoring of proprietary and financial interests that may affect the scientific integrity and balance of content delivered in continuing medical education activities under our auspices.

The University of Virginia School of Medicine requires that all CME activities accredited through this institution be developed independently and be scientifically rigorous, balanced and objective in the presentation/discussion of its content, theories and practices.

All authors/editors participating in an accredited CME activity are expected to disclose to the readers relevant financial relationships with commercial entities occurring within the past 12 months (such as grants or research support, employee, consultant, stock holder, member of speakers bureau, etc.). The University of Virginia School of Medicine will employ appropriate mechanisms to resolve potential conflicts of interest to maintain the standards of fair and balanced education to the reader. Questions about specific strategies can be directed to the Office of Continuing Medical Education, University of Virginia School of Medicine, Charlottesville, Virginia.

The authors/editors listed below have identified no financial or professional relationships for themselves or their spouse/partner: Devendra Amre, MBBS, PhD; Ellis D. Avner, MD; Raymond C. Barfield, MD, PhD; David P. Bick, MD; Laure DeMattia, DO; Kenneth W. Gow, MD; William J. Grossman, MD, PhD; Martin J. Hessner, PhD; Carla Holloway, Acquisitions Editor; Chandy C. John, MD, MS; Robert Kliegman, MD; Eric Kodish, MD; Subra Kugathasan, MD; Anne E. Kwitek, PhD; Eduardo C. Lau, PhD; Mingyu Liang, MB, PhD; James V. Lustig, MD; David A. Margolis, MD; Lawrence Miller, PsyD; Michael Olivier, PhD; Frank Park, PhD; Linda M. Reis, MS; Mark S. Ruttum, MD; John R. Schreiber, MD; Elena V. Semina, PhD; Joseph A. Skelton, MD; Julie-An M. Talano, MD; and, James W. Verbsky, MD, PhD.

The authors/editors listed below identified the following professional or financial affiliations for themselves or their spouse/partner:
Ronald N. Hines, PhD is a consultant for AXCAN Pharma.
Howard J. Jacob, PhD has stock/ownership in PhysioGenix, Inc.
D. Gail McCarver, MD disclosed that her spouse was a consultant and received a consulting fee from Axcan Pharma, Montreal, Canada.
John R. Meurer, MD, MBA has unrestricted CME with GlaxoSmithKline and AstraZeneca.
Russell E. Scheffer, MD is an independent contractor and is on the speaker's bureau for AstraZeneca and Bristol Meyer Squibb, and is an independent contractor for Forest Labs

Disclosure of Discussion of Non-FDA Approved Uses for Pharmaceutical and/or Medical Devices:
The University of Virginia School of Medicine, as an ACCME provider, requires that all authors identify and disclose any "off label" uses for pharmaceutical and medical device products. The University of Virginia School of Medicine recommends that each physician fully review all the available data on new products or procedures prior to clinical use.

TO ENROLL

To enroll in the Pediatric Clinics of North America Continuing Medical Education program, call customer service at **1-800-654-2452** or visit us online at www.theclinics.com/home/cme. The CME program is available to subscribers for an additional fee of $195.00.

PEDIATRIC CLINICS

OF NORTH AMERICA

ELSEVIER
SAUNDERS

Pediatr Clin N Am 53 (2006) xv–xvi

Preface

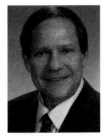
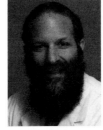

Ellis D. Avner, MD   Robert M. Kliegman, MD
Guest Editors

The development of genomic medicine has ushered in a new era of pediatric practice. The practitioner is faced with an enormous body of new data that are changing the nature of diagnostics, preventative medicine, and therapeutics. A new vocabulary of quantitative trait loci, single nucleotide polymorphisms, polymerase chain reaction (PCR), microarrays, preimplantation genetic diagnosis, pharmacogenomics, proteomics, and functional genomics are now part of clinical practice.

The goal of these two issues of the *Pediatric Clinics* is to translate this new vocabulary into a meaningful framework for the pediatric practitioner. By providing new insights into many pathophysiological processes, genomic medicine has enriched the scientific foundations of pediatrics markedly and has created amazing new approaches to the diagnosis and care provided to patients. For example, instead of using tedious culture methods to identify various viral pathogens, most hospital clinical viral diagnostic laboratories use RNA/DNA-based PCR tests to detect the specific viral genome. These new tests are more specific and sensitive, but more importantly, they are rapid, allowing for a quick definitive diagnosis, shorter periods of unnecessary antibiotic therapy, and a short length of hospitalization.

In the current volume, a talented group of translational investigators initially reviews the methodologies that form the basis of this revolution in clinical practice, and then demonstrates how such scientific advances have improved understanding of disease mechanisms, and diagnostics and therapeutics in numerous common pediatric diseases.

We believe that understanding these new scientific foundations of clinical practice is essential for all pediatric care providers and that this understanding will improve the bedside and ambulatory management and outcomes of pediatric patients.

Ellis D. Avner, MD
Medical College of Wisconsin
Children's Research Institute
Children's Hospital and Health System of Wisconsin
999 North 92nd Street
Milwaukee, WI 53226, USA

E-mail address: eavner@mcw.edu

Robert M. Kliegman, MD
Department of Pediatrics
Medical College of Wisconsin
Children's Research Institute
Children's Hospital and Health System of Wisconsin
999 North 92nd Street
Milwaukee, WI 53226, USA

E-mail address: rkliegma@mail.mcw.edu

ELSEVIER
SAUNDERS

PEDIATRIC CLINICS
OF NORTH AMERICA

Pediatr Clin N Am 53 (2006) 559–577

Preimplantation Genetic Diagnosis

David P. Bick, MD[a,b,c,*], Eduardo C. Lau, PhD[a,c]

[a]Division of Medical Genetics, Department of Pediatrics, Medical College of Wisconsin,
8701 Watertown Plank Road, Milwaukee, WI 53226, USA
[b]Department of Obstetrics and Gynecology, Medical College of Wisconsin,
Milwaukee, WI 53226, USA
[c]Human and Molecular Genetics Center, Medical College of Wisconsin,
Milwaukee, WI 53226, USA

Preimplantation genetic diagnosis (PGD) is a procedure to analyze the genetic make-up of embryos formed through in vitro fertilization (IVF). Based on this analysis embryos are selected for transfer to the uterus to establish a pregnancy. PGD was first accomplished by Alan Handyside in 1990 when his team performed embryo sex determination in families known to carry X-linked diseases [1]. By choosing to have only female embryos transferred to the uterus, these women ensured that their offspring would not be male and thereby eliminated the possibility of bearing an affected male child. Following this initial success, PGD has been used to test for a variety of chromosomal disorders [2], single-gene disorders [3], and recently human leukocyte antigen (HLA) typing of embryos to establish potential donor progeny for hemopoietic stem cell treatment of siblings in need of stem cell transplantation [4].

PGD represents an important adjunct to traditional prenatal testing through amniocentesis or chorionic villus sampling. Although traditional methods can accurately identify fetuses that have chromosome disorders and single-gene disorders during pregnancy, couples must make difficult choices when these tests find an affected fetus. PGD permits couples to avoid the issue of pregnancy termination by initiating pregnancies with unaffected embryos.

This article reviews key aspects of patient management, relevant IVF and PGD procedures, methods used in the genetic analysis, technical difficulties that can affect test results, and indications for PGD. It also examines some of the emerging technologies being introduced into PGD.

---

* Corresponding author. Division of Medical Genetics, Department of Pediatrics, Medical College of Wisconsin, 8701 Watertown Plank Road, Milwaukee, WI 53226.

E-mail address: dbick@mcw.edu (D.P. Bick).

0031-3955/06/$ - see front matter © 2006 Elsevier Inc. All rights reserved.
doi:10.1016/j.pcl.2006.05.006
pediatric.theclinics.com

Patient management

The practice of PGD has evolved significantly over the 15 years since the original reports. During that time many clinical and laboratory procedures have been developed to improve the accuracy and reliability of PGD and to expand the number of conditions that can be tested [5]. The complexity of PGD requires a multidisciplinary team approach that includes reproductive endocrinologists, geneticists, nurses, genetic counselors, embryologists, cytogeneticists, and molecular biologists.

The first step for patients considering PGD is reproductive and genetic counseling. Consultation with a reproductive endocrinologist and nursing staff before embarking on treatment focuses on a discussion of the details of IVF, the risks of medical complications that can occur during ovarian stimulation and oocyte retrieval [6,7], the medications that will be used, the patient experience during an IVF stimulation cycle (often referred to as a "cycle"), the treatment timeline, and the cost. Medical history and laboratory testing of the patient and her male partner before a cycle are used to help predict the probability of success.

Consultation with a geneticist or genetic counselor focuses on an assessment of the genetic risk faced by the patient based on her history, her partner's history, and family history. This information provides the basis for a discussion of the nature, severity, and recurrence risk of the genetic disorders in the family as well as age-related risks. This discussion indicates whether PGD can be helpful for a particular patient's situation and the probability that PGD can identify an unaffected embryo. PGD requires that a DNA test or cytogenetic test exists that can identify the relevant abnormality in a cell derived from an embryo. Details of the test determine the chance that a normal embryo can be identified, the reliability of the test, and the chance of misdiagnosis. It is important that patients weigh PGD against other reproductive options and alternatives such as prenatal diagnosis, gamete donation (use of an egg or sperm donor), remaining childless, accepting the genetic risk without further testing, and adoption.

By combining patient-specific reproductive and genetic information, the reproductive medicine staff can discuss how many oocytes might be retrieved, how many embryos are likely to result, and the outcome of embryo biopsy (removal of one or more cells for analysis). Not all embryos are suitable for biopsy, and some may not survive biopsy. Biopsied cells may not yield a result, may yield ambiguous result, or, rarely, may give inaccurate results. Patients are made aware of the possibility that all embryos may be affected. They are also informed of the probability of a live birth for a given number of transferred embryos, the rate of pregnancy loss, and the risk of multiple births. Prenatal diagnosis is generally recommended to confirm the results of PGD. These discussions take place before and during the cycle to provide patients with a realistic expectation of their chance of success at every step in the process.

Before IVF is started, there is a discussion of the fate of embryos that are not transferred to the uterus. Patients generally cryopreserve appropriate embryos for use in a future cycles should the current cycle fail. Affected and nonviable embryos that are not transferred are discarded, although some couples choose to donate these embryos for research. The central principle that guides this and all other aspects of the PGD process is respect for patient autonomy [8]. At present, patients continue to be able to make these reproductive and genetic decisions despite increasing government regulation of assisted reproductive technologies [9,10].

In vitro fertilization and intracytoplasmic sperm injection

Patients who proceed with PGD are given medications to stimulate the ovaries to produce oocytes and other medications to make the endometrium receptive to embryos transferred into the uterine cavity [11]. During ovarian stimulation ultrasound examination and serum estradiol levels generally are used to assess follicular development [12]. Human chorionic gonadotropin is administered approximately 36 hours before retrieval to complete oocyte maturation [13]. The mature oocytes are retrieved with ultrasound guidance under conscious sedation [14]. Conventional IVF is performed by combining an egg with about 50,000 to 100,000 motile sperm for 12 to 18 hours on the day of retrieval [15], although a smaller number of sperm and a shorter time interval can be successful [16,17].

When PGD is performed following conventional IVF, many sperm cells often are present at the time of embryo biopsy on the third day after retrieval. As a result there is a chance that DNA from sperm cells will contaminate the biopsy and potentially produce erroneous results. This problem has been circumvented by the use of intracytoplasmic sperm injection (ICSI). The ICSI procedure takes a single sperm cell and injects it into the egg to fertilize it, thereby eliminating the risk of contamination with spermatozoan DNA at biopsy [18].

Embryo biopsy

Three methods have been developed to carry out PGD. The most widely used approach tests individual cells (blastomeres) obtained on the third day after in vitro fertilization of the egg at the cleavage stage (approximately eight cells). One or two blastomeres are removed through a hole created in the zona pellucida, and the cells are analyzed (Fig. 1) [19]. Based on this analysis, selected embryos are subsequently transferred to the uterus on day 4 or day 5 after IVF.

An alternative method for carrying out PGD examines the genetic material within the first and second polar bodies, the by-products of meiosis I

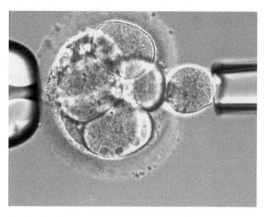

Fig. 1. Removal of a single cell from an embryo. (Courtesy of M. Roesler, MS, Milwaukee, WI.)

and meiosis II, respectively. The polar bodies contain the genetic material that is absent from the female pronucleus that will combine with the male pronucleus to become the zygote. By establishing whether there is an abnormal gene or chromosome arrangement in the polar bodies, it is possible to infer the maternal genetic contribution to the embryo. This method can be used in cases of maternally derived dominant mutations, translocations, and aneuploidy. It cannot be used when paternally derived genetic information is critical to the diagnosis, such as paternally derived dominant mutations, translocations, and aneuploidy [20]. In cases of recessive disorders, it can provide information about the maternal contribution, but not the paternal contribution, and therefore is helpful when the polar body biopsy shows that the embryo received the normal copy of the gene in question. Unlike blastomere biopsy, in which two cells can be studied to replicate data, polar body biopsy data cannot be replicated unless the polar body biopsy is followed by blastomere biopsy.

The third and latest method is blastocyst-stage biopsy [21]. This technique is performed at approximately 5 to 6 days after insemination. The embryo at this stage has differentiated into the trophectoderm, which gives rise to the placenta, and the inner cell mass, which gives rise to the fetus. Laser-assisted biopsy of the human blastocyst using a noncontact infrared laser for drilling of the zona pellucida enables removal of several cells from the trophectoderm layer [22]. It does not expose the embryos to chemicals and does not invade the inner cell mass destined for fetal development. Because several cells can be removed from the trophectoderm for analysis, the accuracy and reliability of PGD is improved. Results are available for a day-6 transfer. In one recent study of 1050 biopsied blastocysts, 93% gave unambiguous results [23]. As blastocyst culture and cryopreservation improve, it is expected that this technique will supplant cleavage stage biopsy and polar body biopsy.

Analysis of genetic material from biopsy

There are a number of different approaches to testing the genetic material derived from PGD. The most commonly used are fluorescence in situ hybridization (FISH) and polymerase chain reaction (PCR). FISH is performed by fixing the cells derived from the biopsy to slides and hybridizing with fluorescently labeled chromosome-specific DNA probes. Individual cells are probed with a mixture of probes (Fig. 2) and then are stripped and probed with a second mixture (Fig. 3), permitting the diagnosis of abnormal cells (Fig. 4) [5]. This approach is used to identify aneuploidy and chromosome rearrangements such as translocations and for sex determination in the setting of X-linked disease and family balancing.

PCR is a DNA-amplification process performed on individual cells derived from the embryo biopsy that results in millions of copies of a few carefully chosen short sequences (loci) within the genome, generally 100 to 500 base pairs in length. To increase the signal from a single cell, the PCR product from the initial amplification can be used in a second PCR reaction to permit the detection of DNA mutations or polymorphic short tandem repeats (STRs) used in linkage analysis. The use of two rounds of PCR is referred to as "nested PCR" [5].

Accuracy of preimplantation genetic diagnosis

PGD is associated with a number of potential pitfalls that can result in misdiagnosis. Single-cell FISH is limited by the number of probes that

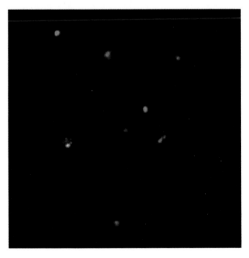

Fig. 2. Fluorescence in situ hybridization of a blastomere. Normal result. Chromosome 13, red; chromosome 18, aqua; chromosome 21, green; chromosome X, blue; chromosome Y, gold. (Courtesy of Peter vanTuinen, PhD, Milwaukee, Wisconsin.)

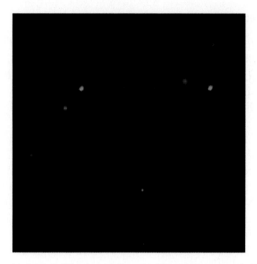

Fig. 3. Fluorescence in situ hybridization of the same blastomere as seen in Fig. 1 with a second set of probes. Normal result. Chromosome 15, red; chromosome 16, aqua; chromosome 22, green. (Courtesy of Peter vanTuinen, PhD, Milwaukee, Wisconsin.)

can be applied simultaneously because the risk of hybridization failure and FISH artifacts increases with increasing numbers of probes [24]. At present, FISH cannot test for aneuploidy of all chromosomes; therefore most programs test for numeric abnormalities involving chromosomes 13, 18, 21, X, and Y, because abnormalities in these chromosomes can result in an affected live-born infant, and also for abnormalities in chromosomes 15, 16,

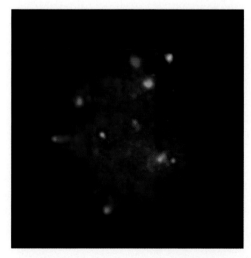

Fig. 4. Fluorescence in situ hybridization of a blastomere. Abnormal result: trisomy 13 and trisomy 21. Chromosome 13, red; chromosome 18, aqua; chromosome 21, green; chromosome X, blue; chromosome Y, gold. (Courtesy of Peter vanTuinen, PhD, Milwaukee, Wisconsin.)

and 22, which are found commonly in spontaneous abortions. Some programs test for additional chromosomes involved in miscarriage or IVF failure [25,26]. Aneuploidy testing with a limited number of FISH probes is often referred to as "aneuploidy screening" or "preimplantation genetic screening" (PGS).

One source of difficulty intrinsic to the early embryo is the presence of mosaicism (presence of two cell lines with different genotypes or karyotypes). Chromosomally normal and abnormal blastomeres can coexist within the same embryo at the early-cleavage stage. In one recent study 28% of embryos had both normal and abnormal cells within the embryo [27]. This study analyzed the copy numbers of 10 chromosomes (1, 7, 13, 15, 16, 18, 21, 22, X, and Y). It is likely that the rate of mosaicism detected would be higher if all chromosomes were analyzed. Mosaicism also can affect the results of testing in single-gene disorders (eg, when the cell studied is trisomic for the chromosome that contains the gene of interest in a single-gene disorder).

Another potential source of error is the PCR used to amplify the targeted loci in the genomic DNA from a single cell. Common artifacts of single-cell PCR include allele dropout (ADO) and preferential amplification (PA) at heterozygous loci leading to misdiagnosis [28,29]. In single-cell PCR, ADO occurs when one allele fails to be amplified. PA occurs when one allele is poorly amplified. In either instance a heterozygous embryo would appear homozygous. In the case of a dominant disorder, an affected embryo will appear normal when the mutant allele is not detected. The use of a fluorescently labeled primer in the second-round PCR reaction has greatly enhanced the sensitivity of PCR product detection, reducing the rate of PA [30]. Blastocyst biopsy is another approach to overcoming ADO and PA. PCR analysis of two to five cells in a tube together markedly reduces rates of PA and ADO [31].

The accuracy of embryo diagnosis also can be improved by combining mutation detection with linkage analysis using STRs [3,32]. The locus containing the mutation along with several closely linked STRs are coamplified in the first-round PCR. This coamplification is followed by a separate amplification of the mutation-containing locus and each of the linked STRs in the second-round PCR. Mutations can be detected by minisequencing [3,33,34], restriction enzyme analysis of PCR products [35], or sequence analysis of single-cell PCR products [29,34,36]. Simultaneous analyses of STRs that are closely linked to the mutation provide independent verification of the results of mutation testing. To avoid meiotic recombination events between the mutation and linked markers, STRs located within or close to the mutation are selected for linkage analysis.

When PCR is performed on a single cell, there is a risk of contamination by previous PCR products (amplicons) or extraneous genomic DNA in the laboratory. Contamination can be minimized by following good laboratory practices as outlined by Thornhill and colleagues [5] and by setting up reagents, first PCR reactions, second PCR reactions, and product analysis in different biosafety cabinets in different rooms of a dedicated PGD laboratory.

Despite the aforementioned precautions, there remains a small risk for inaccurate results. Therefore, confirmation of PGD results by amniocentesis or chorionic villus sampling is recommended.

Indications for preimplantation genetic diagnosis

It is known that the rate of aneuploidy rises with maternal age, as has been shown in live-born children [37], in the midtrimester of pregnancy [38], and in embryos [39]. These data argue strongly for chromosome analysis of embryos in women of advanced maternal age who are using IVF to achieve a pregnancy. Aneuploidy screening in IVF patients of advanced maternal age is the most frequent indication for PGD using FISH [40]. This rationale for PGD extends also to couples who have had a previous child born with a chromosome aneuploidy [41].

IVF patients who have had recurrent miscarriages have been shown to have higher rates of chromosomally abnormal embryos. Aneuploidy screening by PGD reduces the rate of pregnancy loss [25]. Rubio and colleagues [42] found that 26.9% of couples with recurrent miscarriage had chromosomal aberrations in all the embryos in a given cycle and that the percentage of abnormal embryos was similar in subsequent cycles. This finding suggests that once other causes of recurrent miscarriage, such as a chromosome translocation in one member of the couple, have been evaluated, PGD to test for aneuploidy is a valuable diagnostic test in patients experiencing unexplained recurrent miscarriage. Patients who have high rates of aneuploidy can be offered donor eggs rather than proceeding with more IVF cycles using their own eggs.

Among the many causes of male infertility [43] some men who have a severe male-factor condition and a normal karyotype can have chromosomally abnormal sperm. In one such study of 27 men who had oligoasthenoteratospermia and 11 who had nonobstructive azoospermia who underwent testicular sperm extraction, 79% had a significantly increased rate of aneuploidy compared with controls [44]. Aneuploidy screening of embryos has obvious utility in this situation.

Constitutional chromosome abnormalities, notably Klinefelter's syndrome and translocations, can be found in approximately 5% of infertile males [45]; 1.25% women who had secondary infertility [46] and 6% of women who had recurrent miscarriage [47] were found to harbor a chromosome abnormality. Although PGD using aneuploidy screening can be applied to the cases with Klinefelter's syndrome, translocations and other chromosomal rearrangement often require FISH probes that are not among the probes in the typical aneuploidy screening. Translocations, inversions, and other chromosomal rearrangements require the use of FISH probes that are specific to the rearrangement. Despite the technical challenge of customizing the FISH probes to each patient's situation, PGD has been shown to be highly successful in this setting. In one recent study of 45 carriers of balanced translocations, the use of PGD reduced the rate of spontaneous abortions from 87.8% to 17.8% and improved the rate of live births from 11.5% to 81.4% for this cohort [48].

Single-gene disorders represent a large and diverse group of disorders that have been approached with PGD using PCR. Some disorders, such as spinal muscular atrophy [49], are the result of a single mutation that occurs in most affected families, allowing one assay to be used repeatedly. Unfortunately many families harbor mutations that are unique to that family. As a result a customized assay must be developed for each of these families. To validate a diagnostic single-cell PCR protocol before clinical application, extensive preclinical validation on single lymphocytes is necessary to evaluate single-cell amplification efficiencies and ADO rates for all the primers to be used in the procedure. Consequently, some couples requesting PGD must wait several months to permit test development before beginning the cycle. Currently PGD is available for more than 100 different single-gene disorders [20].

PGD testing has been applied to childhood-onset recessive and dominant inherited genetic disorders, such as spinal muscular atrophy [35,49], cystic fibrosis [50], neurofibromatosis types I and II [51], β-thalassemia syndromes [52], myotonic dystrophy [53], spinocerebellar ataxia [54], and retinoblastoma [55], to name a few.

PGD testing also has been developed for a variety of X-linked inherited genetic disorders, including Duschenne/Becker muscular dystrophy [56], hemophilias A and B [33], and fragile X syndrome [57]. When a specific assay for the mutation is not available, PGD to identify female embryos for transfer can be used to eliminate the risk of an affected male. This selection requires that half of the embryos be discarded. The percentage of discarded embryos can be greatly reduced by employing MicroSort (Genetics and IVF Institute, Fairfax, Virginia) to shift the X:Y ratio in the fertilizing sperm population. MicroSort is flow cytometric sperm sorting based on the detection of differential fluorescence emitted by fluorescently stained X and Y chromosome–bearing spermatozoa. Currently in clinical trial, the method averages approximately 90% X- bearing sperm or 75% Y-bearing sperm depending on the sort parameters [58]. When appropriately sorted sperm are used with IVF, a high percentage of the resulting embryos are female [59]. To date, approximately 75% of sorts have been for X-bearing sperm, both to avoid X-linked and X-limited disease and to balance the sex ratio among a family's children. The use of MicroSort sperm has resulted in the birth of more than 700 babies to date. The major congenital malformation rate observed in birth records reviewed to date is 2.1% (David Karabinus, PhD, and Joseph Schulman, MD, personal communication, 2006). The rate of congenital malformations in the general population is 3% to 4% [60].

In recent years late-onset inherited disorders and highly penetrant cancer-predisposition mutations have also been approached using PGD. Because such diseases can present in later life and are not expressed in all cases, the application of PGD to this group of disorders has been controversial [61,62]. Nevertheless, it is an important option for at-risk couples who wish to give birth to unaffected children, because most of these couples would not consider prenatal diagnosis for the disorder. PGD testing has been undertaken for a variety of late-onset inherited genetic disorders including familial adenomatous polyposis coli [63], *BRCA1* and *BRCA2* gene mutations associated with breast and ovarian cancers [61], autosomal dominant polycystic kidney disease (*PKD1* mutations) [64], amyloid precursor protein (*APP*) gene mutations associated with early-onset Alzheimer disease [65], familial amyloid polyneuropathy (*TTR* mutations), [66] and Huntington disease [67].

PGD also permits patients to test for late-onset genetic disorders without knowing their own genotype [68]. Patients at 50% risk of inheriting the autosomal dominant disorder Huntington disease have undertaken PGD to select embryos without knowing whether they have inherited the genetic mutation for this disorder. This nondisclosing Huntington disease PGD permits families to ensure that they will have an unaffected child when they do not wish to know whether they have inherited the mutation [69]. This nondisclosure testing (or exclusion testing) for Huntington disease has raised a number of ethical issues [70–72].

Another novel indication for PGD involves blood group incompatibility such as Kell or Rhesus (Rh) D alloimmunization. Although these disorders can be detected by prenatal diagnosis and treated with intrauterine blood transfusion, the potential complication for the fetus cannot be completely eliminated even after transfusion. Seeho and colleagues [73] describe the first report of an Rh-negative child born to an Rh-sensitized mother after PGD for Rh disease.

When a child is in need of an HLA-matched hematopoietic progenitor cell transplant (HPCT), but no match is available, the affected child's parents can use PGD to conceive a child who is an HLA-matched sibling [4]. The sibling then can act as an umbilical cord blood donor for the child in need of the transplant. The first successful PGD-HLA matching for HPCT involved treatment of a child who had Fanconi anemia in the United States [74], followed by a second successful treatment of Fanconi anemia by an international collaboration [75]. Since then a number other international groups have performed PGD for HLA matching [76,77]. In the United States, PGD testing for HLA matching is available in a number of centers (eg, Reproductive Genetics Institute, Chicago, Illinois; Genesis Genetics Institute, Detroit, Michigan; Children's Hospital & Research Center, Oakland, California; Medical College of Wisconsin/Froedtert Lutheran Memorial Hospital, Milwaukee, Wisconsin).

Dinucleotide repeat microsatellites are the most frequent type STRs in the human genome and are the most commonly used linked markers for

PGD-HLA haplotype analysis [76–78]. Dinucleotide repeat microsatellite markers, however, suffer from PCR artifacts known as repeat slippage, generating multiple extra stutter bands when analyzed. Thus, polymorphic tetra- and tri-nucleotide STRs within and flanking the MHC have been developed as linked probes for HLA haplotype analysis (David Bick, MD, Eduardo Lau, PhD, Milwaukee, Wisconsin, unpublished data, 2005). To exclude the transfer of embryos with recombinant HLA haplotypes, which are generated by meiotic recombination within the HLA region, a panel of STR probes in the flanking regions and within the HLA region are selected for HLA matching.

PGD for HLA matching has been provided for families that have children affected with inherited genetic disorders such as Fanconi anemia, thalassemia, Wiscott-Aldrich syndrome, X-linked adrenoleukodystrophy, X-linked hyper-IgM syndrome, and X-linked hypohidrotic ectodermal dysplasia with immune deficiency [79], as well as sporadic diseases such as aplastic anemia and leukemia [80].

Although PGD for HLA matching can be life saving, the number of families helped through this procedure is small because of the probability of success associated with IVF and the chance of finding a matching embryo [81]. According to published data, 12 clinical pregnancies resulted from 78 transferred embryos [80], and 7 clinical pregnancies resulted from 46 transferred embryos [30]. These data suggest an implantation rate of approximately 15.32% per embryo biopsied on day 3 after conception. In 68 PGD cycles for HLA matching in 49 families, there were only five live births of matched siblings [3].

There is another limitation to the use of PGD in HLA matching. If the affected child inherits a recombinant HLA haplotype from a parent, it is extremely unlikely that that parent will transmit an identical recombinant allele to a potential sibling. The probability of this situation may be as high as 1 in 23 cases [77,78].

Emerging preimplantation genetic diagnosis technologies

FISH analysis of cells from PGD has been used successfully to identify and transfer embryos with normal numbers of the chromosomes assessed. The usefulness of FISH is limited, however, because only a few chromosomes can be detected simultaneously in a single biopsied cell. Complete karyotyping at the single-cell level has been achieved by comparative genomic hybridization (CGH) [82]. CGH detects aneuploidy of any chromosome and can detect partial aneuploidy as well. One study showed that FISH for nine chromosomes would fail to detect 25% of the aneuploidies that were detected using CGH [83]. CGH is a technically challenging method. At the present time embryo biopsy and analysis cannot be completed in time for a blastocyst transfer on day 5 or 6. Therefore, embryos must be cryopreserved after biopsy. Once CGH is completed, appropriate embryos are thawed and transferred. Approximately 75% of embryos survive biopsy, freezing, and thawing, a rate similar to that for unbiopsied embryos [84]. Although this loss of embryos is a drawback to the current process, more rapid CGH procedures that provide a result in time for a blastocyst transfer can be anticipated.

For many couples an IVF cycle will result in more embryos than will be transferred to the uterus at one time. These surplus embryos are cryopreserved and then used in subsequent transfers should the initial fresh transfer fail. It would be reasonable to perform CGH on these embryos before freezing to identify chromosomally normal embryos, because doing so should improve the probability of a pregnancy from cryopreserved embryos. CGH may prove useful in other ways. FISH analysis has not been successful in identifying the cause in women who have experienced recurrent implantation failure. If this failure is related to the particular chromosomes chosen in the published FISH studies, CGH could provide an answer by testing for abnormalities in all chromosomes.

Whole-genome amplification (WGA) from single cells or small numbers of cells by multiple displacement amplification (MDA) [85,86] has started a new era for PGD [31,87,88]. WGA by MDA generates higher uniformity in sequence representation in the amplified DNA than previous methods for WGA [89,90], and the sizes of amplified fragments generated by MDA are greater than 10 kilobases in length. With this approach the first round of amplification from a single cell would be the same for all single-gene disorders, because the entire starting genome is greatly amplified by MDA. The second round of amplification would use PCR designed to detect the particular disorder in question, employing standard molecular methods and conditions because there is abundant DNA resulting from the first round [88]. A discrepancy in genotyping results has been reported for DNA before and after MDA [86,91]. As with PCR analysis of single cells, some preferential amplification or ADO was detected at heterozygous loci using the MDA-based method for single-cell analysis [31,87,88].

Other steps can be used to improve the accuracy and speed the process of PGD. The transition to faster PCR systems (eg, the 9800 PCR System, Applied Biosystems, Foster City, CA) will decrease the time of PCR amplification significantly. Microfluidic chips (eg, Bioanalyzers, Agilent Technologies, Palo Alto, California; LabChip 90 system, Caliper Life Sciences, Hopkinton, Massachusetts) can simplify the analysis by combining DNA separation, sizing, and genotyping of mutations, STRs and insertion/deletion polymorphisms [92–94]. Pyrosequencing, widely used in pharmacogenomics because of its capability for quantitative genotyping of single-nucleotide polymorphisms (SNPs) and highly accurate detection of mutations [95–97], should be able to generate reliable sequencing data for PGD. A more speculative approach could involve gold nanoparticle probes (nanospheres). These probes have enabled direct SNP identification in unamplified human genomic DNA targets [98] as well as direct gene-expression analysis using unamplified total human RNA [99].

In developing human embryos, appropriate gene expression is vital for the regulation of metabolic pathways and key developmental events. It recently was shown that altered gene expression is associated with abnormal morphology in early embryos [100]. It may be possible to select healthy embryos according to gene-expression profiles that can predict viability and implantation potential [100]. Gene-expression profiling using DNA microarrays also can identify aneuploidy in eukaryotic cells [101]. With the invention of highly sensitive molecular detectors (eg, the Trilogy Single Molecule Analyzer, US Genomics, Woburn, Massachusetts), single RNA molecules can be analyzed directly, without amplification [102]. This technique could be applied to the analysis of gene transcription in single embryonic cells.

Use and outcome of preimplantation genetic diagnosis

Although there are no published data detailing the number of centers performing PGD, it is estimated that more than 7000 PGD cycles have been performed worldwide [20]. In the United States, among 101 assisted reproductive medicine programs that carry out 200 or more stimulation cycles per year, 65 offered PGD. Thirty of these programs carry out the analysis of the cells in their own laboratory; the remaining programs send the cells by rapid delivery to another laboratory for analysis (Estil Strawn, MD, David Bick, MD, Kelly Charles, unpublished data, 2005).

The European Society of Human Reproduction and Embryology (ESHRE) PGD Consortium has undertaken a systematic assessment of PGD outcome. The consortium was established in 1997 to collect data concerning reasons for referrals, PGD cycles performed, resultant pregnancies, and outcome of babies born. Although the 66 reporting programs are primarily European, there also are reporting centers in Australia, Argentina, Israel, Korea, Taiwan, and the United States [40]. An analysis of data for the most recently available reporting period, 2002, examines 2219 PGD cycles. Cycle data were divided into PGD for inherited disorders (including chromosome abnormalities such as translocations, sexing for X-linked disease, and monogenic disorders), PGS, and PGD for social sexing (embryo sex determination for nonmedical reasons), called "PGD-SS."

The pregnancy rates per cycle that reached oocyte retrieval for PGD, PGS, and PGD-SS were 18%, 16%, and 21% respectively. These numbers are lower in PGD than would be expected in a routine IVF cycle because embryos diagnosed as affected or abnormal cannot be transferred, resulting in fewer cycles reaching transfer than expected. Further, the PGS rate reflects a mixture of indications for testing. For example, when PGS was used in couples who have severe male-factor infertility, the pregnancy rate was 33%; when PGS was used in couples with advanced maternal age, the pregnancy rate was 12%.

The pregnancy rates per cycle in which embryos were transferred for PGD, PGS, and PGD-SS are 25%, 23%, and 25% respectively [40]. These numbers also seem lower than expected, raising the question of whether biopsy affects an embryo's ability to result in an ongoing pregnancy. Evaluation of embryo survival after biopsy suggests that the removal of one or two cells does not have a significant impact on embryo viability [103]. One possible explanation for a lower pregnancy rate can be found by examining the number of embryos transferred when a transfer is performed. Examination of the ESHRE PGD Consortium data for 2002 [40] finds that there was an average of 1.8 embryos per transfer. The most recent assisted reproductive technology outcome data gathered by the Centers for Disease Control (CDC) [104] indicate that the pregnancy rate after a transfer is 43% for a maternal age comparable to the Consortium data. In the CDC data, however, three or more embryos were transferred in 56% of the transfers. The same CDC data show that the number of embryos transferred dramatically affects that pregnancy rate.

ESHRE PGD Consortium data [40] show that the course and outcome of pregnancies after PGD are comparable to those for pregnancies after IVF with ICSI but without PGD [105]. Embryo biopsy does not seem to affect the course of pregnancy, the baby's characteristics at birth (birth weight, length, gestational age at delivery), or the rate of malformations at birth.

Summary

PGD is an important alternative to standard prenatal diagnosis for genetic disorders. It also can afford families a special opportunity in certain clinical settings such as HLA matching. Low pregnancy and birth rates and the high cost of the procedure, however, make it unlikely that PGD will replace the more conventional methods of prenatal testing. PGD remains a complex combination of different technologies that requires the close collaboration of a team of specialists.

Acknowledgments

The authors thank Kathleen Grande for her assistance in the preparation of the manuscript.

References

[1] Handyside AH, Kontogianni EH, Hardy K, et al. Pregnancies from biopsied human preimplantation embryos sexed by Y-specific DNA amplification. Nature 1990;344:768–70.
[2] Rubio C, Rodrigo L, Perez-Cano I, et al. FISH screening of aneuploidies in preimplantation embryos to improve IVF outcome. Reprod Biomed Online 2005;11(4):497–506.

[3] Fiorentino F, Biricik A, Nuccitelli A, et al. Strategies and clinical outcome of 250 cycles of pre-implantation genetic diagnosis for single gene disorders. Hum Reprod 2006;21(3):670–84.

[4] Verlinksy Y, Rechitsky S, Schoolcraft W, et al. Preimplantation diagnosis for Fanconi ane-mia combined with HLA matching. JAMA 2001;285(24):3130–3.

[5] Thornhill AR, deDie-Smulders CE, Geraedts JP, et al. ESHRE PGD consortium best prac-tice guidelines for clinical preimplantation genetic diagnosis (PGD) and preimplantation genetic screening (PGS). Hum Reprod 2005;20(1):35–48.

[6] Schenker JG. Clinical aspects of ovarian hyperstimulation syndrome. Eur J Obstet Gynecol Reprod Biol 1999;85(1):13–20.

[7] El-Shawarby S, Margara R, Trew G, et al. A review of complications following transvagi-nal oocyte retrieval for in-vitro fertilization. Hum Fertil 2004;7(2):127–33.

[8] Shenfield F, Pennings G, Devroey P, et al, for the ESHRE Ethics Task Force. Taskforce 5: preimplantation genetic diagnosis. Hum Reprod 2003;18(3):649–51.

[9] Rebar RW, DeCherney AH. Assisted reproductive technology in the United States. N Engl J Med 2004;350(16):1603–4.

[10] Katayama ACUS. ART practitioners soon to begin their forced march into a regulated fu-ture. J Assist Reprod Genet 2003;20(7):265–70.

[11] Papanikolaou EG, Kolibianakis E, Devroey P. Emerging drugs in assisted reproduction. Expert Opin Emerg Drugs 2005;10(2):425–40.

[12] Lass A. UK Timing of hCG Group. Monitoring of in vitro fertilization-embryo transfer cycles by ultrasound versus by ultrasound and hormonal levels: a prospective, multicenter, randomized study. Fertil Steril 2003;80(1):80–5.

[13] Ludwig M, Doody KJ, Doody KM. Use of recombinant human chorionic gonadotropin in ovulation induction. Fertil Steril 2003;79:1051–9.

[14] Kwan I, Bhattacharya S, Knox F, et al. Conscious sedation and analgesia for oocyte retrieval during in vitro fertilization procedures. Cochrane Database Syst Rev 2005;(3):CD004829.

[15] Speroff L, Fritz M. Fertilization. In: Clinical gynecologic endocrinology and infertility. 7th edition. Philadelphia: Lippincott Williams & Wilkins; 2005. p. 1215–74.

[16] Suh RS, Zhu X, Phadke N, et al. IVF within microfluidic channels requires lower total num-bers and lower concentrations of sperm. Hum Reprod 2006;21:477–83.

[17] Bungum M, Bungum L, Humaidan P. A prospective study, using sibling oocytes, examin-ing the effect of 30 seconds versus 90 minutes gamete co-incubation in IVF. Hum Reprod 2006;21(2):518–23.

[18] Yanagimachi R. Intracytoplasmic injection of spermatozoa and spermatogenic cells: its bi-ology and applications in humans and animals. Reprod Biomed Online 2005;10(2):247–88.

[19] De Vos A, Van Steirteghem A. Aspects of biopsy procedures prior to preimplantation ge-netic diagnosis. Prenat Diagn 2001;21(9):767–80.

[20] Kuliev A, Verlinsky Y. Place of preimplantation diagnosis in genetic practice. Am J Med Genet 2005;134A:105–10.

[21] De Boer K, MacArthur S, Murray C, et al. First live birth following blastocyst biopsy and PGD analysis. Reprod Biomed Online 2002;4:35.

[22] Kokkali G, Vrettou C, Traeger-Synodinos J, et al. Birth of a healthy infant following tro-phectoderm biopsy from blastocysts for PGD of beta-thalassemia major: case report. Hum Reprod 2005;20(7):1855–9.

[23] McArthur SJ, Leigh D, Marshall JT, et al. Pregnancies and live births after trophectoderm biopsy and preimplantation genetic testing of human blastocysts. Fertil Steril 2005;84(6): 1628–36.

[24] Ruangvutilert P, Delhanty JD, Rodeck CH, et al. Relative efficiency of FISH on metaphase and interphase nuclei from non-mosaic trisomic or triploid fibroblast cultures. Prenat Diagn 2000;20:159–62.

[25] Munne S, Chen S, Fischer J, et al. Preimplantation genetic diagnosis reduces pregnancy loss in women aged 35 years and older with a history of recurrent miscarriages. Fertil Steril 2005; 84(2):331–5.

[26] Kearns WG, Pen R, Graham J, et al. Preimplantation genetic diagnosis and screening. Semin Reprod Med 2005;23(4):336–47.

[27] Baart EB, Martini E, van den Berg I, et al. Preimplantation genetic screening reveals a high incidence of aneuploidy and mosaicism in embryos from young women undergoing IVF. Hum Reprod 2006;21(1):223–33.

[28] Rechitsky S, Verlinsky O, Amet T, et al. Reliability of preimplantation diagnosis for single gene disorders. Mol Cell Endocrinol 2001;183:S65–8.

[29] Hussey ND, Davis T, Hall JR, et al. Preimplantation genetic diagnosis for beta-thalassaemia using sequencing of single cell PCR products to detect mutations and polymorphic loci. Mol Hum Reprod 2002;8:1136–43.

[30] Fiorentino F, Kahraman S, Karadayi H, et al. Short tandem repeats haplotyping of the HLA region in preimplantation HLA matching. Eur J Hum Genet 2005;13(8):953–8.

[31] Handyside AH, Robinson MD, Simpson RJ, et al. Isothermal whole genome amplification from single and small numbers of cells: a new era for preimplantation genetic diagnosis of inherited disease. Mol Hum Reprod 2004;10(10):767–72.

[32] Lewis CM, Pinel T, Whittakeer JC, et al. Controlling misdiagnosis errors in preimplantation genetic diagnosis: a comprehensive model encompassing extrinsic and intrinsic sources of error. Hum Reprod 2001;16(1):43–50.

[33] Fiorentino F, Magli MC, Podini D, et al. The minisequencing method: an alternative strategy for preimplantation genetic diagnosis of single gene disorders. Mol Hum Reprod 2003; 9(7):399–410.

[34] Bermudez MG, Piyamongkol W, Tomaz S, et al. Single-cell sequencing and mini-sequencing for preimplantation genetic diagnosis. Prenat Diagn 2003;23:669–77.

[35] Burlet P, Frydman N, Gigarel N, et al. Improved single-cell protocol for preimplantation genetic diagnosis of spinal muscular atrophy. Fertil Steril 2005;84(3):734–9.

[36] Loeys B, Nuytinck L, Van Acker P, et al. Strategies for prenatal and preimplantation genetic diagnosis in Marfan syndrome (MFS). Prenat Diagn 2002;22:22–8.

[37] Hook EB, Lindsjo A. Down syndrome in live births by single year maternal age interval in a Swedish study: comparison with results from a New York State study. Am J Hum Genet 1978;30:19–27.

[38] Hook EB, Cross PK, Schreinemachers DM. Chromosomal abnormality rates at amniocentesis and in live-born infants. JAMA 1983;249:2034–8.

[39] Munne S, Alikani M, Tomkin G, et al. Embryo morphology, developmental rates, and maternal age are correlated with chromosome abnormalities. Fertil Steril 1995;64:382–91.

[40] Harper JC, Boelaert K, Geraedts J, et al. ESHRE PGD Consortium data collection V: cycles from January to December 2002 with pregnancy follow-up to October 2003. Hum Reprod 2006;21(1):3–21.

[41] Morris JK, Mutton DE, Alberman E. Recurrences of free trisomy 21: analysis of data from the National Down Syndrome Cytogenetic Register. Prenat Diagn 2005;25(12):1120–8.

[42] Rubio C, Pehlivan T, Rodrigo L, et al. Embryo aneuploidy screening for unexplained recurrent miscarriage: a minireview. Am J Reprod Immunol 2005;53(4):159–65.

[43] Schlegel PN. Male infertility: evaluation and sperm retrieval. Clin Obstet Gynecol 2006; 49(1):55–72.

[44] Gianaroli L, Magli MC, Cavallini G, et al. Frequency of aneuploidy in sperm from patients with extremely severe male factor infertility. Hum Reprod 2005;20(8):2140–52.

[45] Foresta C, Garolla A, Bartoloni L, et al. Genetic abnormalities among severely oligospermic men who are candidates for intracytoplasmic sperm injection. J Clin Endocrinol Metab 2005;90(1):152–6.

[46] Papanikolaou EG, Vernaeve V, Kolibianakis E, et al. Is chromosome analysis mandatory in the initial investigation of normovulatory women seeking infertility treatment? Hum Reprod 2005;20(10):2899–903.

[47] Stern C, Pertile M, Norris H, et al. Chromosome translocations in couples with in-vitro fertilization implantation failure. Hum Reprod 1999;14:2097–101.

[48] Verlinsky Y, Tur-Kaspa I, Cieslak J, et al. Preimplantation testing for chromosomal disorders improves reproductive outcome of poor-prognosis patients. Reprod Biomed Online 2005;11(2):219–25.

[49] Fallon L, Harton GL, Sisson ME, et al. Preimplantation genetic diagnosis for spinal muscular atrophy type I. Neurology 1999;53(5):1087–90.

[50] Goosens V, Sermon K, Lissens W, et al. Improving clinical preimplantation genetic diagnosis for cystic fibrosis by duplex PCR using two polymorphic markers or one polymorphic marker in combination with the detection of the deltaF508 mutation. Mol Hum Reprod 2003;9(9):559–67.

[51] Verlinsky Y, Rechitsky S, Verlinsky O, et al. Preimplantation diagnosis for neurofibromatosis. Reprod Biomed Online 2002;4(3):218–22.

[52] Vrettou C, Traeger-Synodinos J, Tzetis M, et al. Real-time PCR for single-cell genotyping in sickle cell and thalassemia syndromes as a rapid, accurate, reliable, and widely applicable protocol for preimplantation genetic diagnosis. Hum Mutat 2004;23(5):513–21.

[53] Sermon K, Seneca S, De Rycke M, et al. PGD in the lab for triplet repeat diseases—myotonic dystrophy, Huntington's disease and fragile-X syndrome. Mol Cell Endocrinol 2001; 183:S77–85.

[54] Drusedau M, Dreesen JCFM, de Die-Smulders C, et al. Preimplantation genetic diagnosis of spinocerebellar ataxia 3 by (CAG)n repeat detection. Mol Hum Reprod 2004;10(1):71–5.

[55] Xu K, Rosenwaks Z, Beaverson K, et al. Preimplantation genetic diagnosis for retinoblastoma: the first reported liveborn. Am J Ophthalmol 2004;137:18–23.

[56] Girardet A, Hamamah S, Dechaud H, et al. Specific detection of deleted and non-deleted dystrophin exons together with gender assignment in preimplantation genetic diagnosis of Duchenne muscular dystrophy. Mol Hum Reprod 2003;9(7):421–7.

[57] Levinson G, Maddalena A, Howard-Peebles PN, et al. Preimplantation genetic screening: an option for families at risk for transmission of the fragile X chromosome. In: Hagerman RJ, McKenzie P, editors. 1992 International Fragile X Conference Proceedings. Dillon (CO): Spectra Publishing Co; 1992. p. 383.

[58] Schulman JD, Karabinus DS. Scientific aspects of preconception gender selection. Reprod Biomed Online 2005;10(Suppl 1):111–5.

[59] Fugger EF, Black SH, Keyvanfar K, et al. Births of normal daughters after MicroSort sperm separation and intrauterine insemination, in-vitro fertilization, or intracytoplasmic sperm injection. Hum Reprod 1998;13(9):2367–70.

[60] Christianson A, Modell B. Medical genetics in developing countries. Annu Rev Genomics Hum Genet 2004;5:219–65.

[61] Wagner JE. Practical and ethical issues with genetic screening. Hematology. In: American Society of Hematology Educational Program. Washington (DC): American Society of Hematology; 2005. p. 498–502.

[62] Harris M, Winship I, Spriggs M. Controversies and ethical issues in cancer-genetics clinics. Lancet Oncol 2005;6:301–10.

[63] Ao A, Wells D, Handyside AH, et al. Preimplantation genetic diagnosis of inherited cancer: familial adenomatous polyposis coli. J Assist Reprod Genet 1998;15(3):140–4.

[64] De Rycke M, Georgiou I, Sermon K, et al. PGD for autosomal dominant polycystic kidney disease type 1. Mol Hum Reprod 2005;11(1):65–71.

[65] Verlinsky Y, Rechitsky S, Verlinsky O, et al. Preimplantation diagnosis for early-onset Alzheimer disease caused by V717L mutation. JAMA 2002;287(8):1018–40.

[66] Almeida VM, Costa PM, Moreira P, et al. Birth of two healthy females after preimplantation genetic diagnosis for familial amyloid polyneuropathy. Reprod Biomed Online 2005; 10(5):641–4.

[67] Moutou C, Gardes N, Viville S. New tools for preimplantation genetic diagnosis of Huntington's disease and their clinical applications. Eur J Hum Genet 2004;12(12):1007–14.

[68] Schulman JD, Black SH, Handyside A, et al. Preimplantation genetic testing for Huntington disease and certain other dominantly inherited disorders. Clin Genet 1996;49(2):57–8.

[69] Stern HJ, Harton GL, Sisson ME, et al. Non-disclosing preimplantation genetic diagnosis for Huntington disease. Prenat Diagn 2002;22(6):503–7.

[70] Spriggs M. Commodification of children again and non-disclosure preimplantation genetic diagnosis for Huntington's disease. J Med Ethics 2004;30(6):538.

[71] Sermon K, De Rijcke M, Lissens W, et al. Preimplantation genetic diagnosis for Huntington's disease with exclusion testing. Eur J Hum Genet 2002;10(10):591–8.

[72] Braude PR, De Wert GM, Evers-Kiebooms G, et al. Non-disclosure preimplantation genetic diagnosis for Huntington's disease: practical and ethical dilemmas. Prenat Diagn 1998;18(3):1422–6.

[73] Seeho SKM, Burton G, Leigh D, et al. The role of preimplantation genetic diagnosis in the management of severe rhesus alloimmunization: first unaffected pregnancy: case report. Hum Reprod 2005;20(3):697–701.

[74] Grewal SS, Hahn JP, MacMillan ML, et al. Successful hematopoietic stem cell transplantation for Fanconi anemia from an unaffected HLA-genotype-identical sibling selected using preimplantation genetic diagnosis. Blood 2004;103(3):1147–51.

[75] Bielorai B, Hughes MR, Auerbach AD, et al. Successful umbilical cord blood transplantation for Fanconi anemia using preimplantation genetic diagnosis for HLA-matched donor. Am J Hematol 2004;77:397–9.

[76] Van de Velde H, Georgiou I, De Rycke M, et al. Novel universal approach for preimplantation genetic diagnosis of beta-thalassemia in combination with HLA matching of embryos. Hum Reprod 2004;19(3):700–8.

[77] Fiorentino F, Biricik A, Karadayi H, et al. Development and clinical application of a strategy for preimplantation genetic diagnosis of single gene disorders combined with HLA matching. Mol Hum Reprod 2004;10(6):445–60.

[78] Verlinsky Y, Rechitsky S, Sharapova T, et al. Preimplantation HLA testing. JAMA 2004; 291:2079–85.

[79] Rechitsky S, Kuliev A, Tur-Kaspa I, et al. Preimplantation genetic diagnosis with HLA matching. Reprod Biomed Online 2004;9(2):210–21.

[80] Kuliev A, Verlinsky Y. Preimplantation HLA typing and stem cell transplantation: report of international meeting, Cyprus, 27–28, March, 2004. Reprod Biomed Online 2004;9(2):205–9.

[81] Qureshi N, Foote D, Walters MC, et al. Outcomes of preimplantation genetic diagnosis therapy in treatment of β-thalassemia: a retrospective analysis. Ann NY Acad Sci 2005; 1054:500–3.

[82] Wilton L, Williamson R, McBain J, et al. Birth of a healthy infant after preimplantation confirmation of euploidy by comparative genomic hybridization. N Engl J Med 2001; 345(21):1537–41.

[83] Wilton L, Voullaire L, Sargeant P, et al. Preimplantation aneuploidy screening using comparative genomic hybridization or fluorescence in situ hybridization of embryos from patients with recurrent implantation failure. Fertil Steril 2003;80(4):860–8.

[84] Jericho H, Wilton L, Gook D, et al. A modified cryopreservation method increases the survival of human biopsied cleavage stage embryos. Hum Reprod 2003;18:568–71.

[85] Lasken RS, Egholm M. Whole genome amplification: abundant supplies of DNA from precious samples or clinical specimens. Trends Biotechnol 2003;21:531–5.

[86] Lu Y, Gioia-Patricola L, Gomez JV, et al. Use of whole genome amplification to rescue DNA from plasma samples. Biotechniques 2005;39(4):511–5.

[87] Hellani A, Coskun S, Benkhalifa M, et al. Multiple displacement amplification on single cell and possible PGD applications. Hum Reprod 2004;10(11):847–52.

[88] Hellani A, Coskun S, Tbakhi A, et al. Clinical application of multiple displacement amplification in preimplantation genetic diagnosis. Reprod Biomed Online 2005;10(3): 376–80.

[89] Lovmar L, Fredriksson M, Liljedahl U, et al. Quantitative evaluation by minisequencing and microarrays reveals accurate multiplexed SNP genotyping of whole genome amplified DNA. Nucleic Acids Res 2003;31:e129.

[90] Zhang L, Cui XF, Schmitt K, et al. Whole genome amplification from a single cell: implication for genetic analysis. Proc Natl Acad Sci U S A 1992;89:5847–51.

[91] Montgomery GW, Campbell MJ, Dickson P, et al. Estimation of the rate of SNP genotyping errors from DNA extracted from different tissues. Twin Res Hum Genet 2005;8(4):346–52.

[92] Sohni YR, Burke JP, Dyck PJ, et al. Microfluidic chip-based method for genotyping microsatellites, VNTRs and insertion/deletion polymorphisms. Clin Biochem 2003;36(1):35–40.

[93] Qin J, Leung FC, Fung Y, et al. Rapid authentication of ginseng species using microchip electrophoresis with laser-induced fluorescence detection. Anal Bioanal Chem 2005;381: 812–9.

[94] Hashimoto M, Barany F, Soper SA. Polymerase chain reaction/ligase detection reaction/ hybridization assays using flow-through microfluidic devices for the detection of low-abundant DNA point mutations. Biosens Bioelectron 2006;21(10):1915–23.

[95] Okada Y, Nakamura K, Wada M, et al. Genotyping of thiopurine methyltransferase using pyrosequencing. Biol Pharm Bull 2005;28(4):677–81.

[96] Soderback E, Zackrisson A-L, Lindblom B, et al. Determination of CYP2D6 gene copy number by pyrosequencing. Clin Chem 2005;51(3):522–31.

[97] Kruckeberg KE, Thibodeau SN. Pyrosequencing technology as a method for the diagnosis of multiple endocrine neoplasia type 2. Clin Chem 2004;50(3):522–9.

[98] Bao YP, Huber M, Wei T-F, et al. SNP identification in unamplified human genomic DNA with gold nanoparticle probes. Nucleic Acids Res 2005;33(2):e15.

[99] Huber M, Wei TF, Muller UR, et al. Gold nanoparticle probe-based gene expression analysis with unamplified total human RNA. Nucleic Acids Res 2004;32(18):e137.

[100] Wells D, Bermudez MG, Steuerwald N, et al. Association of abnormal morphology and altered gene expression in human preimplantation embryos. Fertil Steril 2005;84(2):343–55.

[101] Hughes TR, Roberts CJ, Dai H, et al. Widespread aneuploidy revealed by DNA microarray expression profiling. Nat Genet 2000;25(7):333–7.

[102] Neely LA, Patel S, Garver J, et al. A single-molecule method for the quantitation of microRNA gene expression. Nat Methods 2006;3(1):41–6.

[103] Van de Velde H, De Vos A, Sermon K, et al. Embryo implantation after biopsy of one or two cells from cleavage-stage embryos with a view to preimplantation genetic diagnosis. Prenat Diagn 2000;20:1030–7.

[104] Assisted reproductive technology success rates: national summary and fertility clinic reports. US Department of Health and Human Services, Centers for Disease Control and Prevention, Coordinating Center for Health Promotion, National Center for Chronic Disease Prevention and Health Promotion, Division of Reproductive Health. Atlanta (GA); 2003.

[105] Bonduelle M, Wennerholm UB, Loft A, et al. A multi-centre cohort study of the physical health of 5-year-old children conceived after intracytoplasmic sperm injection, in vitro fertilization and natural conception. Hum Reprod 2005;20:413–9.

ELSEVIER
SAUNDERS

PEDIATRIC CLINICS
OF NORTH AMERICA

Pediatr Clin N Am 53 (2006) 579–590

The Application of Microarray Analysis to Pediatric Diseases

Martin J. Hessner, PhD*, Mingyu Liang, MB, PhD, Anne E. Kwitek, PhD

The Medical College of Wisconsin, 8701 Watertown Plank Road, Milwaukee, WI 53226, USA

Historically, studies to decipher genetic alterations related to human disease have been limited to single genes or proteins. Completion of the Human Genome Project, which began in 1990, has resulted in sequencing of the human genome and the generation of numerous technological, genetic, and bioinformatics resources. These advances have made global transcriptional analysis a reality with the emergence of several approaches that allow investigators to analyze hundreds to thousands of genes in parallel. These techniques include serial analysis of gene expression (SAGE) [1], differential display [2], and DNA microarrays [3–5]. Over the past decade, DNA microarrays have become an extensively applied, mainstream component of biomedical research. The knowledge gained through use of this technology has improved understanding of human biology and disease. DNA microarray technology likely will play an important role in the development of new and effective diagnostic, preventive, and therapeutic approaches [6,7]. This article briefly reviews the state of the technology and its successful translations in pediatric research.

A microarray is essentially a miniaturized high-density dot blot, consisting of thousands or tens of thousands of probes that are immobilized on a two-dimensional solid matrix. Each probe is specific for, and capable of detecting the presence of an RNA transcript in the sample(s) being analyzed. The samples may compare experimental versus control tissue culture cells or diseased versus healthy cells or tissue. The DNA microarray has evolved

---

This work has been supported National Institute of Biomedical Imaging and Bioengineering Grant R01-EB-001421, National Institute of Allergy and Infectious Diseases Grant P01-AI-42380, and National Heart, Lung, and Blood Institute R01-HL-077263.

* Corresponding author.

E-mail address: mhessner@mcw.edu (M.J. Hessner).

doi:10.1016/j.pcl.2006.05.013

into two commonly used formats: spotted cDNA or oligonucleotide arrays [5] and light-directed in situ synthesized oligonucleotide arrays [8,9].

Spotted arrays use high-speed robotics to mechanically or piezoelectrically [10] deposit small volumes of probe solutions onto the array surface. Numerous manufacturers have developed robotic arrayers that enable researchers to construct arrays in their own laboratories. Array construction is technically challenging, and the quality of the array has a direct impact on the reliability of the gene expression data generated [11–18]. Microscope slides, because of their low inherent fluorescence, typically are used to provide the solid support. These are coated with poly-L-lysine, amino silanes or amino-reactive silanes, which enhance surface hydrophobicity to limit spot spreading and to improve adherence of the DNA by providing a positive charge [19,20]. The printed DNA probe can be amplified products from cDNA libraries (typically greater than 200 base pairs [bp]in length) or oligonucleotides (typically 30 to 70 bp in length). As their costs have decreased, oligonucleotides have become the more popular choice over the past few years. Oligonucleotides exhibit numerous advantages over cDNAs in that cumbersome clone library management and amplification can be avoided. Oligonucleotides can be designed to exclude homologous sequences between genes, thereby enhancing specificity. In addition, a given gene can be represented by a set of different oligonucleotides targeting different regions or exons, allowing for the detection of splice variants, or discrimination of closely related genes. After printing, the DNA is cross-linked to the support using ultraviolet irradiation, followed by a blocking step using succinic anhydride to reduce the positive charge at unoccupied sites on the slide surface so that labeled sample targets do not bind nonspecifically to the array.

After the array is prepared, RNA samples are extracted from the two tissues that are to be compared. For spotted arrays, these typically are labeled differentially during reverse transcription with cyanine dye-tagged nucleotides, yielding cDNAs that are labeled with either Cy3 or Cy5. The dye-labeled cDNA targets then are cohybridized to the same array. The advantage of cohybridization is that the comparison is direct and avoids experimental variation potentially introduced by hybridizing a single sample to a single array. After hybridization, the array is washed, then analyzed with a fluorescence scanner (Fig. 1). Specially designed software is used to determine the relative amounts of an mRNA species in the original two samples for every gene on the array, this typically is defined as a normalized intensity ratio between the two fluorophores for each array element [5,16,19,21,22].

Many laboratories do not have the equipment, expertise, or desire to create their own custom arrays. This has created a large demand for commercially prepared microarrays. The Affymetrix GeneChip (Affymetrix, Santa Clara, California), the most widely used commercial system, uses an in situ synthesized oligonucleotide array and highly optimized protocols that allow investigators to rapidly generate reliable expression data. In situ synthesized oligonucleotide arrays use ultraviolet light passed through a series

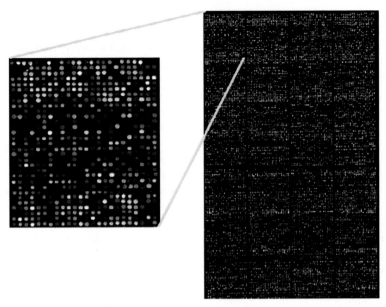

Fig. 1. Competitive hybridization between the Jurkat human acute T cell leukemia cell line (Cy5-labeled) and the melanoma cell line UACC-903 (Cy3-labeled) cDNA labeled though subsequent incorporation of Cy5 or Cy3-dUTP. Hybridized to a 20,000 probe human cDNA array. Software depicts transcripts equally represented in both channels as yellow. Transcripts over-represented in the Jurkat (Cy5) sample are depicted as red, whereas transcripts over-represented in UACC-903 (Cy3) are represented in green.

of photolithographic chrome/glass masks to deprotect photolabile phosphoramidite deoxynucleosides [23] and direct the synthesis of the oligonucleotide on the glass support used during hybridization. This approach obviates the requirement of hydrolyzing the oligonucleotide from its synthetic support and reattaching it to the array, as is the case with spotted oligonucleotides arrays. A maskless light-directed oligonucleotide array fabrication technology has been developed [24] and is being commercialized by NimbleGen (Madison, Wisconsin). This may offer a more cost-effective means of fabricating custom arrays. An important distinction between spotted arrays and in situ synthesized arrays is the number of samples hybridized to the array. A single RNA is hybridized to a single Affymetrix GeneChip, and comparisons between samples are made in silico. This approach relies on highly controlled commercial fabrication methods and well-defined laboratory methodologies so that comparisons can be made across arrays. This is an advantage when conducting large experiments involving many samples, because comparison of any two samples does not require cohybridization, which depending on the study design, can reduce greatly the number of arrays required.

Regardless of the format selected, image processing, image analysis, and data mining are computationally intensive, resulting in massive amounts of information that must be managed properly and ultimately interpreted within the context of the biological question being investigated. After the hybridized image is acquired, it is converted into spot intensity and intensity ratio measures. This large body of data typically is stored and managed in spreadsheet form for further analysis. These data then undergo normalization, an essential step that adjusts the data for systematic nonbiological effects arising from technical variation and measurement error. The overall goal of normalization is to remove the effects of such noise, while maintaining the structure of the data and the ability to detect genes that exhibit statistically significant expression differences between the samples under examination. Initial enthusiasm for global gene expression analysis was dampened after it was realized that such massive datasets produced many false false-positive results and that conventional statistical methods to exclude the null hypothesis were inadequate. This has prompted development of many different analytical approaches for sensitive detection of gene expression changes while providing a measure of statistical significance and likelihood of error. The final output of a gene expression study is generally a table listing the fold change of the experimental sample versus control for up to tens of thousands of genes with various types of confidence measures. Interpreting the biological meaning of gene expression experiments can be challenging; however, numerous tools have been developed to assist investigators. Clustering [25], which groups genes on the basis of similar expression patterns with the assumption that they are co-coordinately regulated or possibly part of the same signaling pathway, was one of the first tools developed and widely used to interpret microarray data [25]. Other widely used, related methods to discover patterns of gene expression common to a particular physiological state include supervised clustering, principle component analysis, self-organizing maps, and linear discriminant analysis. More recently, software such Expression Analysis Systematic Explorer (EASE) [26] and Onto-Express [27] have facilitate the biological interpretation of gene lists by providing statistical methods for discovering the most over-represented biological themes using gene ontology databases, generating gene annotation tables, and enabling automated linking to online analysis tools.

With this background, this article reviews some of the advances this technology has enabled in the study of pediatric diseases. Many of the first significant observations were in the area of oncology, where new insights, not possible with previous conventional approaches, have been made. Now reports are emerging in other fields, including metabolic diseases and autoimmunity. Many of these investigations have used in vitro systems or animal models. Significant human studies, however, are beginning to emerge. These contributions have contributed to our understanding of the pathophysiology of complex pediatric disorders. Examples from research in the fields of hematology/oncology/metabolic disorders and autoimmune disorders are presented.

Hematology/oncology

In 1999, Lander published a commentary that compared the results of microarray technology with the underlying order of elements in the periodic table, permitting organisms to be characterized by the order and structure of their gene sequence and regulation [28]. In this perspective, he discussed the potential of microarrays to study RNA expression or DNA variation at a global level rather than at a gene-by-gene level, providing critical insight into systems biology. Furthermore, the ability to identify specific global expression patterns within complex human disease epitomized personalized medicine, so that ideally therapies could be selected/tailored to the individual patient's genome to maximize effectiveness and minimize negative adverse effects.

In the field of pediatric oncology, methods to classify cancer cell types initially relied on tumor cell morphology, and then on a few specific genetic markers or cytogenetic abnormalities. As useful as these approaches have been, and in some cases still are, they fail to distinguish many cancer cell types and cannot always identify critical chromosomal rearrangements. Acute lymphoblastic leukemia (ALL) is the most common childhood leukemia, with nearly 4000 new diagnoses per year. Survival of childhood ALL has increased dramatically during the past last 40 years (from approximately 15% survival to nearly 80%) [29]; however, this success has come not from new drugs or prognostic markers, but from empirically determined improvements in use and combination of existing drug therapies [30]. In part because of disease heterogeneity, treatment failures still occur, and patients still may experience negative adverse effects. The ability to better identify and classify specific cancers and cancer subtypes through the use of global expression profiling offers the potential of more targeted therapies.

Toward this goal, a pivotal study reported the first application of microarray technology for the classification and prediction of cancer types involving pediatric ALL and acute myeloid leukemia (AML) [31]. The goal of this study was twofold. First, could gene expression profiling determine a molecular signature that could distinguish ALL from AML, without a priori knowledge of the genes affected? Second, could this signature then be used to predict tumor class? Thirty-eight tumor samples (27 ALL and 11 AML) were examined for gene expression levels using Affymetrix oligonucleotide chips and analyzed using unsupervised clustering. Fifty genes were selected whose clustered expression patterns significantly differed between the two leukemias. Subsequent cross-validation testing was performed, removing one sample at a time from the sample set and determining in which group the tumor was predicted. From this analysis, they were able to predict the class of 36 of the 38 tumors, all of which matched the clinical diagnosis. To test whether this 50-gene predictor set could classify tumor class accurately, they attempted to classify 34 independent tumor samples. The 50-gene expression signature could classify 29 of the 34 samples with 100%

accuracy. This study was a true proof of principle that microarray analysis might be sufficiently accurate to classify tumor types as a clinical diagnostic tool.

Many studies subsequently have followed and determined signatures of different ALL subclasses [32–34], subtypes that respond differently to various treatments [29,35,36]. Key genes were identified that correlated tumor type with prognosis and response to treatment [37–39] and identified a minimal set of genes that could assign disease class accurately. It is notable that in each of these studies, no single gene was an accurate predictor. The multiple gene signature resulting from microarray studies provides the most accurate (greater than 95% compared with approximately 90% accuracy for combined morphology, immunophenotyping, and cyogenetics and molecular genetics) and promising diagnostic tool to date [30]. Numerous issues, however, must be resolved before gene expression profiles will become standard clinical diagnostic tools. Validation and reproducibility across broad tissue sources stored under differing conditions and cost-effectiveness [40] are major limitations.

An additional application of microarray technology in the area of oncology is the development of a sensitive and global assay for loss of heterogeneity (LOH). In this type of array application, patient-derived DNA (instead of RNA) is hybridized to the array. Traditionally, LOH was identified using karyotyping and more recently comparative genomic hybridization or microsatellite analysis. The recent release of high-density single nucleotide polymorphism (SNP) arrays, however, offers a new high-throughput and comprehensive means to assess tumors for LOH. One such study has applied the Affymetrix 10k SNP array to LOH studies on tumors from 10 male ALL patients [41]. This study assessed 11,555 SNPs evenly distributed across the genome in tumor and normal tissue from the same patient to identify allele loss (seen as homozygotes) compared with normal tissue (seen as heterozygotes). Results were compared with both karyotype and microsatellite data. The study demonstrated that SNP arrays may be a feasible alternative to traditional methods. Additionally, they may be able to detect smaller regions of LOH, and they require less starting biological material and are less labor intensive [41].

Metabolic disorders

Respiratory chain complex I deficiency, the most common disorder of energy generation, is known to be genetically heterogeneous. The disorder results from different mutations in different patient groups affecting many nuclear or mitochondrial genes encoding complex I subunits. Kirby and colleagues used DNA microarray to study two patients with lethal neonatal mitochondrial complex I deficiency sharing a nuclear complementation group, and found NDUFS6 to be substantially underexpressed in cell lines obtained from those patients [42]. NDUFS6 is a complex I subunit gene that previously had not been associated with complex I deficiency. Subsequent PCR and sequence analyses revealed the presence of homozygous mutations that caused splicing abnormalities or deletions in both patients [42].

DNA microarrays have been used rather extensively in pediatric research, mainly for the purpose of identifying abnormal genomic regions, sequences, or arrangements associated with pediatric diseases. An early study using a chromosome 11 microarray correctly mapped the gene responsible for congenital hyperinsulinism, sulfonylurea receptor (SUR1), to a 2-Mb region [43]. Janecke and colleagues used a whole-genome microarray analysis of SNPs to identify a founder haplotype and define a critical interval of 1.53 cM on chromosome 14q23.3-q24.1 that contained the gene associated with autosomal recessive childhood-onset severe retinal dystrophy [44]. Subsequently, mutations in RDH12, a gene located in the genomic region identified by the microarray analysis and encoding a retinol dehydrogenase, were found to be associated with this form of retinal dystrophy. Wiszniewski and colleagues used a microarray to screen for mutations in ABCA4, a retinal-specific member of the ATP-binding cassette (ABC) family, in patients who had autosomal recessive retinitis pigmentosa, the most severe retinal dystrophy associated with ABCA4 mutations [45]. They then expressed ABCA4 with the identified missense mutations in the photoreceptors of *Xenopus laevis* tadpoles through transgenesis, and found that these mutations, likely through protein misfolding, caused retention of ABCA4 in the photoreceptor inner segment and complete absence of functional ABCA4 in its normal location, the outer segment. They further found that patients with different retinal dystrophies harboring two misfolding alleles exhibited early age of onset (5 to 12 years) of retinal disease.

Autoimmune disorders

Juvenile idiopathic arthritis (JIA) encompasses a group of diseases affecting approximately 250,000 children in the United States. The diseases are classified by their type of presentation: oligoarthritis, polyarthritis, or systemic-onset JIA (SoJIA) [46]. SoJIA patients account for approximately 10% of arthritis cases beginning in childhood, and SoJIA often poses challenges to pediatric rheumatologists because of chronicity and associated disability. The pathogenic mechanism of SoJIA is not well-understood, although increased levels of interleukin (IL)-6 have been reported to correlate with the systemic activity of the disease and with the development of arthritis [47]. Recently, Pascual and colleagues [48] used DNA microarrays to create a paradigm shift by implicated IL-1 as a major mediator of the inflammatory cascade. Briefly, peripheral blood mononuclear cells (PBMCs) were isolated from healthy individuals and analyzed after differential incubation with autologous or SoJIA serum for gene expression signatures (using the HG U133A Affymetrix GeneChip array, which possesses 22,283 probe sets). In healthy PBMCs, SoJIA patient serum induced transcription of numerous genes related to innate immunity, including several members of the IL-1 cytokine/cytokine receptor family (IL-1b, IL-1R1, and IL-1R2), and chemokines involved in the chemotaxis of neutrophils (CXCL1, CXCL3, CXCL5, CXCL6). When directly comparing the expression profiles of SoJIA patient PBMCs versus healthy controls, many of the transcripts that were induced by SoJIA sera were present in SoJIA PBMCs, including IL-1b and the IL-1 decoy receptor (IL-1R2), CXCL1, and CCR1. These were consistent with the neutrophilia and monocytosis observed in patients who had SoJIA. These investigators then further analyzed increased expression of IL-1b at the protein level, finding that upon activation, SoJIA PBMCs released large amounts of IL-1b. To respectively treat the systemic manifestations and arthritis, most patients who have SoJIA require treatment with corticosteroids and methotrexate (MTX) for prolonged periods [49]. These findings, however, suggested that SoJIA patients have a dysregulation of IL-1 production, prompting these investigators to hypothesize that patients who have SoJIA may benefit from IL-1 antagonist treatment. Nine patients possessing active disease that was resistant to conventional aggressive treatment achieved a complete or partial remission when treated with a commercially available rIL-1Ra. The identification of IL-1 as a major mediator of the inflammatory cascade, and the use of IL-1Ra may prevent severe, deforming arthritis and the need for prolonged use of corticosteroids in pediatric patients.

Systemic lupus erythematosus (SLE) is a systemic autoimmune disease that affects multiple organs, including the skin, vessels, kidneys, and central nervous system. Children represent approximately 20% of all patients who have SLE. Patients exhibit B and T lymphopenia and polyclonal hypergammaglobulinemia, with high titers of autoantibodies targeting nuclear components, DNA, and nucleosomes [50–52]. Like many autoimmune disorders, the pathogenic mechanism remains elusive; however, evidence supports the interaction of environment (eg, viral infections) and an array of susceptibility genes. Treatment of SLE typically involves nonspecific immunosuppression (glucocorticoids and chemotherapy). Bennett and colleagues [53] used Affymetrix U95AV2 oligonucleotide microarrays, which interrogate 12,561 human genes, to examine the gene expression signatures of PBMCs isolated from children who had active SLE. Briefly, PBMCs from three pediatric cohorts (nine healthy children, 30 SLE patients, and 12 patients who had juvenile chronic arthritis) were evaluated. When comparing patients who had SLE with healthy controls, a striking predominance of genes known to be up-regulated in response to type I interferon (IFN) and a smaller group of neutrophil-specific genes was observed in the SLE patients. This gene expression signature was not observed in patients who had juvenile chronic arthritis, indicating that the pattern of gene expression distinguishes SLE from healthy individuals and from other autoimmune diseases.

Type 1 diabetes mellitus (T1DM) is a polygenic autoimmune disease that targets the insulin-producing pancreatic β cells. Because most patients possess an 80% to 90% loss in β cell mass at diagnosis, it is not possible to capture the disease-initiating events, even if it were possible to obtain the tissues relevant for study of the autoimmune process (ie, pancreatic islets or pancreatic lymph nodes). Therefore, immunopathogenic mechanisms of T1DM have been elucidated largely through animal models, specifically the BioBreeding (BB) rat and the nonobese diabetic (NOD) mouse. To better understand immune processes during development of T1DM, the authors' laboratory has conducted gene expression profiling of pancreatic lymph nodes of BB rats during the prediabetic period [54]. These array-based studies have revealed innate immune activity, in particular that of mast cells and eosinophils [9], and have led to several novel observations, including the finding that before insulitis (infiltration of mononuclear cells into the islets of Langerhans), BB rats are predisposed to T1DM in that their pancreatic β cells recruit innate cells through the expression of chemokine eotaxin. The identification of innate immunity through gene expression studies in SLE [53], SoJIA, and studies in the BB rat [48] is consistent with a growing body of evidence implicating the innate immune system, specifically granulocytes and mast cells, as important initiators and propagators of autoimmune diseases [55]. In multiple sclerosis (MS) or its mouse model, experimental allergic encephalomyelitis (EAE), development of disease has been correlated with the number or distribution of mast cells, and in animal models drugs inhibiting mast cell degranulation (such as cromolyn) have reduced disease severity [55,56]. Gene expression profiling of brain lesion autopsy samples from patients who have MS has revealed presence of high numbers of mast cell transcripts [57]. Mast cells and granulocytes also have been implicated in other autoimmune disorders, including rheumatoid arthritis and bullous pemphigoid, where mast cell inhibiting agents have been found to have therapeutic effects [55]. These studies showcase how global gene expression technologies have been used to gain new insight into autoimmunity and highlight the fact that autoimmune diseases involve the interplay of the adaptive and innate immune systems. This presents new insights into disease pathophysiology and identifies new therapeutic targets for treatment and prevention of these disorders [58].

Microarray analysis is an evolving technology with potential pitfalls. This technology, however, permits a global view of disease. Perhaps the greatest advantage of high-throughput gene expression analysis is the potential to detect unsuspected changes in gene expression and provide novel insights into disease mechanisms.

References

[1] Velculescu VE, Zhang L, Vogelstein B, et al. Serial analysis of gene expression. Science 1995; 270(5235):484–7.
[2] Liang P, Pardee AB. Differential display of eukaryotic messenger RNA by means of the polymerase chain reaction. Science 1992;257(5072):967–71.

[3] Lockhart DJ, Dong H, Byrne MC, et al. Expression monitoring by hybridization to high-density oligonucleotide arrays. Nat Biotechnol 1996;14(13):1675–80.

[4] Chee M, Yang R, Hubbell E, et al. Accessing genetic information with high-density DNA arrays. Science 1996;274(5287):610–4.

[5] Schena M, Shalon D, Davis R, et al. Quantitative monitoring of gene expression patterns with complementary DNA microarray. Science 1995;270:467–70.

[6] Debouck C, Goodfellow PN. DNA microarrays in drug discovery and development. Nat Genet 1999;21(Suppl 1):48–50.

[7] Diehn M, Alizadeh AA, Brown PO. Examining the living genome in health and disease with DNA microarrays. JAMA 2000;283(17):2298–9.

[8] Fodor SP, Read JL, Pirrung MC, et al. Light-directed, spatially addressable parallel chemical synthesis. Science 1991;251(4995):767–73.

[9] Fodor SP, Rava RP, Huang XC, et al. Multiplexed biochemical assays with biological chips. Nature 1993;364(6437):555–6.

[10] Ramakrishnan R, Dorris D, Lublinsky A, et al. An assessment of Motorola CodeLink microarray performance for gene expression profiling applications. Nucleic Acids Res 2002; 30(7):e30.

[11] Hacia JG, Collins FS. Mutational analysis using oligonucleotide microarrays. J Med Genet 1999;36(10):730–6.

[12] Hessner MJ, Wang X, Hulse K, et al. Three color cDNA microarrays: quantitative assessment through the use of fluorescein-labeled probes. Nucleic Acids Res 2003;31(4):e14.

[13] Hessner MJ, Wang X, Khan S, et al. Use of a three-color cDNA microarray platform to measure and control support-bound probe for improved data quality and reproducibility. Nucleic Acids Res 2003;31(11):e60.

[14] Hessner MJ, Meyer L, Tackes J, et al. Immobilized probe and glass surface chemistry as variables in microarray fabrication. BMC Genomics 2004;5(1):53.

[15] Hessner MJ, Singh VK, Wang X, et al. Utilization of a labeled tracking oligonucleotide for visualization and quality control of spotted 70-mer arrays. BMC Genomics 2004;5(1):12.

[16] Wang X, Ghosh S, Guo S-W. Quantitative quality control in microarray image processing and data acquisition. Nucleic Acids Res 2001;29:E75–82.

[17] Wang X, Hessner MJ, Wu Y, et al. Quantitative quality control in microarray experiments and the application in data filtering, normalization and false positive rate prediction. Bioinformatics 2003;19(11):1341–7.

[18] Wang X, Jiang N, Feng X, et al. A novel approach for high quality microarray processing using third-dye array visualization technology. IEEE Transactions on Nanoscience 2003; 2(4):193–201.

[19] Schena M, Shalon D, Heller R, et al. Parallel human genome analysis: microarray-based expression monitoring of 1000 genes. Proc Natl Acad Sci U S A 1996;93(20):10614–9.

[20] Duggan D, Bittner M, Chen Y, et al. Expression profiling using cDNA microarrays. Nat Genet 1999;21:10–4.

[21] Hegde P, Qi R, Abernathy K, et al. A concise guide to cDNA microarray analysis. Biotechniques 2000;29(3):548–50.

[22] Eisen M, Brown P. DNA arrays for analysis of gene expression. Methods Enzymol 1999;303: 179–205.

[23] Pease AC, Solas D, Sullivan EJ, et al. Light-generated oligonucleotide arrays for rapid DNA sequence analysis. Proc Natl Acad Sci U S A 1994;91(11):5022–6.

[24] Singh-Gasson S, Green RD, Yue Y, et al. Maskless fabrication of light-directed oligonucleotide microarrays using a digital micromirror array. Nat Biotechnol 1999;17(10): 974–8.

[25] Eisen MB, Spellman PT, Brown PO, et al. Cluster analysis and display of genome-wide expression patterns. Proc Natl Acad Sci U S A 1998;95(25):14863–8.

[26] Hosack DA, Dennis G Jr, Sherman BT, et al. Identifying biological themes within lists of genes with EASE. Genome Biol 2003;4(10):R70.

[27] Draghici S, Khatri P, Bhavsar P, et al. Onto-Tools, the toolkit of the modern biologist: Onto-Express, Onto-Compare, Onto-Design and Onto-Translate. Nucleic Acids Res 2003;31(13): 3775–81.

[28] Lander ES. Array of hope. Nat Genet 1999;21(Suppl 1):3–4.

[29] Holleman A, Cheok MH, den Boer ML, et al. Gene-expression patterns in drug-resistant acute lymphoblastic leukemia cells and response to treatment. N Engl J Med 2004;351(6):533–42.

[30] Carroll WL, Bhojwani D, Min DJ, et al. Childhood acute lymphoblastic leukemia in the age of genomics. Pediatr Blood Cancer 2006;46(5):570–8.

[31] Golub TR, Slonim DK, Tamayo P, et al. Molecular classification of cancer: class discovery and class prediction by gene expression monitoring. Science 1999;286(5439):531–7.

[32] Moos PJ, Raetz EA, Carlson MA, et al. Identification of gene expression profiles that segregate patients with childhood leukemia. Clin Cancer Res 2002;8(10):3118–30.

[33] Ross ME, Zhou X, Song G, et al. Classification of pediatric acute lymphoblastic leukemia by gene expression profiling. Blood 2003;102(8):2951–9.

[34] Yeoh EJ, Ross ME, Shurtleff SA, et al. Classification, subtype discovery, and prediction of outcome in pediatric acute lymphoblastic leukemia by gene expression profiling. Cancer Cell 2002;1(2):133–43.

[35] Cario G, Stanulla M, Fine BM, et al. Distinct gene expression profiles determine molecular treatment response in childhood acute lymphoblastic leukemia. Blood 2005;105(2):821–6.

[36] Lugthart S, Cheok MH, den Boer ML, et al. Identification of genes associated with chemotherapy cross-resistance and treatment response in childhood acute lymphoblastic leukemia. Cancer Cell 2005;7(4):375–86.

[37] Liang DC, Shih LY, Huang CF, et al. CEBPalpha mutations in childhood acute myeloid leukemia. Leukemia 2005;19(3):410–4.

[38] Tartaglia M, Martinelli S, Iavarone I, et al. Somatic PTPN11 mutations in childhood acute myeloid leukaemia. Br J Haematol 2005;129(3):333–9.

[39] Xu F, Taki T, Yang HW, et al. Tandem duplication of the FLT3 gene is found in acute lymphoblastic leukaemia as well as acute myeloid leukaemia but not in myelodysplastic syndrome or juvenile chronic myelogenous leukaemia in children. Br J Haematol 1999;105(1): 155–62.

[40] Simon R. Roadmap for developing and validating therapeutically relevant genomic classifiers. J Clin Oncol 2005;23(29):7332–41.

[41] Irving JA, Bloodworth L, Bown NP, et al. Loss of heterozygosity in childhood acute lymphoblastic leukemia detected by genome-wide microarray single nucleotide polymorphism analysis. Cancer Res 2005;65(8):3053–8.

[42] Kirby DM, Salemi R, Sugiana C, et al. NDUFS6 mutations are a novel cause of lethal neonatal mitochondrial complex I deficiency. J Clin Invest 2004;114(6):837–45.

[43] Cheung VG, Gregg JP, Gogolin-Ewens KJ, et al. Linkage-disequilibrium mapping without genotyping. Nat Genet 1998;18(3):225–30.

[44] Janecke AR, Thompson DA, Utermann G, et al. Mutations in RDH12 encoding a photoreceptor cell retinol dehydrogenase cause childhood-onset severe retinal dystrophy. Nat Genet 2004;36(8):850–4.

[45] Wiszniewski W, Zaremba CM, Yatsenko AN, et al. ABCA4 mutations causing mislocalization are found frequently in patients with severe retinal dystrophies. Hum Mol Genet 2005; 14(19):2769–78.

[46] Wallace CA, Levinson JE. Juvenile rheumatoid arthritis: outcome and treatment for the 1990s. Rheum Dis Clin North Am 1991;17(4):891–905.

[47] de Benedetti F, Massa M, Robbioni P, et al. Correlation of serum interleukin-6 levels with joint involvement and thrombocytosis in systemic juvenile rheumatoid arthritis. Arthritis Rheum 1991;34(9):1158–63.

[48] Pascual V, Allantaz F, Arce E, et al. Role of interleukin-1 (IL-1) in the pathogenesis of systemic onset juvenile idiopathic arthritis and clinical response to IL-1 blockade. J Exp Med 2005;201(9):1479–86.

[49] Adebajo AO, Hall MA. The use of intravenous pulsed methylprednisolone in the treatment of systemic-onset juvenile chronic arthritis. Br J Rheumatol 1998;37(11):1240–2.

[50] Arce E, Jackson DG, Gill MA, et al. Increased frequency of pre-germinal center B cells and plasma cell precursors in the blood of children with systemic lupus erythematosus. J Immunol 2001;167(4):2361–9.

[51] Amoura Z, Piette JC, Chabre H, et al. Circulating plasma levels of nucleosomes in patients with systemic lupus erythematosus: correlation with serum antinucleosome antibody titers and absence of clear association with disease activity. Arthritis Rheum 1997;40(12):2217–25.

[52] Rubin RL, Tang FL, Chan EK, et al. IgG subclasses of autoantibodies in systemic lupus erythematosus, Sjogren's syndrome, and drug-induced autoimmunity. J Immunol 1986;137(8): 2528–34.

[53] Bennett L, Palucka AK, Arce E, et al. Interferon and granulopoiesis signatures in systemic lupus erythematosus blood. J Exp Med 2003;197(6):711–23.

[54] Hessner MJ, Wang X, Meyer L, et al. Involvement of eotaxin, eosinophils, and pancreatic predisposition in development of type 1 diabetes mellitus in the BioBreeding rat. J Immunol 2004;173(11):6993–7002.

[55] Benoist C, Mathis D. Mast cells in autoimmune disease. Nature 2002;420(6917):875–8.

[56] Seeldrayers PA, Yasui D, Weiner HL, et al. Treatment of experimental allergic neuritis with nedocromil sodium. J Neuroimmunol 1989;25(2–3):221–6.

[57] Lock C, Hermans G, Pedotti R, et al. Gene–microarray analysis of multiple sclerosis lesions yields new targets validated in autoimmune encephalomyelitis. Nat Med 2002;8(5):500–8.

[58] Bach JF, Bendelac A, Brenner MB, et al. The role of innate immunity in autoimmunity. J Exp Med 2004;200(12):1527–31.

PEDIATRIC CLINICS
OF NORTH AMERICA

Pediatr Clin N Am 53 (2006) 591–619

Pharmacogenomics and the Future of Drug Therapy

Ronald N. Hines, PhD[a,b], D. Gail McCarver, MD[a,b],*

[a]Department of Pediatrics, Section of Clinical Pharmacology,
Pharmacogenetics and Teratology, Medical College of Wisconsin,
8701 Watertown Plank Road, Milwaukee, WI 53226, USA
[b]Children's Research Institute, Children's Hospital and Health Systems,
P.O. Box 1997, Milwaukee, WI 53201, USA

Completion of the human genome project and its potential for radically altering the practice of medicine has led to great anticipation and excitement, and some trepidation, in the lay public and scientific community. Of the potential human genome applications, many believe that pharmacogenomics may represent one of the first success stories, and in fact, some successes have been seen. The promise of pharmacogenomics is individualized therapy such that the selection of medication and its dose would be improved by knowledge of the individual patient's genetic constitution. This contrasts with the current empirical approach that relies on a combination of the physician's familiarity with therapeutic choices and dosing information based on age, body weight, and if appropriate, renal clearance. Pharmacogenomics also offers the promise of improved drug design based on knowledge of the drug candidate's chemistry, the molecular characteristics of the target, and the factors determining drug disposition. Finally, pharmacogenomics can be used to streamline drug development by stratifying clinical trial subjects by genotype, thereby increasing the likelihood and degree of an efficacious response without toxicity and enhancing overall success rates. Ultimately, it is hoped that the application of pharmacogenomics to clinical practice would increase therapeutic responsiveness from the current average of 50% to 75% [1] and dramatically reduce the incidence of adverse drug reactions. The latter are estimated at 2 million per year in the United States, including 100,000 deaths [2]. This article provides some background regarding the history and development of pharmacogenomics that also illustrates important principles. Perhaps more importantly, the promises and

* Corresponding author.
E-mail address: gmccarve@mcw.edu (D.G. McCarver).

0031-3955/06/$ - see front matter © 2006 Elsevier Inc. All rights reserved.
doi:10.1016/j.pcl.2006.05.008

pediatric.theclinics.com

challenges of pharmacogenomics are examined, particularly within the context of pediatric therapeutics.

Historical perspective and important principles

Pharmacogenomics is defined as the study of inherited variation in drug disposition and response. The field focuses on genetic polymorphisms, which are defined as Mendelian traits that exist in a population in at least two phenotypes, neither of which is rare (ie, occurring at greater than 1% frequency. Note that this definition specifies that the phenotype (ie, the outward consequences of the genotype), is what is being measured. The emphasis on phenotype rather than genotype extends from the field's history in that, until very recently, pharmacogenomics was driven by clinical observations rather than molecular approaches. Further, pharmacogenomics is much older than one might expect based on the current level of interest and hyperbole. Often quoted as the first documented observation of an adverse drug reaction and cautionary note, Pythagaros described interindividual variability in the incidence of hemolytic anemia in response to the ingestion of fava beans in 510 BC [3]. Although still not elucidated completely, favism is thought to be caused in part to genetic variation in acid phosphatase 1 (*ACP1*) among individuals also deficient in glucose-6-phosphate dehydrogenase (*G6PD*), the latter an X-linked trait [4]. Favism also illustrates another important and apparently universal principal in pharmacogenomics, that is that the frequency of a particular genetic polymorphism and the underlying causative genotype frequently vary significantly from one population to another [5].

In their classic study of alkaptonuria, Garrod and Oxon [6] were the first to suggest that chemical imbalances, such as alkaptonuria and cystinuria, were not caused by disease per se, but instead, were caused by individual differences in chemical metabolism (ie, chemical individuality), and further, that the most likely explanation for the observed incidence of such disorders was Mendelian inheritance. These authors also suggested that other such chemical abnormalities likely existed that failed to exhibit an overt phenotype, but would be apparent with careful chemical analysis. Thus, they were the first to describe another important principle of pharmacogenomics; phenotypes often are only observed upon exposure to a particular chemical or drug. Proof that such chemical individuality is inherited as a Mendelian trait, and also that distinct ethnic differences existed in the patterns of inheritance, was reported by Snyder [7] in his description of an inherited differences in the ability to taste phenylthiocarbamide. It was not until 1957, however, that Motulsky [8] suggested that drug-induced toxicity and equally or more importantly, failed efficacy at normal therapeutic doses, was caused by innocuous genetic differences that lead to enzyme deficiencies. Two years later, Vogel [9] was the first to suggest the term pharmacogenetics, defining it as "the study of the role of genetics in drug response."

The discovery that isoniazid was an effective chemotherapeutic agent against *Mycobacterium tuberculosis* [10] led to the widespread use of this drug. Subsequently, considerable interindividual variation in isoniazid metabolic inactivation was noted, and the frequency of the inactivation phenotype was found to exhibit a bimodal distribution (ie, rapid and slow inactivators). The first large study associating drug response with the inactivation phenotype was reported by Evans and colleagues [11], wherein peripheral neuropathy was associated with the slow inactivator phenotype, while failed efficacy was more common in rapid inactivators. Four years later, Evans and White [12] demonstrated that the isoniazid genetic polymorphism was caused by differences in hepatic *N*-acetyltransferase (NAT) and that the same trait was responsible for interindividual differences in the metabolism of sulfamethazine and hydralazine, but not sulfanilamide or *p*-aminobenzoic acid. It was not until 1991, however, that three, single nucleotide polymorphisms (SNPs) in the *NAT2* locus (*NAT2*5*, 341T > C, I114T; *NAT2*6*, 590G > A, R197Q, and *NAT*7*, 857G > A, G286E) were shown to account for more than 90% of the observed variation in isoniazid acetylation in at least Asian and non-Latino white populations [13]. A fourth variant, *NAT2*14*, 191G > A, R64Q, is rare in Asian and non-Latino white populations, but is present at a 7% to 12% allelic frequency in African and African American populations [14].

The *N*-acetylation polymorphism illustrates several principles that often are overlooked. First, the significance of the *N*-acetylation polymorphism only became clinically relevant when a susceptible drug was put into widespread use. Second, the clinical significance of the polymorphism is dependent on the therapeutic index of the drug. Clearly, the variation in isoniazid inactivation would not have received nearly as much attention if the drug's therapeutic window was such that toxicity was not induced by the higher plasma levels associated with the slow acetylation phenotype or if a robust bacteriostatic response was still observed with the rapid acetylation phenotype. Third, the initial metabolic disposition of isoniazid is limited to a single major pathway, eliminating possible compensation or masking of the phenotype by alternative metabolic pathways. Finally, a pronounced difference in pharmacological activity is exhibited between the parent drug, isoniazid, and its initial metabolite, acetylisoniazid. If the metabolite were as active as the parent compound, the clinical relevance of the *NAT* polymorphism would have been minor at best.

Unique to pediatrics, numerous examples exist wherein a deficient phenotype results not from a genetic variation, but instead, from the ontogeny of important pharmacokinetic or pharmacodynamic parameters. For example, low levels of *CYP3A4* expression in the neonate and young infant [15,16] lead to deficiencies in the ability to clear cisapride [17,18] and result in increased risk for adverse effects associated with the parent drug. This phenomenon contributed substantially to the decision to withdraw this drug from the market. Another example, delayed onset of *FMO3* expression in young children [19], was likely a significant contributing factor to the cases of transient trimethylaminuria reported by Mayatepek and Kohlmüeller [20]. Finally, Tateishi and colleagues [21] showed that theophylline elimination did not achieve adult levels until at least 3 months of age, consistent with the earlier report of delayed onset of *CYP1A2* expression [22]. Thus, many instances exist wherein children must grow into their genotype. This and other important pharmacogenomic principles illustrated by the historical perspective highlighted are summarized in Box 1.

Early success stories

During the ensuing decades, multiple clinically relevant pharmacogenomic difference have been identified and characterized. In each of these, variation in drug response was associated with one or more variant alleles at a particular genetic locus. With the advent of molecular biology approaches, the pace of discovery of genetic differences has quickened; however, delineation of the function of these loci is a slower process. Although many examples could be given, these have been reviewed in several articles [23–25], and as such, only three specific examples are presented that have particular relevance to pediatric clinical practice

- Cytochrome P4502D6 (*CYP2D6*) variation and its influence on response to a host of drugs being used in pediatric psychotherapy and pain management
- Genetic variation at the thiopurine methyltransferase (*TPMT*) locus as a major underlying cause of the variation observed in thiopurine therapy for childhood cancer and several inflammatory/immune-related diseases

---

Box 1. Important pharmacogenomic principles

- The frequency of a particular genetic polymorphism and the underlying causative genotype frequently varies significantly from one population group to another.
- Variant genotypes are usually innocuous, in that phenotypes are observed only upon exposure to a particular chemical or drug.
- Temporal changes in gene expression can result in phenotypes inconsistent with genotype.
- Clinical relevance is determined by:
  - Widespread use
  - Narrow therapeutic index
  - Limited alternative clearance pathways
  - Absence of alternative drugs
  - Differential pharmacological activity or toxicity between parent drug and metabolite

---

- Cytochrome P4502C9 (*CYP2C9*) and vitamin K oxidoreductase complex 1 (*VKORC1*) variation and their impact on the response to anticoagulation therapy

CYP2D6 and response to debrisoquin

One of the best studied polymorphisms is that of *CYP2D6*, a genetic variant discovered following the clinical observation of unusual subject sensitivity to the hypotensive effects of the adrenergic blocking agent, debrisoquin [26,27]. Given that the plasma levels of unchanged drug correlated with response, investigators concluded that variation in metabolism was likely the responsible mechanism. Using the metabolic ratio of the parent drug to its 4-hydroxy metabolite, investigators identified a bimodal distribution with 7% to 10% of non-Latino whites deficient in metabolic ability. Based on family and twin studies, poor metabolism was shown to have a genetic basis, with poor metabolizers being homozygous for a recessive allele. Population studies showed that this poor metabolizer phenotype was present in 5% to 10% of non-Latino whites, 5% of African Americans, but only 1% to 2% of Asians. Debrisoquin was not approved for use in the United States, but the disposition of many clinically important drugs also is impacted by *CYP2D6* variants, many of which are used in pediatric patients. These include beta blockers such as S-metoprolol and propafenone; antidepressants such as amitriptyline, clomipramine, desipramine, imipramine, and fluoxetine; antipsychotics such as haloperidol and thioridazine; and the opioid codeine. Extensive efforts have been made to identify and characterize variant *CYP2D6* alleles. Over 102 *CYP2D6* variant haplotypes have been identified, with half of these exhibiting a functional impact on gene function. When one looks at causative variants, however, only 28 have been identified, most of which are SNPs. For example, 14 variant *CYP2D6* haplotypes have been identified, all containing a single SNP, 1846G > A. This SNP causes a splicing defect, resulting in a complete loss of activity in all of the 14 variant haplotypes. Of the 28 causative variants, 20 result in a complete loss of activity (most either because of a frame shift or splicing defect) and are causative of the poor metabolic phenotype in individuals homozygous for any combination of these alleles. Five result in decreased activity that is substrate-dependent and are causative for an intermediate metabolic phenotype. Thus far, three variants result from gene duplication events causing an ultrafast metabolic phenotype associated with marked increases in metabolic activity and decreased efficacy following standard drug dosing in homozygous individuals.

Thiopurine methyltransferase and thiopurine therapy

The thiopurine drugs, 6-mercaptopurine, thioguanine, and azathioprine, are used widely for treating various disorders, including childhood acute lymphoblastic leukemia (ALL), inflammatory bowel disease, rheumatoid arthritis, systemic lupus erythromatosus, and in transplantation. In all instances, the thiopurine drugs require metabolic activation to thioguanine nucleotides to elicit their cytotoxic pharmacological effect. Metabolic activation is a multi-step process initiated by the enzyme, hypoxanthine guanine phosphoribosyl transferase (HGPRT), leading to intracellular thioguanine nucleotides. This activation pathway, however, competes with inactivation by thiopurine methyltransferase (TPMT) and xanthine oxidase. Weinshilboum and Sladek [28] first demonstrated that the variation in response to thiopurines was caused by *TPMT* genetic differences based on their measurements of enzyme activity in red blood cells. The distribution of activity in nearly 300 subjects, and family studies, demonstrated that the trait was autosomal-codominant with the low-activity allele exhibiting a 6% frequency. With the molecular characterization of the gene, 10 different variant alleles have been identified, but only three, *TPMT*2, *TPMT*3A,* and *TPMT*3C,* account for nearly two-thirds of the variance in enzyme activity levels. Each of these variants results in protein products that are targeted for degradation, resulting in low enzyme levels. As has been observed for many of the drug-metabolizing enzyme polymorphisms, considerable differences in allelic frequency exist between different ethnic/racial groups. The *TPMT*2* allele is observed at a frequency of 0.2% to 0.5% in non-Latino whites and African Americans, but it is absent in Asian groups. The most frequent variant allele among non-Latino whites is *TPMT*3A,* with a frequency between 3% and 6%, whereas the *TPMT*3C* allele is most common among African and Asian populations, at frequencies between 2% and 8%. Reflecting the admixture within African Americans, the *TPMT*3A* exhibits a frequency of about 1%, whereas the *TPMT*3C* exhibits a frequency of 2% to 3% in this population [29]. More recently, a variable number of tandem repeat (VNTR) polymorphisms have been identified in the *TPMT* promoter that also contribute to the variance in enzyme levels [30,31].

TPMT genotype has been shown to correlate dramatically with toxicity in several diseases. Studies in Japan and the United States revealed that rheumatic disease patients heterozygous for any one of the deficient *TPMT* alleles (*TPMT*2, TPMT*3A,* or *TPMT*3C*) were forced to terminate azathioprine treatment within a month because of leukopenia, whereas most individuals homozygous for the reference allele (*TPMT*1*) were able to complete the entire treatment regimen [32,33]. In a British study, tolerance of long-term 6-mercaptopurine maintenance therapy in ALL patients who were heterozygous for a variant *TPMT* allele was 89%, the same as for those who were homozygous for the reference, high-activity enzyme. A single *TPMT*3A* patient, however, was able to stay on therapy for only 47% of the maintenance period [34]. In two studies from the United States, 65% of patients referred for thiopurine toxicity exhibited either TPMT deficiency (homozygous for the *TPMT*3A* allele) or intermediate TPMT activity (heterozygous *TPMT*3A/*3C* allele). Based on the frequency of these variants in the general population, the expected number of patients would have been only 10%. Among 180 ALL patients, erythrocyte thioguanine nucleotide levels were inversely proportional to TPMT activity. To avoid toxicity in this study, dose lowering was required in 100% of the homozygous TPMT-deficient patients, in 35% of the heterozygous variant TPMT patients, and in 7% of the homozygous reference TPMT patients. The dose adjustments allowed all patients to receive full protocol doses of other chemotherapeutics and also maintain high thioguanine nucleotide levels [35]. Based on this study and others, current standard practice is to initiate thiopurine therapy using doses reduced by 85% to 90% for patients who are homozygous *TPMT* variant and by 35% for those who are *TPMT* heterozygotes. Demonstrating a TPMT effect in the opposite direction, when azathioprine is used in combination therapy to prevent allograft rejection after renal transplantation in pediatric patients, high TPMT activity is associated with an increased risk for rejection [36].

Because of the strong associations with adverse outcome, many health centers now routinely assess *TPMT* genotype or TPMT erythrocyte phenotype before initiating thiopurine therapy for most if not all indications. Further, a pharmacoeconomic study by Tavadia and colleagues [37] suggests that the cost of *TPMT* screening would be cost-neutral if one assumes only patients homozygous for *TPMT* deficient alleles will experience myelosuppression. Thus, screening would be cost-beneficial, as some patients who are heterozygous for *TPMT*-deficient alleles also would exhibit thiopurine toxicity. Thus, *TPMT* represents a clear example in which pharmacogenomic testing before therapy has been shown to significantly improve patient safety and reduce health care costs.

CYP2C9, VKORC1 and anticoagulant therapy

Coumarin-based therapy is used widely in adult and pediatric patients for preventing and treating thromboembolism. Warfarin acts by inhibiting *VKORC1*, necessary for the recycling of reduced vitamin K that in turn is necessary for the post-translational γ-carboxylation and activation of several clotting factors. Because of its narrow therapeutic index and the seriousness of bleeding complications caused by excessive dosing, initiation of warfarin therapy requires careful monitoring of the prothrombin time with international normalized ratio (INR) target values of 2 to 3. Maintenance of effective therapy is difficult because of significant influences from diet, age, other drugs, and disease state [38,39]. Genetic differences, however, also contribute substantially to the greater than tenfold interindividual difference in warfarin response. Warfarin clearance is mediated primarily by hepatic *CYP2C9*-mediated hydroxylation [40]. Although 11 *CYP2C9* alleles have been associated with reduced or complete loss of activity, all but two of these alleles appear to be rare and of questionable significance when considering population health. In contrast, *CYP2C9*2* (R144C) and *CYP2C9*3* (I359L) occur at allelic frequencies of approximately 12% and 8%, respectively, in non-Latino white populations, although they are much less frequent in African Americans or Asians. Numerous studies from several groups have demonstrated an association between various warfarin therapeutic endpoints and both *CYP2C9*2* and **3* genotypes, including dose requirements during the induction phase of therapy [41], warfarin maintenance dose [42–44], risk for bleeding complications [42,45], and risk for overanticoagulation [45]. It was clear from the variation observed within each genotype group, however, that other loci were making a substantial contribution to the variation in warfarin response.

With the discovery of the *VKORC1* gene and its unequivocal identity as the pharmacological target for warfarin [46,47], there was immediate interest in determining whether variation in *VKORC1* might contribute to interindividual differences in warfarin response. In an initial study by D'Andrea and colleagues [48], the *VKORC1* gene was resequenced in 147 patients receiving warfarin and who previously were characterized for *CYP2C9* genotype. A significant association was observed between a transition variation in intron 1 (1173C > T), wherein a higher daily warfarin dose was observed in patients who were homozygous for the reference sequence (7.0 plus or minus 3.0 mg, n = 54) compared with those who were either heterozygotes (5.1 plus or minus 2.5 mg, n = 69) or homozygous for the variant (3.7 plus or minus 1.6 mg, n = 24). The effect of this variant on gene function, however, was not apparent. Together, the *VKORC1* and *CYP2C9* genetic variants accounted for approximately 35% of the observed variability in warfarin response in this study group. Rieder and colleagues [49] independently identified 10 common (greater than 5%) noncoding *VKORC1* SNPs in a cohort of 186 patients previously characterized for *CYP2C9* variants and anticoagulation-related outcomes. These 10 SNPs were used to infer five common haplotypes (greater than 5%) (H1, H2, H7, H8, and H9) in the 186-patient cohort, and at least one of three population-specific DNA diversity panels consisting of non-Latino white Americans, African Americans, or Asian Americans. Using multiple linear regression analysis adjusted for clinically important covariates, four of the five common haplotypes were associated independently with warfarin maintenance dose. H1 and H2 haplotypes were associated with a low dose requirement (2.9 and 3.0 mg, respectively) whereas H7 and H9 were associated with a higher maintenance dose (6.0 and 5.5 mg, respectively). Applying phylogenetic clustering, the five haplotype groups fell into two groups, group A consisting of haplotypes H1 and H2, and group B consisting of haplotypes H7, H8, and H9 (Fig. 1A). Assigning the 186-patient cohort to *VKORC1* haplotype groups (A/A, A/B, or BB), and either reference *CYP2C9* or variant *CYP2C9* (**2* or **3*) genotype, a significant impact of both *VKORC1* haplotype and *CYP2C9* genotype was apparent, with about 25% of the variation in required warfarin dose being accounted for by *VKORC1* haplotype and 6% to 10% by *CYP2C9* genotype (Fig. 1B). These findings were replicated in an independent cohort of 357 patients (Fig. 1C). Given that all of the identified variants were noncoding, Rieder and colleagues [49] examined a possible effect on *VKORC1* mRNA levels in 51 human liver samples and showed a threefold higher steady-state level of *VKORC1* mRNA in haplotype B/B versus haplotype A/A individuals, suggesting an effect on transcription. *VKORC1* haplotype frequencies differed significantly among the three population panels examined, with the frequency of the group A haplotypes (predictive of low warfarin dose requirement) being highest in Asian Americans (89%), lowest in African Americans (14%), and in between in non-Latino white Americans (37%). This observation may explain partially the variability in warfarin response observed in the Asian population in the absence of significant variant *CYP2C9* allele frequencies. The large effect size of the combined *CYP2C9* and *VKORC1* haplotype on interindividual differences in warfarin response combined with the relative genetic frequencies among several US populations provides a strong argument for implementing these genetic tests before initiating anticoagulation therapy with this drug.

Pharmacogenetics versus pharmacogenomics

Although there may be additional drugs developed whose pharmacokinetic or pharmacodynamic properties are influenced substantially by variation at one or two genetic loci, it is recognized that pharmacogenomics exhibits more parallels with complex disease in that variation more likely will be explained by the sum of smaller contributions from multiple genetic loci. This realization has led many to argue for the application of genome-wide scans to identify candidate genes that might underlie observed phenotypic variation. Although such screening was cost-prohibitive only a few years ago, rapid advances in screening technologies, advances in mapping of SNPs, and development of a genome-wide haplotype map (HapMap project) and the resulting identification of SNP tags, quickly are reducing the costs of such endeavors. The number of cases needed to effectively demonstrate such small effect sizes, however, remains an obstacle to most investigators, and in fact, represents a strong argument for multi-center collaborative studies. Are there alternative approaches that remain viable in pharmacogenomics? In fact, investigators in this field are fortunate to often have available a relatively rich pharmacokinetic and pharmacodynamic knowledge base resulting from drug development. Thus, it would appear the most productive approach would be to take advantage of the existing knowledge base to identify several pharmacokinetic or pharmacodynamic candidate genes or pathways likely to be involved in interindividual differences in drug response and direct initial studies at these targets. Whole genome scans then might be reserved for those instances when lack of knowledge results in a substantial amount of the variation in response not being explained by the identified candidate genes. Thus, a combined, but tiered and prioritized approach would be applied. Are there instances where such an approach has proven successful? One of the best examples is the progress being made in our understanding of the pharmacogenomics of asthma therapy, although this also serves as an example where genome-wide scanning may prove beneficial.

Pharmacogenomics approach toward asthma treatment

Asthma is a pediatric disease of increasing concern that includes hypersensitivity of the bronchus, inflammation, and reversible airway obstruction. Already affecting nearly 300 million patients worldwide, strong evidence suggests an alarming increase in prevalence. The disease also is consuming an increasing fraction of health care expenditures; nearly $12.6 billion were spent in 1998, with medication costs representing the largest component [50]. Adverse drug reactions remain a serious problem, with failed efficacy [51,52] and safety concerns [53–55] being observed with all three major therapeutic modalities (ie, the β$_2$-adrenergic receptor (ADRB2) agonists, the

A

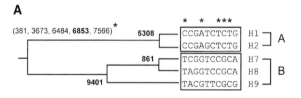

B

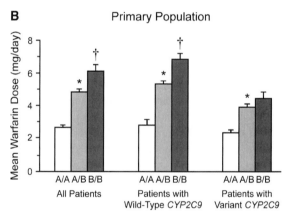

C

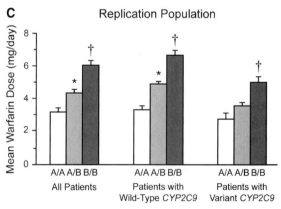

leukotriene antagonists, and inhaled corticosteroids). Does available information suggest asthma treatment would benefit from a pharmacogenomics approach? Consistent with genetic variation in the pharmacodynamics of asthma therapy, substantial interindividual differences in forced expiratory volume at one second (FEV_1) and the concentration of methacholine causing a 20% decrease in FEV_1 (PC_{20}) are observed in response to therapy [56]. Evidence also would suggest both phenotypic traits exhibit a strong genetic component [51,57,58]. These data, along with the prevalence and seriousness of the disease, suggest that asthma therapy would benefit from a pharmacogenomic approach. Further, the multiple therapeutic approaches and complexity of the disease itself suggest that multiple candidate genes must be included.

Corticosteroid signaling pathway

Corticosteroids are known to produce a potent anti-inflammatory response, and as such, they represent the most effective and commonly used drugs for chronic asthma therapy. These drugs, however, also are known to have serious adverse effects [59]. Corticosteroid-based drugs act primarily by binding to and activating the glucocorticoid receptor, a member of the large nuclear hormone receptor family of ligand-activated transcription factors. The activated receptor up-regulates a group of anti-inflammatory genes such as the lipocortins, the type II interleukin-1 receptor, and the secretory leukocyte proteinase inhibitor. Equally, if not more importantly, the glucocorticoid receptor also down-regulates proinflammatory genes by interacting directly with activator protein-1 (AP-1) and nuclear factor κB (NFκB) and inhibiting their activity [60]. The large interindividual differences

◄————————————————————————————————

Fig. 1. Effect of *VKORC1* haplotype combination on clinical warfarin dose. (*A*) Common haplotypes (H1, H2, H7, H8, and H9) were clustered with use of the UPGMA method (unweighted pair group method with arithmetic mean); they formed two distinct evolutionarily distant groups, designated A (comprising H1 and H2) and B (comprising H7, H8, and H9). Eight single-nucleotide polymorphisms (SNPs) are labeled at the nodes of the tree, and four SNP sites (shown in boldface) were used to discriminate between each branch and to distinguish groups A and B. Asterisks indicate correlated SNP sets that were associated significantly with warfarin dose. Group A was associated with a low warfarin dose, and group B was associated with a high warfarin dose. (*B*) Patients in the primary population were genotyped and assigned a *VKORC1* haplotype combination (A/A, A/B, or B/B). The patients were classified further according to *CYP2C9* genotype (the reference or either the *2 or *3 variant). The total numbers of patients having a group A combination, a group B combination, or both were 182 (all patients), 124 (reference *CYP2C9*), and 58 (variant *CYP2C9*). Four patients could not be assigned to group A or to group B. (*C*) Three hundred fifty-seven patients from the replication sample were genotyped and grouped as were those in the primary patient population; 233 had reference *CYP2C9* and 124 variant *CYP2C9*. The asterisks in the bottom two panels denote $P < .05$ for the comparison with combination A/A, and the daggers $P < .05$ for the comparison with combination A/B. The T bars represent standard errors. (*From* Rieder MJ, Reiner AP, Gage BF, et al. Effect of VKORC1 haplotype on transcriptional regulation and warfarin dose. New Engl J Med 2005;352(22):2285–93; © 2005 Massachusetts Medical Society; with permission.)

observed in response to corticosteroid therapy, including instances of frank resistance [56,61], is consistent with genetic variation contributing to differences in response. Acknowledging the complexity of the pathways involved in effecting corticosteroid therapy, Tantisira and colleagues [62] selected 14 candidate genes involved in glucocorticoid synthesis, binding, signaling, and metabolism most likely to influence therapeutic response. One hundred thirty-one SNPs that oversampled exonic information, but included at least one SNP per 10 kilobase pairs, were used to initially screen 415 adult asthmatics. Because of sample size limitations, only non-Latino whites were included in the analysis to avoid problems with population stratification. Individual SNPs were tested for association with the change in FEV_1 as a phenotypic outcome over an 8-week period using general linear regression. Four SNPs from three genes, corticotropin-releasing hormone 1 (*CRHR1*), Fc fragment of IgE, low affinity II, the receptor for CD23A (*FCER2*), and the glucocorticoid receptor (*NR3C1*) exhibited a statistically significant association ($P < .05$). No attempt was made to adjust for multiple comparisons, making it likely that false positives were present in this subset of SNPs. The four identified SNPs, representing *CRHR1, FCER2,* and *NR3C1,* then were used to screen 201 patients from the Childhood Asthma Management Program (CAMP). A single SNP within *CRHR1* intron 2 was associated positively with an improvement in FEV_1 after 8 weeks of therapy ($P = .006$). In the initial adult patients, individuals homozygous for the reference allele (allelic frequency approximately 70%) exhibited a 5.49% plus or minus 1.40% mean change in FEV_1 compared with 13.28% plus or minus 3.11% for those individuals homozygous for the variant allele. Similarly, patients from the CAMP study who were homozygous for the reference allele exhibited a mean change in FEV_1 of 7.57% plus or minus 1.5%, while those homozygous for the variant allele exhibited a change of 17.80% plus or minus 6.77%. Given the recognized value of using haplotype versus individual SNP analysis, Tantisira and colleagues [62] determined that three *CRHR1* SNPs distinguished four possible common haplotypes in the study populations (H1-H4) that occurred at frequencies of 0.46%, 0.27%, 0.21%, and 0.05%, respectively. The H2 haplotype was associated significantly with an enhanced response to inhaled corticosteroid therapy. H2 homozygous individuals exhibited a twofold enhanced response in the adult study and a threefold enhanced response in the CAMP study compared with individuals homozygous for H1, H3, or H4. Although these studies were very promising and clearly demonstrated a role for genetics in explaining interindividual differences in response to inhaled corticosteroids, the *CRHR1* variant explained less than 5% of the overall variation in therapeutic response. Thus, this study confirms the need to examine multiple candidate genes, but also argues for a more objective, global approach for this particular therapeutic regimen. These investigators were unable to replicate their findings in a third study population of 224 adult asthmatics. Likely reasons were the small effect size and limited study population, along with the fact that none of the SNPs used likely were causative for the phenotype, but rather, were in imperfect linkage disequilibrium.

A mouse model in which the TBX21 transcription factor has been knocked out, spontaneously develops airway inflammation and hyperresponsiveness similar to that observed in asthmatic patients [63]. An examination of the *TBX21* human ortholog revealed a single common *TBX21* nonsynonymous SNP in which a glutamine is substituted for histidine at amino acid position 33 (H33Q). Recruiting children from the CAMP cohort, Tantisira and colleagues [64] tested the effect of the *TBX21* variant on the efficacy of long-term inhaled corticoid steroid therapy. About 30% of the study group were randomized into a steroid arm, while the remaining patients were on a nonsteroid placebo or nedocromil arm. Further, the actual analysis was restricted to non-Latino white children to avoid population stratification and the low sample representation from other population groups. No difference was observed between the placebo or nedocromil arm, and as such, these two groups were pooled into a nonsteroid arm for analysis. Five children in the steroid arm were heterozygote for the *TBX21* H33Q variant; none were homozygous as expected. Although there was no association of the H33Q variant on changes in FEV_1, a significant association was observed with changes in PC_{20} over 4 years. After adjustment for age, gender, and baseline lung function, patients heterozygous for the *TBX21* H33Q variant showed nearly a fourfold enhancement in the mean log-transformed PC_{20} value, while patients homozygous for the H33 allele only showed a 1.2-fold enhancement. The mean log-transformed change in PC_{20} for patients homozygous for the H33 allele in the nonsteroid group was 0.66, and there was no effect of the H33Q variant in this study group. Unfortunately, attempts to identify a mechanism whereby the H33Q variant might impact TBX21 function were unsuccessful. Further, like *CRHR1*, the *TBX21* variant only explains a few percent of the variability observed response to inhaled corticosteroids.

ADBR2 signaling pathway agonists

ADRB2 is a G_S-protein coupled receptor that signals through adenylate cyclase to increase protein kinase A activity and induce a rapid relaxation of the airway smooth muscle. Despite the well-recognized and long-documented interindividual variability in response, ADRB2 agonists remain the most commonly used therapy for treating acute asthmatic episodes [50]. Early *ADRB2* resequencing efforts using DNA from 51 asthmatic and 56 normal subjects identified nine SNPs, four of which were nonsynonymous [65]. Of these four, only two were common, 46G > A (R16G) and 79C > G (Q27E), with the variant allele exhibiting frequencies between 40% and 60% and 20% and 40%, respectively. This initial study did not report any differences in SNP frequencies between cases and controls, likely because of the limitations of a relatively small and heterogeneous study population. Several follow-up studies that varied in design and in general, also used limited sample sizes, reported inconsistent results regarding an association between *ADRB2* variants and therapeutic response as measured by FEV_1. In a longitudinal study of 269 children, however, Martinez and colleagues [66] demonstrated that patients homozygous for the R16 allele were 5.3 times (95% confidence interval [CI] 1.7,17.7) and heterozygotes 2.3 times (1.3,4.2) more likely to respond to albuterol than patients homozygous for the G16 allele. No association was observed with the Q27E variant. Consistent with these results, Lima and colleagues [67] reported a significantly greater response to albuterol in individuals homozygous for the R16 allele versus either heterozygous individuals or individuals homozygous for the G16 allele. In addition to the difference in immediate response, the R16G variation appears to impact a second phenotypic outcome (ie, ligand-dependent desensitization of ADRB2 or tachyphylaxis). Several investigators have reported a positive association between the R16 allele and increased susceptibility to tachyphylaxis [68–70], although these studies are somewhat controversial, and further studies are needed [71].

Because the likelihood of multiple polymorphisms resulting in combinatorial affects within a given locus, it increasingly is recognized that association studies with haplotypes rather than single SNPs will be a more accurate and sensitive approach. Drysdale and colleagues [72] were the first to report such an analysis involving *ADRB2*. Thirteen SNPs were identified, which clustered into 12 haplotypes with considerable ethnic and racial differences in haplotype frequencies. These investigators observed that mean changes in FEV_1 were associated significantly with haplotype pairs, but not with individual SNPs. Over twofold differences were observed. Haplotype 4, consisting of a variant position at nucleotide 46G > A (G16R), with the remaining 12 positions matching the reference sequence, was associated with a depressed response to albuterol. In contrast, haplotype 2, consisting of variants at position -1023G > A, -468C > G, -367T > C, -47T > C (C19R in the ADRB2 leader peptide sequence), -20T > C, and 79C > G (Q27E), was associated with increased responsiveness. Using family studies and a subset of the 13 SNPs that would delineate the most common haplotypes, Silverman and colleagues [73] observed similar results.

Studies to examine other members of the ADRB2 signaling transduction cascade and their possible contribution to interindividual differences in therapeutic response also have been initiated, although much remains to be done. Nine mammalian isoforms of adenylate cyclase have been identified (ADCY1-9). Of these, ADCY9 is expressed widely in skeletal muscle, brain, kidney, lung, liver, and heart and is thought to be a major component of the ADRB2 signaling cascade. Small and colleagues [74] undertook an *ADCY9* SNP discovery project and identified a 2312A > G base transition that results in an I772M amino acid substitution within the C1 cytoplasmic domain, thought to be critical for adenylate cyclase catalytic activity. The affect of this variant on human ADRB2 agonist signaling in vivo remains to be determined, but the M772 variant did exhibit a substantially decreased activity in response to isoproterenol in an HEK293 cell-based assay. Although preliminary, these studies suggest that other candidate genes along this signaling cascade may play a role in explaining the variability in response to ADRB2 agonists. Delineating these additional genes likely will improve the ability to predict efficacy, and avoid adverse effects with these drugs.

Leukotriene pathway antagonists

The third and most recently developed therapeutic arm for asthma is the leukotriene antagonists. Leukotrienes are synthesized from arachidonic acid in human mast cells, basophils, eosinophils, and macrophages by 5-lipoxygenase (ALOX5) and 5-lipoxygenase activating protein (FLAP) with the initial, unstable product being LTA_4. LTA_4 is converted to cysteinyl leukotrienes by the sequential action of LTC_4 synthase (LTC4S, a glutathione S-transferase) to form LTC_4, γ-glutamyl transpeptidase to produce LTD_4, and finally, dipeptidase to produce LTE_4. These three cysteinyl leukotrienes (LTC_4, LTD_4 and LTE_4) account for the activity originally characterized as slow reacting substance of anaphylaxis (SRS-A). Their release into the extracellular space is mediated primarily by the ABC transporter, MRP1 (ABCC1) [75]. The cysteinyl leukotrienes are highly effective bronchoconstrictors, with activities 100- to 10,000-fold more potent than histamine. In addition, the cysteinyl leukotrienes cause vasodilation and increased vascular permeability and stimulate mucous secretion. At least one of the compounds, LTD_4, also is a potent chemoattractant for eosinophils. Thus, the cysteinyl leukotrienes produce many of the principle characteristics of the asthmatic lung. Finally, these compounds have been found at increased levels in the bronchial lavage fluid and urine of asthmatics and were further increased after an acute asthmatic attack [76,77]. The activity of the cysteinyl leukotrienes is mediated by the cysteinyl leukotriene receptor 1 (*CYSLTR1*), a member of the seven membrane-spanning G-protein coupled receptor family, which when activated, results in increased intracellular calcium mobilization. *CYSLTR1* is expressed widely. It however, is localized to the peribronchial and peri-bronchiolar smooth muscle cells, but not the epithelial cells lining the airway lumen. Expression also has been observed in the spleen, macrophages, and peripheral blood leukocytes [78–80]. Further, up-regulation of *CYSLTR1* has been reported in tissue from stable asthma patients with further increases in expression in patients suffering acute attacks [81]. Both CYSLTR1 antagonists (eg, pranlukast, zafirlukast, and montelukast) and an ALOX5 inhibitor (zileutron) have been approved for asthma treatment.

Early studies to identify genetic variants within the *ALOX5* gene identified a VNTR polymorphism within the promoter, resulting in changes in the number of binding sites for the transcription factors Sp1 and early growth response factor-1 (Egr-1). The dominant *ALOX5* allele contained five repeats (an approximate 80% allelic frequency), while minor alleles were identified containing deletions of one or two of the repeats or the addition of a single repeat. In vitro, each of these polymorphisms results in a 20% to 35% decrease in *ALOX5* promoter activity [82]. The possible association of the *ALOX5* VNTR polymorphism with the response to ABT-761, a zileutron-like ALOX5 inhibitor, was examined in 114 patients taking high dose ABT-761 versus 107 patients receiving placebo. Patients homozygous for the major allele or heterozygous for one of the minor variant alleles demonstrated an approximate 20% change in FEV_1 at the end of the treatment period. In contract, 10 patients homozygous for the minor allele did not benefit from the ABT-761 therapy, similar to that observed with patients receiving placebo [83]. Although this study represented the first demonstration of a genetic variant impacting the cysteinyl leukotriene pathway, the frequency of this variant would suggest it only accounts for a small percentage of the variation seen in response to the drugs targeting this pathway.

Eosinophils in the asthmatic airway represent the major source of LTC4 synthase (LTC4S), and as such, of cysteinyl leukotrienes in these patients [84]. A -444A > C transversion in the *LTC4S* promoter, postulated to result in the creation of an activator protein 2 (AP2) site and perhaps increased gene expression [85], was tested for its possible contribution to variation in response to zafirlukast [86]. Consistent with the variant allele resulting in increased *LTC4S* expression, calcium ionophore-stimulated eosinophils from normal subjects with at least one variant allele produced approximately three times more LTC_4 compared with stimulated eosinophils isolated from homozygous reference normal subjects. In patients who had asthma, zafirlukast treatment for 2 weeks was associated with increased FEV_1 in patients with at least one variant allele (n = 13) compared with patients homozygous for the reference allele (n = 10). These findings were corroborated in a study of Japanese asthmatics participating in a pranlukast trial [87]. Individuals with at least one variant allele (n = 16) exhibited a mean FEV_1 improvement of 14.3% plus or minus 5.3% after 4 weeks of therapy, compared with 3.1% plus or minus 2.4% among patients homozygous for the reference allele (n = 31). More recent studies, however, have called into question the validity of the associations with the *LTC4S* -444A > C promoter polymorphism. In a retrospective analysis of eight randomized, placebo-controlled trials involving patients who had mild-to-moderate asthma, no association was observed between genotype and bronchial hyper-responsiveness to adenosine monophosphate (PD_{20}) or methacholine (PC_{20}), changes in FEV_1, exhaled nitric oxide, or eosinophilia [88]. Independently, Kedda and colleagues [89] failed to find any association between the *LTC4S* polymorphism and chronic asthma severity or aspirin intolerance. Further, the polymorphism had no functional effect on the *LTC4S* promoter in vitro.

Most recently, Lima and colleagues [90] took a polygenic approach, examining possible associations between multiple genetic variants within several leukotriene pathway candidate genes and interpatient variability in montelukast response. Patients were recruited from a randomized, double-masked, parallel-designed American Lung Association Asthma Clinical Research Center Network trial comparing the efficacy of placebo (n = 86), theophylline (n = 77), and montelukast (n = 88) in patients who had poorly controlled mild-to-moderate persistent asthma. Outcome measures included change in FEV_1 after 6 months of montelukast treatment and the binary risk of having an asthma exacerbation event during the treatment period. A total of 28 SNPs in $ALOX5$, LTA_4 hydroxylase ($LTA4H$), $LTC4S$, $MRP1$, and $CYSLT1R$, and the $ALOX5$ repeat promoter polymorphism were included in the study. To avoid issues of population stratification, the association analyses were restricted to non-Latino whites in the montelukast arm (n = 61). Positive associations were found between individual SNPs in the $ALOX5$ and $MRP1$ genes and changes in FEV_1 ($P < .05$). Individuals with at least one of the variant $ALOX5$ VNTR promoter polymorphisms or at least one of the variant $LTC4S$ -444A>C promoter polymorphisms had a 73% or 80% reduced risk, respectively, for asthma exacerbations compared with individuals homozygous for the reference genotype. In contrast, individuals heterozygous or homozygous for a single $LTA4H$ SNP had a 4.0- to 4.5-fold increased risk for asthma exacerbation. Of interest, the direction of the effect observed with the $ALOX5$ VNTR is opposite to that expected based on earlier studies [82,83]. Further, the association observed with the $LTC4S$ -444A>C variant is consistent with some studies [86,87], but not others [88,89]. To their credit, the study design by Lima and colleagues [90] acknowledged the likely effect of multiple genetic variants contributing to the interindividual differences in therapeutic response. The problem of a small sample size, however, which was exacerbated by the need to avoid issues of population stratification, represented a significant limitation. In addition, these investigators failed to adjust their results for multiple comparisons, arguing it was more important not to dismiss differences that could be real. Thus, as acknowledged by the investigators, this study, and most, if not all of those highlighted previously, remains exploratory and illustrates the need for larger, multi-center studies.

Future prospects and challenges

The integration of pharmacogenetics into medicine is occurring in two spheres, the first being the pharmaceutical industry, wherein integration is occurring in the context of both preclinical drug development and clinical trials. Within this sphere, pharmacogenomic knowledge and technology are changing the types of available drugs, both because of their role in preclinical drug development and because of their ability to bring to market drugs that would otherwise be viewed as too dangerous or not sufficiently efficacious. The second sphere of integration is in clinical practice, wherein pharmacogenomic knowledge will change how drugs are prescribed. Generally, the pace of integration in the first sphere has been quicker than in the latter.

Preclinical drug development

The number of drugs surviving the development process has been disappointing recently. In addition, the number of truly blockbuster new drugs has been at an extreme low. The development of high-throughput screening technologies with high-density SNP maps set the stage to allow human disease-associated drug targets to be identified, and the stratification of clinical trials to reduce attrition. Thus, with the completion of the human genome project, it is estimated that the pharmaceutical industry has seen an increase from about 500 drug targets to about 5000 to 6000 gene target classes, with each class consisting of multiple specific genes. Examples of such target classes include nuclear hormone receptors and G-protein coupled receptors. Targets are being identified through case-control studies in which specific candidate genes are tested for association with a well-defined human disease, or in which whole human genome scanning is used for association [91]. Such studies require well-validated SNPs, and importantly, the availability of DNA from well-phenotyped patients and controls. The latter is generally the limiting factor. Nevertheless, such an approach is being used and sufficiently valued that some companies are incorporating DNA collections into all new phase 2 studies. An increase in the number and quality of new drugs and increased success from new targets may be the most substantial early impact of pharmacogenomic information.

The importance of correct phenotypic assessment in the development of new targets and clinical trials cannot be overstated. Phenotypic heterogeneity is a serious pitfall that is likely to result in false-positive and false-negative associations, even if the appropriate genes are selected for inclusion, and sufficient power is achieved. Problems of phenotypic heterogeneity are more common with complex diseases and diseases for which diagnostic assessment is based on subjective criteria. The use of large retrospective medical record databases also is fraught with such problems, but even more carefully collected databases may result in data that are insufficiently complete or objective for use in pharmacogenomic studies. Similarly, the clinical measurement of therapeutic response must be sufficiently objective and quantified in a standardized format. In general, short-term adverse events typically are documented more objectively in existing databases than chronic endpoints. Thus, using pharmacogenomics to define the inherited risk of long-term adverse toxicity is even more challenging. One might argue that these problems are not unique for pharmacogenomic studies, but rather true for all clinical trials. Nevertheless, the issue of valid phenotypic determination represents a challenge to the field. This is particularly true if whole genome scanning is to be used, as this approach requires a large number of subjects, making it more difficult to achieve cost-effectiveness.

Most candidate drugs that reach phase 1 safety testing fail in early phase 2, that is, during the development phase in which efficacy must be shown in a relatively small number of subjects with disease. One of the most exciting contributions of pharmacogenomic profiling is the ability to differentiate patient groups that are most likely to respond. Glaxo Smith Kline (Research Triangle Park, North Carolina) has shared with the US Food and Drug Administration (FDA) and the public its proof-of-concept pipeline data on this subject [92]. The company evaluated an antiobesity medication in its pipeline on 49 subjects and 40 placebo-treated controls. About 20% of the population were hyper-responders. Importantly, the hyper-responsive phenotype cosegregated with three SNPs that had been identified from a panel of 21 candidate genes. Those who were homozygous for genes that predicted nonresponse were clinically the least responsive. Individuals heterozygous for the predictive genes also had a shift in their weight loss curve compared with placebo controls, but not as great as subjects who were homozygous for the variant genotype predicting a hyper-response. Clearly, if individuals were selected without pharmacogenomic prescreening, the company may have decided it was not cost-effective to carry the drug forward. Thus, this project proved the concept that a candidate gene approach, if well-structured, can cost-effectively improve drug development. This approach also represents a substantial shift from the previous drug development paradigm of developing blockbuster drugs that can be prescribed broadly for common chronic disorders. On the negative side of the argument, there is some ethical concern that such information may leave some groups of patients as therapeutic orphans. Nevertheless, some pharmaceutical companies are using pharmacogenetic strategies early in drug development. With such a strategy, personalized medicine may not meet the challenge of a therapy designed for each individual patient, but rather the more economically viable alternative of developing therapies that target specific population subsegments.

Additional examples of pharmacogenomics in drug development are largely retrospective. One well-known example is trastuzumab, a monoclonal antibody against the ERBB2 (HER2) receptor. Retrospective analysis of the original breast cancer trials of this drug demonstrated an increased efficacy in those who overexpress the ERBB2 receptor. The availability of a diagnostic test for this receptor allowed the drug to progress to approval and into clinical use. Moreover, this process identified the ERBB2 receptor as a target, a byproduct of the pharmacogenomic studies that may be particularly important given that trastuzumab is only partially effective [93].

Clinical trials

Multiple questions must be addressed before the successful integration of pharmacogenomics into clinical trials. The preeminent issue is determining the predictive value of a specific genotype for efficacy or toxicity. Congruity between genotype, gene expression, and enzyme activity in vitro or in vivo is needed. If the concordance between genotype and gene expression is relatively low, because of either post-transcriptional induction or environmental interactions (eg, drug–drug interactions or age), genotype data not only may be noninformative, it may be misleading.

A second important question is which SNPs of a given pathway, process, or disease should be selected for inclusion? Some have suggested that only SNPs or haplotypes occurring at greater than 5% frequency in one or more populations be included. For some genes, however, multiple alleles that occur at relatively rare frequencies (less than 1%) substantially impact function. One solution is that low-frequency but high-impact alleles be grouped into a single phenotype, and all individuals with any of the included alleles be studied as a group.

A third issue is determining the implications of the SNP's evaluation to the general population. In that regard, how should ethnicity be evaluated within the context of clinical trials? Clearly, results of trials within one ethnic group may be of little value for another ethnic group, as gene frequencies are likely to differ across population groups. For relatively simple processes, however, for which all relevant genetic loci are known (eg, many drug-metabolizing enzymes), studies can be conducted in a single ethnic group and the impact to others inferred from the relative allelic frequencies. The more difficult situation is pharmacogenomic studies in which either the relevant disease genes or genes impacting drug disposition are not well-defined. In such cases, the impact cannot be inferred, and either testing of each ethnic group or whole genome scanning association studies are needed.

There is hope that pharmacogenomic testing will improve patient safety, both in clinical trails and in clinical practice. Because of the rarity of most adverse events, the most informative periods for safety assessment are phase 2 and postmarketing surveillance. A proof-of-concept paper has demonstrated the utility of pharmacogenomics with tranilast, an antirestenosis drug in adults. About 12% of the 11,500 phase 3 patients treated with tranilast developed hyperbilirubinemia. Candidate gene assessment identified that a *UGT1A1* repeat polymorphism was highly associated with this adverse effect [94]. The tranilast phase 3 data also were used to demonstrate that if a large control population is used, only a relatively small number of subjects exhibiting an adverse event, that is 10 to 30, would be needed to verify the SNP association [95]. Of course, the ease of detection is dependent on the strength of the association between the gene and the adverse event, the ease of detection of the adverse event, and the degree to which it is similar across multiple genetic backgrounds. If several genes are involved, more patients would be needed.

It has been debated whether medications withdrawn from the market will be rescued using pharmacogenetic approaches. Pharmaceutical representatives have argued that this is unlikely, because DNA from patients would need to have been collected before a drug's withdrawal, and there would need to be a financial incentive, as most compounds would be off-patent. An example of such a possible rescue drug in pediatrics might be the prokinetic agent, cisapride, a drug commonly used in pediatrics that was withdrawn because of prolongation of the QT interval, a trait now linked to certain genetic loci, and drug interactions that now are better defined.

A practical problem has been that the resources for both types of drug development studies are segregated. In addition, on average, it costs about $3 million to carry out one study. Although both the pharmaceutical industry and academia currently have competency in SNP validation and high throughput screening, the former generally has greater resources. The pharmaceutical industry also has expertise with chemical screening and regulatory compliance. Patient collections of DNA, however, which are typically the rate-limiting factor, are housed largely within academia. Importantly, it is clear that the process of characterizing patient phenotype in a validated fashion is time- and cost-intensive, and to some degree, prohibitive. In part to address this issue, a public-private partnership between the National Institutes of Health (NIH), the foundation of NIH (a nonprofit foundation established by Congress to support the mission of the NIH), Pfizer (New York, New York), and Affymetrix (Santa Clara, California) is being created to accelerate genetic association studies. This new partnership, the Genetic Association Information Network (GAIN), has $5 million from Pfizer to support management cost, and $15 million from Pfizer for laboratory support to determine the genetic contributions to five common diseases. Affymetrix, a leading company in genetic biotechnology, will provide the laboratory resources for studies of two additional common diseases. It is likely that additional unique public–private partnerships will be needed to address the scope and sample size of gene–environment studies.

Clinical practice

In spite of the tremendous amount of information known about the genetic basis for variable drug response, it has, as yet, had little impact on day-to-day clinical practice. The acceptance of pharmacogenomic testing into mainstream medical practice is likely to take place gradually. Several issues have precluded quick translation into practice, including the lack of readily available clinical service laboratories that can perform such tests quickly and cost-effectively, a paucity of trained health care providers who can interpret the test data and the associated clinical pharmacology, and the question of whether insurers will pay for such testing. Moreover, multiple ethical issues present ongoing challenges. The number of approved drugs with a reference to genetic testing in their labeling information, however, is increasing. As of 2004, 22 drugs had reference to such testing within the labeling information, some of which was considered sufficient to guide therapeutic decision making [96]. In 2005, the FDA published a guidance document for industry on the submission of genotyping data for drug-metabolizing enzymes. Some have estimated that in the next 5 to 10 years, as many as 10% to 20% of newly approved drugs will involve genetic testing. The introduction of testing likely will be disease- and context-specific.

For each indication, health care providers (both prescribers and insurers) and FDA regulators will want to know how substantial the impact of testing will be, in terms of the prevention of failed efficacy and adverse drug reactions. Of course, before use in routine clinical diagnostics, the genes selected must be shown in retrospective and prospective studies to be of sufficient value to be cost-effective. Retrospective data analysis of the efficacy, adverse events, and costs of therapy for psychiatry patients treated with substrates for the well-studied *CYP2D6* polymorphism suggests that genotyping can reduce costs [97].

Many practitioners have questioned and will question whether pharmacogenetic testing is more effective than their current practice of careful monitoring. As noted previously, the field most advanced in using pharmacogenetics is oncology, both in the evaluation of disease-related targets, such as mutated oncogenes, and in evaluation of genes for drug metabolism. This relates, in part, to the fact that most chemotherapeutic agents have either a narrow or nonexistent therapeutic window, such that even a small improvement in the ability to refine therapy may have a large impact on patient outcome.

Ethical issues

Some have argued that pharmacogenetics is challenged by unique ethical issues. Such a posture, that is, that genetic tests are categorically distinct from tests that do not concern DNA, has been called genetic exceptionalism. Most of the ethical issues, however, are the same fundamental ethics issues present in all clinical research or patient care: autonomy and respect for persons, beneficence, nonmaleficence, and justice. As such, genetic exceptionalism is refuted by well-recognized ethicists [98].

Autonomy

Considerable discussion has occurred regarding whether an individual patient's access to particular medicines could be limited or abolished based on efficacy or toxicity probability-based on pharmacogenetic testing. To date, no regulatory action excluding a patient from therapy-based on pharmacogenetic testing has been reported. It is possible, however, that such regulatory actions may be reasonable in the future. In this regard, pharmacogenetic testing does not differ from nongenetic testing that may identify patients for whom the potential benefit does not outweigh the risk. If a drug is not indicated based on an individual patient's evidence, there is no ethical justification for prescribing it. In such a scenario, the principle of nonmaleficence has greater weight than autonomy. It is improbable, however, that a drug will have a 0% chance of efficacy or 100% chance of toxicity [1]. If the outcome is sufficiently serious and no other therapies available, it is unlikely that treatment will be withheld.

The difficulty lies in deciding to what degree should testing be required before therapy can be used. Should this decision be regulated or simply left to health care providers to resolve in discussion with patients? Currently, most drug selection is done on the basis of physician assessment of multiple pieces of data, mostly nongenetic, and conveyance of an opinion of that information to the patient. If a patient does not have the characteristics for which the medicine was licensed, the drug still can be prescribed as off-label prescribing. The health care provider has a greater degree of accountability for any problems that arise from the unlabeled use of the drug. It is unlikely that pharmacogenetic testing will change the process to a great degree. The health care provider will need to include pharmacogenetic data in weighing the risk–benefit equation in a context-specific manner that includes discussion of the information with the patient. The question of the degree to which the genetic associations must be reproducible is also similar to all other testing. Similar to nongenetic testing, physicians will have to decide what predictive value is acceptable. Because most drugs are not labeled for use in children, most prescribing by pediatric providers is off-label.

The right of a patient to refuse pharmacogenetic testing is also an issue that has been raised, but that too should be similar to other clinical testing. Simply put, with relatively few extreme exceptions, the patient retains a degree of autonomy. Thus, similar to nongenetic testing, the critical issue will be whether the evidence is strong enough for regulatory agencies or health care providers to deny therapy on the basis of testing. Some would argue that the provider (either practitioner or insurer) is not obligated to use therapy without complete information. What strength of association is required for this principle to apply? At what point is the ethical issue of autonomy trumped by the obligation to assure nonmaleficence? These same issues are present with nongenetic testing.

Pharmacogenetic testing is available through direct-to-consumer advertising, particularly on the Internet. This process should be banned, similar to other medical testing that requires appropriate professional assessment of the application of the data. Currently, there is no regulatory oversight of this Internet marketing of direct-to-consumer medical testing.

Privacy and confidentiality

Mishandling of access to tests and samples is clearly an issue for all types of medical testing, both genetic and nongenetic. Pharmacogenomics, similar to other genetic testing, carries the added burden of dealing with the impact of testing on other family members who have not consented to testing [99]. In addition, pharmacogenetic research requires large repositories of biological specimens that are linked to personal health information, a process that must have ethical safeguards in place to protect patients. In this regard, the development of independent brokers who hold deidentified information for dispersal has become an accepted approach to address this concern.

Justice and discrimination

The current expectation of evidenced-based patient care involves health care providers using data to differentiate which patients are treated optimally with specific therapies. In this regard, pharmacogenetic testing is not different from other clinical testing. Notably, as with other testing, evidence is used to select those patients most likely to benefit and those for whom the probability of benefit does not exceed the likelihood of adverse events. Prescribing based on enhanced scientific evidence using pharmacogenetics should increase the objectivity and thus minimize wrongful discrimination based on subjective stereotypes or racial/ethnic identification. There is some concern, however, that the inverse may occur. That is, that the failure to use pharmacogenetic information to increase the chance of efficacy or minimize toxicity will be more likely among socially disadvantaged groups. Just as with other aspects of patient care, financial access to testing and information or education regarding testing may become an issue of social equity. In this regard, differential public education and public trust of health care providers can be a source of injustice. Such issues, however, are not unique to pharmacogenetics. To date, no evidence exists that unethical discrimination has occurred or will occur using pharmacogenetic testing. On an individual treatment level, discrimination based on ethnicity would be expected to be uncommon, because about 95% of genetic variation is within rather than between ethnic groups.

In contrast, equity in drug development may be vulnerable to such discrimination. The potential ability of pharmacogenetics to generate orphan patients (ie, those with the wrong genes), who have no treatment options, is of some concern. This is particularly worrisome if such genetic differences are linked to ethnic groups for which higher rates of poverty are well-recognized. Similarly, there is concern that the generation of orphan drugs may impact socially disadvantaged ethnic groups if potentially valuable medicines are dropped, because the market is known a priori to be small or not lucrative. These concerns may be overstated, however, as the likelihood of broad-scale discrimination is unlikely, as most genetic differences occur within rather than between ethnic groups.

Cost and other practicalities

Pharmacogenetic testing will impact informed drug selection, not just at the level of individual patients, but at the level of insurance programs and health systems formularies. For providers and insurance companies, the issue will be whether the added benefits are worth the costs. What about a drug that is only slightly more effective than standard therapy? What if a test only improves the predictability for a small minority of the population? Again, these issues are the same as those observed with other clinical tests and generally will require case-by-case context-based solutions. It has been assumed that in the long term, greater efficacy will result in greater cost-efficacy. This is likely to be true, because drug costs are only a fraction of total health care costs. Improved health outcomes based on the application of pharmacogenomics to clinical practice would be expected to result in larger savings in hospitalization and procedure costs. It also may be true, however, that pharmacogenetic information may lead to a greater level of expectation and an increased complexity in health care delivery. Additionally, it may require more provider time and lead to more ambitious end points and more use of services. Thus, although individual studies suggest cost effectiveness [100], the long-term broad implication for health care costs is not defined.

In summary, integration of pharmacogenetics into practice will require public and provider education. As with other medical testing, legal and regulatory safeguards are needed. Most of the ethical issues are not different from those of nongenetic testing. Answers to the question of which patient should get which drug, and at what dose will not be easy, but the enhanced approach provided by pharmacogenetic data ultimately will be incorporated into decision making at multiple levels.

References

[1] Spear BB, Heath-Chiozzi M, Huff J. Clinical application of pharmacogenetics. Trends Mol Med 2001;7(5):201–4.

[2] Lazarou J, Pomeranz BH, Corey PN. Incidence of adverse drug reactions in hospitalized patients: a meta-analysis of prospective studies. J Am Med Assoc 1998;279(15):1200–5.

[3] Meletis J, Konstantopoulos K. Favism—from the avoid fava beans of Pythagoras to the present. Haema 2004;7(1):17–21.

[4] Bottini E, Bottini FG, Borgiani P, et al. Association between ACP1 and favism: a possible biochemical mechanism. Blood 1997;89(7):2613–5.

[5] Porter IH, Boyer SN, Watson-Williams EJ, et al. Variation of glucose-6-phosphate dehydrogenase in different populations. Lancet 1964;42:895–9.

[6] Garrod AE, Oxon MD. The incidence of alkaptonuria: a study in chemical individuality. Lancet 1902;2:1616–20.

[7] Snyder LH. Studies in human inheritance. IX. The inheritance of taste deficiency in man. Ohio J Sci 1932;32:436–8.

[8] Motulsky AG. Drug reactions, enzymes and biochemical genetics. J Am Med Assoc 1957; 165(7):835–7.

[9] Vogel F. Moderne probleme der humangenetik. Ergeb Inn Med Kinderheilkd 1959;12: 52–125.

[10] Selikoff IJ, Robitzek EH, Ornstein GG. Treatment of pulmonary tuberculosis with hydrazide derivatives of isonicotinic acid. J Am Med Assoc 1952;150(10):973–80.

[11] Evans DA, Manley KA, McKusick VA. Genetic control of isoniazid metabolism in man. BMJ 1960;5197:485–91.

[12] Evans DAP, White TA. Human acetylation polymorphism. J Lab Clin Med 1964;63(3): 394–403.

[13] Blum M, Demierre A, Grant DM, et al. Molecular mechanism of slow acetylation of drugs and carcinogens in humans. Proc Natl Acad Sci U S A 1991;885:237–41.

[14] Hein DW. N-acetyltransferase 2 polymorphism: effects of carcinogen and haplotype on urinary bladder risk. Oncogene 2006;25(11):1649–58.

[15] Lacroix D, Sonnier M, Moncion A, et al. Expression of CYP3A in the human liver. Evidence that the shift between CYP3A7 and CYP3A4 occurs immediately after birth. Eur J Biochem 1997;247:625–34.

[16] Stevens JC, Hines RN, Gu C, et al. Developmental expression of the major human hepatic CYP3A enzymes. J Pharmacol Exp Ther 2003;307(2):573–82.

[17] Tréluyer JM, Rey E, Sonnier M, et al. Evidence of impaired cisapride metabolism in neonates. Br J Clin Pharmacol 2001;52(4):419–25.

[18] Pearce RE, Gotschall RR, Kearns GL, et al. Cytochrome P450 involvement in the biotransformation of cisapride and racemic norcisapride in vitro: differential activity of individual CYP3A isoforms. Drug Metab Dispos 2001;29(12):1548–54.

[19] Koukouritaki SB, Simpson P, Yeung CK, et al. Human hepatic flavin-containing monooxygenase 1 (*FMO1*) and 3 (*FMO3*) developmental expression. Pediatr Res 2002;51(2):236–43.

[20] Mayatepek E, Kohlmüeller D. Transient trimethylaminuria in childhood. Acta Paediatr 1998;87(11):1205–7.

[21] Tateishi T, Asoh M, Yamaguchi A, et al. Developmental changes in urinary elimination of theophylline and its metabolites in pediatric patients. Pediatr Res 1999;45(1):66–70.

[22] Sonnier M, Cresteil T. Delayed ontogenesis of CYP1A2 in the human liver. Eur J Biochem 1998;251(3):893–8.

[23] Leeder JS. Pharmacogenetics and pharmacogenomics. Pediatr Clin North Am 2001;48(3): 765–81.

[24] Wilkinson GR. Drug metabolism and variability among patients in drug response. N Engl J Med 2005;352(21):2211–21.

[25] Bomgaars L, McLeod HL. Pharmacogenetics and pediatric cancer. Cancer J 2005;11(4): 314–23.

[26] Mahgoub A, Dring LG, Idle JR, et al. Polymorphic hydroxylation of debrisoquine in man. Lancet 1977;2(8038):584–6.

[27] Gonzalez FJ, Skoda RC, Kimura S, et al. Characterization of the common genetic defect in humans deficient in debrisoquin metabolism. Nature 1988;331(6155):442–6.

[28] Weinshilboum RM, Sladek SL. Mercaptopurine pharmacogenetics: Monogenic inheritance of erythrocyte thiopurine methyltransferase activity. Am J Hum Genet 1980;32(5): 651–62.

[29] McLeod HL, Siva C. The thiopurine S-methyltransferase gene locus—implications for clinical pharmacogenomics. Pharmacogenomics 2002;3(1):89–98.

[30] Spire-Vayron de la Moureyre C, Debuysere H, Mastain B, et al. Genotypic and phenotypic analysis of the polymorphic thiopurine S-methyltransferase gene (TPMT) in a European population. Br J Pharmacol 1998;125(4):879–87.

[31] Yan L, Zhang S, Eiff B, et al. Thiopurine methyltransferase polymorphic tandem repeat: genotype-phenotype correlation analysis. Clin Pharmacol Ther 2000;68(2):210–9.

[32] Black AJ, McLeod HL, Capell HA, et al. Thiopurine methyltransferase genotype predicts therapy-limiting severe toxicity from azathioprine. Ann Intern Med 1998;129(9):716–8.

[33] Ishioka S, Hiyama K, Sato H, et al. Thiopurine methyltransferase genotype and the toxicity of azathioprine in Japanese. Intern Med 1999;38(12):944–7.

[34] McLeod HL, Coulthard S, Thomas AE, et al. Analysis of thiopurine methyltransferase variant alleles in childhood acute lymphoblastic leukaemia. Br J Haematol 1999;105(3): 696–700.

[35] Relling MV, Hancock ML, Rivera GK, et al. Mercaptopurine therapy intolerance and heterozygosity at the thiopurine S-methyltransferase gene locus. J Natl Cancer Inst 1999; 91(23):2001–8.

[36] Dervieux T, Medard Y, Baudouin V, et al. Thiopurine methyltransferase activity and its relationship to the occurrence of rejection episodes in paediatric renal transplant recipients treated with azathioprine. Br J Clin Pharmacol 1999;48(6):793–800.

[37] Tavadia SM, Mydlarski PR, Reis MD, et al. Screening for azathioprine toxicity: a pharmacoeconomic analysis based on a target case. J Am Acad Dermatol 2000;42(4):628–32.

[38] Andrew M, Marzinotto V, Brooker LA, et al. Oral anticoagulation therapy in pediatric patients: a prospective study. Thromb Haemostas 1994;71(3):265–9.

[39] Kamali F, Khan TI, King BP, et al. Contribution of age, body size, and CYP2C9 genotype to anticoagulant response to warfarin. Clin Pharmacol Ther 2004;75(3):204–12.

[40] Rettie AE, Korzekwa KR, Kunze KL, et al. Hydroxylation of warfarin by human cDNA-expressed cytochrome P-450: a role for P-4502C9 in the etiology of (S)-warfarin-drug interactions. Chem Res Toxicol 1992;5(1):54–9.

[41] Peyvandi F, Spreafico M, Siboni SM, et al. CYP2C9 genotypes and dose requirements during the induction phase of oral anticoagulant therapy. Clin Pharmacol Ther 2004;75(3): 198–203.

[42] Aithal GP, Day CP, Kesteven PJL, et al. Association of polymorphisms in the cytochrome P450 CYP2C9 with warfarin dose requirement and risk of bleeding complications. Lancet 1999;353(9154):717–9.

[43] Taube J, Halsall D, Baglin T. Influence of cytochrome P450 CYP2C9 polymorphisms on warfarin sensitivity and risk of over-anticoagulation in patients on long-term treatment. Blood 2000;96(5):1816–9.

[44] Veenstra DL, Blough DK, Higashi MK, et al. CYP2C9 haplotype structure in European American warfarin patients and association with clinical outcomes. Clin Pharmacol Ther 2005;77(5):353–64.

[45] Higashi MK, Veenstra DL, Kondo LM, et al. Association between CYP2C9 genetic variants and anticoagulation-related outcomes during warfarin therapy. J Am Med Assoc 2002; 287(13):1690–8.

[46] Rost S, Fregin A, Ivaskevicius V, et al. Mutations in VKORC1 cause warfarin resistance and multiple coagulation factor deficiency type 2. Nature 2004;427(6974):537–41.

[47] Li T, Chang CY, Jin DY, et al. Identification of the gene for vitamin K epoxide reductase. Nature 2004;427(6974):541–4.

[48] D'Andrea G, D'Ambrosio RL, Di Perna P, et al. A polymorphism in the VKORC1 gene is associated with an interindividual variability in the dose–anticoagulant effect of warfarin. Blood 2005;105(2):645–9.

[49] Rieder MJ, Reiner AP, Gage BF, et al. Effect of VKORC1 haplotypes on transcriptional regulation and warfarin dose. N Engl J Med 2005;352(22):2285–93.

[50] Tantisira KG, Weiss ST. The pharmacogenetics of asthma: an update. Curr Opin Mol Ther 2005;7(3):209–17.

[51] Drazen JM, Silverman EK, Lee TH. Heterogeneity of therapeutic responses in asthma. Br Med Bull 2000;56(4):1054–70.

[52] Szefler SJ, Phillips BR, Martinez FD, et al. Characterization of within-subject responses to fluticasone and montelukast in childhood asthma. J Allergy Clin Immunol 2005;115(2): 233–42.

[53] Kennedy MJ, Carpenter JM, Lozano RA, et al. Impaired recovery of hypothalamic-pituitary-adrenal axis function and hypoglycemic seizures after high-dose inhaled corticosteroid therapy in a toddler. Ann Allergy Asthma Immunol 2002;88(5):523–6.

[54] Dunlop KA, Carson DJ, Shields MD. Hypoglycemia due to adrenal suppression secondary to high-dose nebulized corticosteroid. Pediatr Pulmonol 2002;34(1):85–6.

[55] Lanes SF, Garcia Rodriguez LA, Huerta C. Respiratory medications and risk of asthma death. Thorax 2002;57(8):683–6.

[56] Malmstrom K, Rodriguez-Gomez G, Guerra J, et al. Oral montelukast, inhaled beclomethasone, and placebo for chronic asthma. A randomized, controlled trial. Montelukast/ Beclomethasone Study Group. Ann Intern Med 1999;130(6):487–95.

[57] Wilk JB, Djousse L, Arnett DK, et al. Evidence for major genes influencing pulmonary function in the NHLBI family heart study. Genet Epidemiol 2000;19(1):81–94.

[58] Palmer LJ, Burton PR, James AL, et al. Familial aggregation and heritability of asthma-associated quantitative traits in a population-based sample of nuclear families. Eur J Hum Genet 2000;8(11):853–60.

[59] Murphy S, Bleecker ER, Boushey H, et al. Guidelines for the diagnosis and management of asthma. Highlights of the expert panel. NHLBI National Asthma Education and Prevention Program. Bethesda (MD): NIH Publications. 1997;2:1–153.

[60] Leung DY, Bloom JW. Update on glucocorticoid action and resistance. J Allergy Clin Immunol 2003;111(1):3–22.

[61] Szefler SJ, Martin RJ, King TS, et al. Significant variability in response to inhaled corticosteroids for persistent asthma. J Allergy Clin Immunol 2002;109(3):410–8.

[62] Tantisira KG, Lake S, Silverman ES, et al. Corticosteroid pharmacogenetics: association of sequence variants in CRHR1 with improved lung function in asthmatics treated with inhaled corticosteroids. Hum Mol Genet 2004;13(13):1353–9.

[63] Finotto S, Neurath MF, Glickman JN, et al. Development of spontaneous airway changes consistent with human asthma in mice lacking T-bet. Science 2002;295(5553):336–8.

[64] Tantisira KG, Hwang ES, Raby BA, et al. TBX21: a functional variant predicts improvement in asthma with the use of inhaled corticosteroids. Proc Natl Acad Sci U S A 2004; 101(52):18099–104.

[65] Reihsaus E, Innis M, MacIntyre N, et al. Mutations in the gene encoding for the beta 2-adrenergic receptor in normal and asthmatic subjects. Am J Respir Cell Mol Biol 1993;8(3):334–9.

[66] Martinez FD, Graves PE, Baldini M, et al. Association between genetic polymorphisms of the beta 2-adrenoceptor and response to albuterol in children with and without a history of wheezing. J Clin Invest 1997;100(12):3184–8.

[67] Lima JJ, Thomason DB, Hohamed MHN, et al. Impact of genetic polymorphism of the β2-adrenergic receptor on albuterol bronchodilator pharmacodynamics. Clin Pharmacol Ther 1999;65(5):519–25.

[68] Israel E, Drazen JM, Liggett SB, et al. The effect of polymorphisms of the beta(2)-adrenergic receptor on the response to regular use of albuterol in asthma. Am J Respir Crit Care Med 2000;162(1):75–80.

[69] Dishy V, Sofowora GG, Xie HG, et al. The effect of common polymorphisms of the β2-adrenergic receptor on agonist-mediated vascular desensitization. N Engl J Med 2001;354(14):1030–5.

[70] Israel E, Chinchilli VM, Ford JG, et al. Use of regularly scheduled albuterol treatment in asthma: genotype-stratified, randomised, placebo-controlled cross-over trial. Lancet 2004; 364(9444):1505–12.

[71] Tattersfield AE, Hall IP. Are beta(2)-adrenoceptor polymorphisms important in asthma—an unraveling story. Lancet 2004;364(9444):1464–6.

[72] Drysdale CM, McGraw DW, Stack CB, et al. Complex promoter and coding region β2-adrenergic receptor haplotypes alter receptor expression and predict in vivo responsiveness. Proc Natl Acad Sci U S A 2000;97(19):10483–8.

[73] Silverman EK, Kwiatkowski DJ, Sylvia JS, et al. Family-based association analysis of beta(2)-adrenergic receptor polymorphisms in the childhood asthma management program. J Allergy Clin Immunol 2003;112(5):870–6.

[74] Small KM, Brown KM, Theiss CT, et al. An Ile to Met polymorphism in the catalytic domain of adenylyl cyclase type 9 confers reduced beta2-adrenergic receptor stimulation. Pharmacogenetics 2003;13(9):535–41.

[75] Lam BK, Owen WF Jr, Austen KF, et al. The identification of a distinct export step following the biosynthesis of leukotriene C4 by human eosinophils. J Biol Chem 1989;264(22): 12885–9.

[76] Holgate ST, Bradding P, Sampson AP. Leukotriene antagonists and synthesis inhibitors: new directions in asthma therapy. J Allergy Clin Immunol 1996;98(1):1–13.

[77] Busse WW. Leukotrienes and inflammation. Am J Respir Crit Care Med 1998;157:S210–3.

[78] Lynch KR, O'Neill GP, Liu Q, et al. Characterization of the human cysteinyl leukotriene CysLT1 receptor. Nature 1999;399(6738):789–93.

[79] Sarau HM, Ames RS, Chambers J, et al. Identification, molecular cloning, expression, and characterization of a cysteinyl leukotriene receptor. Mol Pharmacol 1999;56(3):657–63.

[80] Figueroa DJ, Breyer RM, Defoe SK, et al. Expression of the cysteinyl leukotriene 1 receptor in normal human lung and peripheral blood leukocytes. Am J Respir Crit Care Med 2001; 163(1):226–33.

[81] Zhu J, Qiu YS, Figueroa DJ, et al. Localization and upregulation of cysteinyl leukotriene-1 receptor in asthmatic bronchial mucosa. Am J Respir Cell Mol Biol 2005;33(6):531–40.

[82] In KH, Asano K, Beier D, et al. Naturally occurring mutations in the human 5-lipoxygenase gene promoter that modify transcription factor binding and reporter gene transcription. J Clin Invest 1997;99(5):1130–7.

[83] Drazen JM, Yandava CN, Dube L, et al. Pharmacogenetic association between ALOX5 promoter genotype and the response to antiasthma treatment. Nat Genet 1999;22(2):168–70.

[84] Cowburn AS, Sladek K, Soja J, et al. Overexpression of leukotriene C4 synthase in bronchial biopsies from patients with aspirin-intolerant asthma. J Clin Invest 1998;101(4): 834–46.

[85] Sanak M, Simon HU, Szczeklik A. Leukotriene C4 synthase promoter polymorphism and risk of aspirin-induced asthma. Lancet 1997;350(9091):1599–600.

[86] Sampson AP, Siddiqui S, Buchanan D, et al. Variant LTC(4) synthase allele modifies cysteinyl leukotriene synthesis in eosinophils and predicts clinical response to zafirlukast. Thorax 2000;55(Suppl 2):S28–31.

[87] Asano K, Shiomi T, Hasegawa N, et al. Leukotriene C4 synthase gene A(-444)C polymorphism and clinical response to a CYS-LT(1) antagonist, pranlukast, in Japanese patients with moderate asthma. Pharmacogenetics 2002;12(7):565–70.

[88] Currie GP, Lima JJ, Sylvester JE, et al. Leukotriene C4 synthase polymorphisms and responsiveness to leukotriene antagonists in asthma. Br J Clin Pharmacol 2003;56(4):422–6.

[89] Kedda MA, Shi J, Duffy D, et al. Characterization of two polymorphisms in the leukotriene C4 synthase gene in an Australian population of subjects with mild, moderate, and severe asthma. J Allergy Clin Immunol 2004;113(5):889–95.

[90] Lima JJ, Zhang S, Grant A, et al. Influence of leukotriene pathway polymorphisms on response to montelukast in asthma. Am J Respir Crit Care Med 2006;173(4):379–85.

[91] Debouck C, Metcalf B. The impact of genomics on drug discovery. Annu Rev Pharmacol Toxicol 2000;40:193–207.

[92] Roses AD. Pharmacogenetics and drug development: the path to safer and more effective drugs. Nat Rev Genet 2004;5(9):645–56.

[93] Noble ME, Endicott JA, Johnson LN. Protein kinase inhibitors: insights into drug design from structure. Science 2004;303(5665):1800–5.

[94] Danoff TM, Campbell DA, McCarthy LC, et al. A Gilbert's syndrome UGT1A1 variant confers susceptibility to tranilast-induced hyperbilirubinemia. Pharmacogenomics J 2004; 4(1):49–53.

[95] Xu CF, Lewis KF, Yeo AJ, et al. Identification of a pharmacogenetic effect by linkage disequilibrium mapping. Pharmacogenomics J 2004;4(6):374–8.

[96] Zineh I, Gerhard T, Aquilante CL, et al. Availability of pharmacogenomics-based prescribing information in drug package inserts for currently approved drugs. Pharmacogenomics J 2004;4(6):354–8.

[97] Chou WH, Yan FX, de Leon J, et al. Extension of a pilot study: impact from the cytochrome P450 2D6 polymorphism on outcome and costs associated with severe mental illness. J Clin Psychopharmacol 2000;20(2):246–51.

[98] Lipton P, Afshar H, Bobrow M, et al. Pharmacogenetics. Ethical issues. London: Nuffield Council on Bioethics; 2003. p. 1–103.

[99] The troubled helix: Social and psychological implications of the new human genetics. Cambridge: Cambridge University Press; 1996.

[100] Hughes DA, Vilar FJ, Ward CC, et al. Cost-effectiveness analysis of HLA B*5701 genotyping in preventing abacavir hypersensitivity. Pharmacogenetics 2004;14(6):335–42.

PEDIATRIC CLINICS
OF NORTH AMERICA

ELSEVIER
SAUNDERS

Pediatr Clin N Am 53 (2006) 621–638

Gene Therapy: Future or Flop

Frank Park, PhD[a,b,*], Kenneth W. Gow, MD[c]

[a]Department of Medicine, Kidney Disease Center, Medical College of Wisconsin,
8701 Watertown Plank Rd., HRC 4100, Milwaukee, WI 53226, USA
[b]Department of Physiology, Medical College of Wisconsin, 8701 Watertown Plank Rd.,
HRC 4100, Milwaukee, WI 53226, USA
[c]Department of Surgery, Division of Pediatric Surgery, Emory University School of Medicine,
2015 Uppergate Drive, Atlanta, GA 30322, USA

Exciting new advancements in the field of molecular genetics have begun to identify novel candidate genes that may be involved in many inherited or acquired disorders [1,2]. As a result, the field of gene therapy has erupted allowing scientists and clinicians to explore the possibility of treating disorders at the genomic level. The basic principle of gene therapy is to transfer exogenous wild-type genes using various vector systems into specific cell types within the human body to correct a pathologic disorder. The discovery of a singular "holy grail" vector has yet to be found, however. The ideal vector would have many, if not all, of the following components: be easy to produce, infect both dividing and nondividing cells, have regulatable gene expression, be immunologically inert, permit tissue-specific targeting, contain an accommodating packaging limit to incorporate large expression cassettes, and have site-specific integrating ability without producing adverse effects. It is unlikely that this type of vector will be found, so specific vectors will need to be tailor-made to adequately modify relevant cells to provide the needed therapeutic correction.

Currently, gene therapy vectors either are based on simple nucleic acid sequences or derived from unique viruses. The predominant use for gene therapy vectors has been to insert exogenous genes into particular cell types for overexpression of the therapeutic gene product. At this time, nucleic acid (also known as "naked DNA") based technology is a poor man's version of a gene transfer system. Formulations with lipids, electrical currents, and extremely high physical pressures have been combined with naked DNA to

---

* Corresponding author. Medical College of Wisconsin, Department of Medicine, Kidney Disease Center, 8701 Watertown Plank Rd., HRC 4100, Milwaukee, WI 53226.
E-mail address: fpark@mcw.edu (F. Park).

enhance its transfection efficiency in vivo, but the level of genetic modification lags behind most viral vectors [3]. For this reason, our review will focus on the development of viral-based vector systems, which are state-of-the-art in the field of gene therapy. Researchers have attempted to harness the power of viruses in hopes of using their efficient ability to hijack cells for gene expression of therapeutic molecules.

Although therapy for most pediatric diseases has continued to improve, progress in some areas has reached a plateau using standard therapy. To this end, many believe that gene therapy may offer hope as a specific means to provide therapeutic intervention. The biology of pediatric patients poses unique challenges with regard to the development of gene therapy vectors, however. Unlike mature adults in whom the cells are fully differentiated and relatively quiescent, most of the cells in young children are in varying states of differentiation and proliferation, which requires the transferred genes to be propagated into the daughter cells. Otherwise, the viral vector will be lost as the cells begin to divide and proliferate. At present, there remains a paucity of virus-based vector systems that have the capability of integrating into the genome following cell entry other than retroviruses.

We address the applicability of several viral vector systems as they would pertain to clinical pediatric use, discuss the potential role of an emerging new field of nucleic acid gene therapy based on RNA, and summarize how the field of gene therapy has dealt with different pediatric diseases using the various gene therapy tools.

Viral vector development: from infectious agents to vehicles of therapy

Many of the early clinical trials used gene therapy vectors because of their availability and convenience, because the prevailing thought was that one size fits all. For this reason, many of the clinical trials did not have a useful outcome other than providing some information regarding their safety in humans. With an increasing number of different viruses being developed as gene therapy tools, however, the ability to fashion a specific vector for a particular disease will become possible.

In general, the basic design of all viral vectors is similar in that they are composed of two or more fragments of the native viral genome. One fragment will contain the viral gene sequence in which the coding region has been replaced with the expression cassette of the gene of interest and the terminal repeats, which have short noncoding sequences found at the ends of the viral genome. These terminal repeats contain elements that are necessary for replication, packaging, or integration of the viral DNA into the genome. The other fragment, which may be further broken into several more pieces, contains the viral coding region that is necessary for the vector to function effectively by providing the viral proteins in trans necessary for packaging and assembly during vector production.

Presently, viral vectors can be categorized as either integrating (eg, oncoretroviruses and lentiviruses) or nonintegrating (eg, adenoviruses [Ad] and adeno-associated viruses [AAV]). Each of these viral vector systems has distinct properties and we will discuss their potential applications for pediatric diseases.

Integrating viral vectors

The overall development of gene therapy was initiated through the design of retroviruses based on Moloney leukemia virus (MLV). Conceptually, the retrovirus would be an ideal genetic modifier in pediatric diseases because of its innate ability to stably integrate into the host genome [4]. Copies of the integrated provirus therefore will be able to propagate into the daughter cells following parental cell division, and only the termination of the cells bearing the retroviral cassette will result in a loss of gene expression.

The design of the retroviral vectors is fairly straightforward in that much of the viral gene required for replication is deleted. This allows only the cells exposed to the retroviral vectors to express the therapeutic payload without producing dangerous recombinant progeny. This issue is crucial in the design of all retroviral vectors that will be targeted for use in the clinics. The two main classes of retroviral vectors currently being used are derived from both gamma-retroviruses (also known as oncoretroviruses) and lentiviruses.

Oncoretroviral vectors

Oncoretroviral vectors based on murine MLV are single-stranded RNA viruses that have been studied heavily in many clinical studies, including the very first gene therapy study using severe combined immunodeficiency-adenosine deaminase deficiency (SCID-ADA) children, which involved the insertion of the adenosine deaminase (ADA) gene [5]. In recent years, this vector system has been found to be extremely limited in its ability to transduce cells in vivo, because nuclear membrane dissolution is needed for integration to occur efficiently [6].

For this reason, researchers have addressed this limitation by using this vector system predominantly for ex vivo applications. Ironically, the ex vivo approach using MLV-based vectors to modify hematopoietic stem cells became the first successful breakthrough for gene therapy in which young children who had a genetic mutation in the gamma-c gene were treated to correct their immune systems [7]. Unfortunately, a serious setback occurred shortly after this initial breakthrough in 2001 tempering the excitement within the gene therapy community. At that time, 3 of the 11 children developed T-cell leukemogenesis, with one succumbing [8–11]. The clinical studies were halted to review the complications thoroughly, and it was decided ultimately that the leukemogenesis was attributed to a phenomenon known as insertional mutagenesis. In this study, the promoter activity of the retroviral long-terminal repeat (LTR), a region of viral DNA needed for recognition and integration into the genomic DNA, was found to provide the transcriptional machinery needed for the activation of a neighboring oncogene, which turned out to be the *LMO2* proto-oncogene [9,10]. Even though most of the children survived without the appearance of oncogenesis, the potential for insertional mutagenesis will likely cause clinicians to avoid using oncoretroviral vector-based vectors in future trials especially with the discovery of newer forms of retroviral vectors based on nononcogenic retroviruses.

Lentiviral vectors

One newly developed retroviral vector system derived from human immunodeficiency virus type 1 (HIV-1), also known as lentivirus, has been found to retain its ability to integrate into the genome, and its integration efficiency can be enhanced by cell division similar to MLV-based vectors. There are several differences that make lentiviral vectors more attractive than MLV-based vectors, however. First, investigators have demonstrated that terminally differentiated cells in vivo, such as neurons and hepatocytes, are readily transduced by lentiviral vectors, but not MLV-based vectors [12–14]. Second, the lentiviral vector packaging capacity can be up to ~18 kb, which should provide sufficient room to incorporate many large genes [15]. Third, the tropism of the lentiviral vectors can be altered by changing the envelope proteins that coat the vector in a process known as pseudotyping [16–19]. Fourth, the promoter activity of the LTR can be silenced in a process known as self-inactivation, or SIN, without markedly affecting the viral titer [20]. Fifth, lentiviral vectors integrate into genomic areas that are not within the promoter region or into sites that are far in proximity to the start site of the expressed genes, unlike MLV-based vectors, which are found to integrate close to the promoter regions of genes [21]. Finally, lentiviral vectors are derived from immunodeficiency viruses, in which infected patients rarely develop tumor formation attributable to the integration of the virus, unlike the predecessor retroviral vectors based on MLV, which are predisposed to causing oncogenesis.

Another important aspect to emphasize is the ability of lentiviral vectors to increase transduction efficiency when target cells are stimulated to undergo hyperplasia either by drug [22] or surgical methods [14,23,24] before the application of the lentiviral vectors. Moreover, investigators have demonstrated an age-dependent enhancement in lentiviral vector transduction in which early postnatal administration of lentiviral vectors can mediate higher transduction into the liver and other organs compared with late postnatal administration [25,26].

For pediatric gene therapists, the enhanced ability of lentiviral vectors to integrate into the target cell genome can be exploited, because many pediatric diseases involve cells that are slowly or rapidly proliferating. In addition, lentiviral vectors have been shown to transduce hematopoietic stem cells more efficiently than MLV-based vectors [27,28], which is an important issue for ex vivo applications using these vectors. It is likely that all future retroviral vectors will switch over to the lentiviral vector system, depending on its safety profile in humans.

Currently, the first clinical trial using lentiviral vectors involves the transduction of hematopoietic stem cells to express antisense RNA sequences against HIV genes [29,30]. Although encouraging findings were observed in the phase I/II clinical trial, the main point of the trial was to examine several important safety factors concerning the lentiviral vector, such as the potential for insertional mutagenesis, the possible production of replication-competent lentiviruses, and vector mobilization [30]. A second ex vivo phase I/II gene therapy clinical trial has been initiated in France to determine the safety and efficacy of lentiviral vector-transduced CD34$^+$ hematopoietic stem cells to treat patients with either sickle cell disease or β-thalassemia [31]. Although neither clinical trial will involve young children, these studies should validate the usefulness of lentiviral vectors as a therapeutic tool in the field of pediatrics, particularly for AIDS, monogenic disorders, and other pathologies involving proliferating target cells.

Nonintegrating viral vectors

In this section, we discuss the usefulness of nonintegrating viral vectors based on Ad and AAV for gene therapy applications.

Adenoviral vectors

Ad vectors are large (36 kb), non-enveloped, double-stranded DNA viruses that have been extremely well studied for a wide variety of gene therapy applications because of their ease to propagate into high titers, their broad tropism, and their extremely efficient ability to transduce different cell types in vivo [32]. The Ad vector system has been hampered, however, by its transient gene expression because it resides within the transduced cell as an episome. Vector persistence is not a priority for every pediatric disease, so the transient gene expression provided by Ad vectors is not a major concern.

On the other hand, the host immune response that is elicited against Ad vectors following their administration has been the major limitation in their use for therapeutic application. Dose-dependent toxicity and immune system activation can lead to, at a minimum, the elimination of the transduced cells containing the Ad vector, resulting in the loss of gene expression [33,34]. More seriously, it can produce devastating results, as highlighted by the untimely death in 1999 of a teenager who was enrolled in a clinical trial at the University of Pennsylvania for the treatment of ornithine transcarbamylase deficiency, a monogenic liver disorder [35]. As a result, the enthusiasm to use early-generation Ad vectors has diminished for clinical applications dealing with genetic disorders.

Early-generation Ad vectors still play a prominent role in the treatment of cancer, however. Much of the early cancer gene therapy involved the transduction of Ad vectors into different cancer cells to express genes that would help to overcome the genetic abnormalities that lead the cell toward a state of malignancy. A classic example would be the restoration of p53 function in anaplastic Wilms tumors [36], which would restore the cell cycle checkpoints and facilitate apoptosis in cells that already have withstood inordinate genetic damage. In this case, the cytotoxicity associated with the Ad vectors would not be a major concern, because the goal is to eliminate the tumorigenic cells by delivering a "killer" gene. Moreover, the activation of the immune system by the Ad vector may only enhance the likelihood of eliminating the transduced tumorigenic cells.

Another important technological advance has been the generation of novel tropism-modified Ad vectors to increase the targeting into normally resistant tumorigenic cells and expand the usefulness of Ad vectors for additional types of cancers [37–39].

Other researchers have continued to make design modifications in the Ad vector system to reduce its immunogenicity by removing all of its viral genes in hopes of using this system for other genetic disease models. This helper-dependent or "gutless" adenoviral vector has been tested recently in various animal models, including hemophilia B [40,41] and muscular dystrophy [42]. Ehrhardt and colleagues [40,41] demonstrated that gutless Ad vector administration produced physiologic levels of human coagulation factor IX without any evidence of cellular pathology or elevated liver enzyme activity. Another group of investigators used the increased packaging size of the gutless Ad vectors ($\sim$30 kb instead of $\sim$8 kb in early-generation Ad vectors) to incorporate the dystrophin gene to phenotypically restore $\sim$40% of the skeletal muscle contractility in muscular dystrophic (*mdx*) mice compared with their wild-type counterparts [42]. Unfortunately, similar to its earlier predecessors, the transgene expression remained short lived, such that 95% of its original therapeutic levels were diminished by 6 months after treatment [40]; this phenomenon may continue to hamper the usefulness of this vector system for genetic diseases requiring persistent gene expression.

Adeno-associated viral vectors

The other commonly used nonintegrating virus was discovered initially as a contaminant of adenovirus, and was named adeno-associated virus (AAV). AAV vectors were categorized initially as an integrating vector system [43,44], but recent studies have demonstrated that the integration frequency is low in vivo (eg, <10% of the persistent vector genomes integrate into hepatocytes) [45]. Currently AAV vectors are considered largely nonintegrating.

AAV vectors are derived from a small (4.7 kb), nonpathogenic, single-stranded DNA virus. The first AAV vector that was designed from AAV serotype 2 (AAV2) was found to be devoid of toxicity in small and large animal models, unlike adenoviral vectors [46]. Ironically, even though minimal integration occurs using AAV vectors, this vector system has been capable of maintaining persistent transgene expression. Similar to other viral vector systems, AAV2 vectors can transduce with equal efficiency into quiescent and dividing cells [47]. Several characteristics of this vector system may limit its usefulness for many genetic disorders, including its small packaging size ($\sim$5 kb), its restricted tissue tropism, and its relatively low transduction efficiency in vivo [46,48].

In general, AAV2 vectors have been well suited for diseases in which the target cells are largely quiescent with a slow rate of turnover, because it has been shown that slowly or rapidly dividing cells lead to the loss of the AAV vector genome because of its low integration frequency [45]. For this reason, much of the clinical use of AAV2 vectors in the past few years has been through the study of monogenic disorders, in particular hemophilia B [49,50]. The early outlook for AAV-mediated clinical gene therapy for hemophilia B was promising, but an unexpected immune response against the AAV2 vector was detected in two patients resulting in the termination of the clinical trial [51]. No vector-related immune responses were detected previously in any of the animal studies performed using AAV2 vectors, so one of the defining lessons learned from this trial was that human clinical trials are essential to validate the safe translation of the results found in animal models using gene therapy vectors.

Investigators currently are working to discover new serotypes of AAV in hopes of expanding the limited tropism of the virus and finding a serotype that would have minimal immune responsiveness [52–55]. Grimm and colleagues [54] demonstrated improved transgene expression using AAV2 vector genomes packaged with alternative AAV capsids. Nakai and coworkers [55] expanded on this finding and demonstrated that helper proteins from AAV serotype 8 could significantly enhance the transduction of AAV2 vector genomes into a wide numbers of cells that normally were refractory to AAV2 entry following intravenous administration in adult mice, including endothelial, smooth muscle, and neuronal cells. The capsid proteins from alternative serotypes, such as AAV7 and AAV8, would likely result in minimal humoral response in most patients, because the pre-existing exposure would be rare, resulting in few patients having neutralizing antibodies against them, unlike AAV2 [56].

Overall, it would appear that current experimentation in the field of AAV should expand the clinical use of this vector system into cell types normally refractory to AAV2, although it may remain limited to diseases in which the target cells undergo minimal proliferation.

Nucleic acid technology

Nucleic acid–based gene therapy involves the transfer of modified RNA or DNA molecules into cells. DNA-based therapy involves a circular form of DNA known as a plasmid that contains a gene encoding for a protein with known therapeutic benefit in combination with sequences that direct expression within a cell. Even with lipid formulations, the transfection efficiency into cells in vivo is extremely low [3], so the current state-of-the-art gene transfer vectors are derived from viruses.

Cutting-edge research in the field of nucleic acids has turned to the more unstable partner, RNA, to develop other novel methods to express normal gene sequences by repairing the cellular mutant mRNA (trans-splicing RNA), or conversely, knockdown gene expression within the cells (RNA interference). These RNA-based technologies are still in the developmental phase and cannot function without being incorporated into a vector system, but they will play an important complementary role in the development of future gene therapy applications.

Knockdown of gene expression

RNA interference

Until recently, the primary focus of gene therapy applications has been the incorporation of a normal gene sequence back into a recipient cell to produce a gain-of-function phenotype. The lack of a reliable, effective method to selectively knockdown pathologically active genes toward normal levels was not readily available. A new biologic phenomenon known as RNA interference (RNAi) has been discovered to specifically inhibit transcript functionality and lead to downregulated gene expression [57].

The concept of RNAi in eukaryotes was believed to originate as an RNA-mediated intracellular surveillance mechanism to protect the organism from genomic invaders, such as transposable elements and viral infections. Apparently, this system evolved to specify sequence-specific chromosomal modifications and to regulate expression of a significant fraction of endogenous genes through the recognition of small interfering RNA molecules (siRNA). The mechanism of RNAi is based on its ability to selectively inhibit either in the cytoplasm using short complimentary RNA oligonucleotide duplexes or in the nucleus using a short hairpin RNA (shRNA) molecule. Ultimately, either type of RNA duplex will lead to the specific targeting of gene transcripts for downregulation.

Gene therapy will not be limited only to treating loss-of-function disorders but also has applications in diseases characterized by aberrant gene expression. These include pediatric tumors or the replication of a virus, such as is found in pediatric AIDS. Recent studies have studied the design of rational RNAi molecules to specifically knock down β-catenin to inhibit the proliferation of hepatic tumors in vitro [58]. Others have used the RNAi technology to specifically target oncogenic fusion genes in leukemias and lymphomas [59]. For pediatric AIDS, many approaches have been investigated in which anti–HIV-1 genes are introduced to target cells to confer resistance to HIV-1 infection or replication into HIV-1–susceptible cells [29,30,60,61]. As discussed earlier, antisense RNA is being tested currently in lentiviral vectors to inhibit the replication of HIV [29,30]. As the specificity and efficacy of RNAi becomes more refined in the next few years, however, it is likely that this approach will replace these other methods to inhibit HIV replication [62]. It is likely that the RNAi mechanism will become the dominant technology for treatments involving genetic inhibition.

RNA repair

Trans-splicing technology

This technology is based on the biology of mRNA processing, which involves the removal or splicing out of intronic (or intervening) sequences, so that the exons (or expressed reading frames) can be "cut-and-pasted" together allowing for the translation of the gene product. If exon sequences contain a mutation or deletion resulting in the production of a nonfunctional protein, the theory is that it can be replaced with a lab-engineered wild-type sequence to restore the ability of the cell to produce a normal functioning protein.

Although there are currently several RNA-based repair systems under investigation the most clinically promising is the spliceosome-mediated RNA trans-splicing technology. The elements of this technology contain the spliceosome, are endogenously expressed mutant pre-mRNA target transcripts, and the engineered pre-mRNA trans-splicing molecules [63,64]. The cell supplies the former two molecules, whereas the latter RNA molecule is designed in the lab. In the presence of all three components, the spliceosome will mediate the attachment of the genetically engineered pre-mRNA trans-splicing molecule with the native mutant portion of the target pre-mRNA sequence. The replacement of the mutant portion of the pre-mRNA should allow the newly corrected mRNA to translate biologically functional proteins. As an added benefit, the levels of the newly corrected mRNA will depend on normal cellular regulation of its endogenous promoter, which would be more ideal than using other viral or cellular promoters with constitutive activity.

Early studies found highly inefficient RNA repair using the trans-splicing RNA mechanism in different models of monogenetic disorders, including hemophilia A, cystic fibrosis, and Duchenne muscular dystrophy [65–67]. Recently, increased efficiencies in this approach were observed following the incorporation of this RNA repair system into AAV vectors. Partial correction of the transmembrane conductance ability of the chloride channel was achieved in polarized human cystic fibrosis epithelial cells in vitro [67]. Moreover, the insertion of the mini-dystrophin gene into the skeletal muscle of *mdx* mice, a model for Duchenne muscular dystrophy, was found to correct the dystrophic phenotype in vivo [66]. Although further enhancements are needed to maximize the efficiency of the trans-splicing mechanism, the recent in vivo studies using the trans-splicing technology, particularly in monogenic disorders that affect individuals at a young age, demonstrate the potential of this novel method as a viable gene correction application.

In utero gene therapy: Can this be the next big step in pediatric gene therapy?

The treatment of many severely debilitating or lethal genetic disorders during fetal development has the potential to enhance the quality of life of the fetus upon birth. Moreover, the accessibility to specific sites postnatally for genetic manipulation may be extremely challenging.

For this approach to become clinically feasible, it is clear that an integrating vector system will be needed, because previous studies have shown the ineffectiveness of episomal vectors, including Ad and AAV vectors that produced only transient gene expression following in utero administration [68,69]. Because it is imperative that the vector propagates into differentiating cells during development, the currently available vectors that can address this criterion are either retroviral or lentiviral vectors. Recent studies by Waddington and colleagues [70] have demonstrated highly efficient lentiviral vector transduction into a wide number of organs following in utero administration into immune-competent mice and that prolonged expression of a secretable protein marker, coagulation factor IX, was achieved [71]. This finding was encouraging, because it is known that mature mice administered lentiviral vectors in vivo produce an immune response against the transduced cells and a humoral response to the secreted protein leading to the gradual loss of expression [72]. It is likely that the immune system was at an immature state during the period of lentiviral vector administration, so the immune system evolved to consider the vector and its expressed transgene as self-, nonimmunogenic antigens rather than foreign entities.

As pediatric genetic screening programs expand to include more diverse genes [73], in utero gene therapy may be another option for families otherwise faced with abortion or birth of a severely debilitated child. Currently, several diseases are being considered for in utero approaches, including hemophilia B, ornithine transcarbamylase deficiency, phenylketonuria, fragile X syndrome, and familial hypercholesterolemia. The risk factors need to be weighed over the therapeutic potential, however, such as limiting the gene transfer to only somatic cells that will make up the fetal body and not the germ cells leading to future inheritance issues, including the mother. It is clear that the potential of in utero gene therapy remains on the horizon in the treatment of genetic diseases that have lethal or severely debilitating phenotypes at birth.

Current drawbacks of gene therapy: What can we do to fix them?

First, we must prevent the activation of the immune system against the gene therapy vector, and second, we must develop a strategy to integrate gene therapy vectors into regions of the DNA that will not promote insertional mutagenesis. We will address these two issues in the following sections and suggest possible ways to circumvent these problems.

Immune response by the host against the vector or the expressed transgene

One of the main culprits preventing gene therapy from succeeding is the immune response that is mounted against the vector or the expressed transgene following cellular transduction. The body has adapted to the invasion of pathogens, such as viruses or their components, by immediately developing an innate immune response. Subsequently, the body develops a secondary adaptive immune response, which includes a cell-mediated response mechanism involving cytotoxic T lymphocytes (CTL) and natural killer cells [35,74,75] or a humoral response characterized by the production of neutralizing antibodies specific to the de novo expression of the transgene product or the vector [72,76]. Ultimately, the process of adaptive immunity not only contributes to the elimination of vectors and transduced cells from the body but will develop a memory response that thwarts future administration of the vector or transgene.

As discussed earlier, the importance of vector-related immune responses arose in public awareness in 1999 following a death attributed to an intense immune response mediated by the presence of the Ad vector proteins [35]. This casualty has resonated within the gene therapy field, and methods are being studied to promote tolerance against the gene therapy vectors to prevent this type of response in future trials.

Inhibition of costimulatory pathways

Strategies attempting to inhibit costimulatory pathways, such as CD40/CD40L and CD28-CD80/CD86 interactions, involving T cells and antigen-presenting cells (APCs) have been designed as a means to suppress the anti-vector immune response. Kay and coworkers [77] found that blockade of the CD40/CD40L pathway using CTLA4-Ig could increase the duration of transgene expression in mice injected with Ad vectors, and similar immune response suppression was achieved against AAV using CTLA4-Ig in combination with nasal instillation of AAV [78]. Even under the best conditions, however, this approach will only treat the existing problem but will not address the underlying mechanism driving the immune system toward vector elimination.

Tolerogenic dendritic cells

For this reason, an alternative approach has been postulated in which immature, inactivated dendritic cells are genetically manipulated to promote tolerance. Dendritic cells are robust immune professional antigen-presenting cells and play a pivotal role in either T-cell activation or tolerance induction. Previous studies used the dendritic cells as a means to induce tolerance toward self- or transplantation-antigens [79,80], and recent studies have promoted tolerance induction by modifying dendritic cells using lentiviral vectors [81]. At present, this method has the ability only to blunt the response in animals without pre-existing exposure to the vector, but further research in dendritic cell biology should provide the necessary information needed to overcome the pre-existing immunity. Moreover, this approach would have the same limitation as the approach to inhibit the costimulatory pathways, in that two separate complex drugs would need to be administered to the animal to produce the desired result; this issue could limit these approaches in the clinics.

Viral vectorology

Alterations in the viral vector could help to weaken the anti-vector immune response by removing the antigenic proteins in the capsids found in Ad and AAV as described earlier. The replacement of the capsid proteins from alternative serotypes, such as AAV7 and AAV8, would minimize the humoral response in most patients [53,56], whereas designing Ad vectors based on group B adenovirus serotype 35 would be beneficial because most humans have no neutralizing antibodies to this serotype [82].

Another change in the vector would be to switch the internal promoter that drives the transgene expression. In a recent study by Follenzi and colleagues [72], replacing a viral promoter isolated from the cytomegalovirus with a liver-specific albumin promoter significantly reduced the CTL response in the liver. Similar findings have been observed using other viral vectors, including AAV [83], using liver-specific promoter, although this may not be a universal solution because muscle-specific promoters could not reduce the adaptive immune response [84].

Insertional mutagenesis

Random integration by gene therapy vectors based on MLV resulted in severe adverse effects in young children enrolled in a recent clinical trial performed in France [9,10]. The following are possible methods that may be used to minimize the likelihood of insertional mutagenesis in future clinical trials using integrating vectors.

Vector modifications

One simple method would be to use alternative viruses, such as immunodeficiency viruses, that are not predisposed to triggering oncogenesis. As described earlier, lentiviral vectors can be modified with SIN technology to minimize the promoter activity and prevent oncogenic sequence transcription following integration. Current clinical trials using lentiviral vectors contain the SIN technology [29–31], and if this modification is not sufficient then future design changes will require the incorporation of strong stop and polyadenylation signals to increase the safety of the vector [85].

Suicide gene therapy

Another approach would be to insert a suicide gene, such as thymidine kinase or cytosine deaminase, to eliminate transformed cells following vector integration. Conceptually, this approach has been applied to other viral vector systems, including adenovirus, as a potential therapeutic to treat various cancers [86,87]. In a recent study, however, Painter and coworkers [88] cloned the human telomerase promoter driving the herpes simplex virus thymidine kinase gene into an advanced generation SIN lentiviral vector to transduce tumorigenic cell lines. The purpose of this study was to demonstrate that a single copy of a lentiviral vector could produce sufficient expression of the suicide gene to convert enough of the administered prodrug substrate, ganciclovir, into a cytotoxic compound to eliminate the lentiviral vector-transduced tumor cells. Additional potency of this suicide gene therapy approach could be enhanced by combining ganciclovir with other drugs, such as gemcitabine, a mechanism-based inhibitor of ribonucleotide reductase [89]. This method requires further proof-of-concept testing to determine whether telomerase activity actually will awaken from its slumber if a normal transduced cell becomes oncogenic, but this concept may prove to be an important tool in future integrating vector systems.

Site-specific integration

The third and most novel approach that will fundamentally change the landscape of gene therapy is the identification of a method to insert vectors into a predetermined site within the genome. An integrase protein was isolated from *Streptomyces* phage ΦC31 by the Calos laboratory at Stanford University, which could recognize pseudo *attP* sites in the mammalian genome and catalyze the genomic integration of naked DNA containing *attB* sites [90]. Studies using naked DNA approaches have demonstrated specific genomic integration, albeit at an extremely low frequency, to correct monogenic disorders in mice in vivo [91–93].

An alternative site-specific integrating strategy was presented in an elegant study by Tan and coworkers [94], who fused a polydactyl zinc-finger DNA binding element for E2C to the integrase protein from HIV to bias the normally random integration of the retroviral genome toward a more specific site near the E2C-binding region, which has a known 18-bp recognition sequence. The rate-limiting step for both of these approaches is the low efficiency in locating and integrating into the specific sites, so technical advances in this area will be needed to increase the efficiency and demonstrate that this approach can be applied to viral vectors for targeting into specific sites without promoting oncogenesis.

Final perspective on gene therapy

As each year passes, newer and more efficient viral and nonviral vector systems will be developed. Ongoing research supports the concept that no single vector system will be unilaterally applied for the treatment of the every pediatric disease. In reality, hybrid vector systems will be designed whereby two or more different viral vectors or nucleic acid–based components will be combined to generate a gene delivery system that can modify cells in vivo to provide regulatable transgene expression in a safe and nontoxic manner. With this in mind, the short-term future of gene therapy may produce few landmark breakthroughs as gene therapists apply new vector systems and attempt to elucidate their impact on human toxicity and immune system activation. The success that has occurred even with the limited knowledge of how vectors function in humans would suggest that the future for gene therapy remains bright, and it is likely that gene therapy vectors will become commonplace as a therapeutic tool for pediatric and other genetic diseases and disorders.

References

[1] Feigin RD. Prospects for the future of child health through research. JAMA 2005;294: 1373–9.

[2] Rimoin DL, Hirschhorn K. A history of medical genetics in pediatrics. Pediatr Res 2004;56: 150–9.

[3] Wolff JA, Budker V. The mechanism of naked DNA uptake and expression. Adv Genet 2005;54:3–20.

[4] Xu L, Yee JK, Wolff JA, et al. Factors affecting long-term stability of Moloney murine leukemia virus-based vectors. Virology 1989;171:331–41.

[5] Blaese RM, Culver KW, Miller AD, et al. T lymphocyte-directed gene therapy for ADA-SCID: initial trial results after 4 years. Science 1995;270:475–80.

[6] Miller DG, Adam MA, Miller AD. Gene transfer by retrovirus vectors occurs only in cells that are actively replicating at the time of infection. Mol Cell Biol 1990;10:4239–42.

[7] Cavazzana-Calvo M, Hacein-Bey S, de Saint Basile G, et al. Gene therapy of human severe combined immunodeficiency (SCID)-X1 disease. Science 2000;288:669–72.

[8] Baum C, von Kalle C, Staal FJ, et al. Chance or necessity? Insertional mutagenesis in gene therapy and its consequences. Mol Ther 2004;9:5–13.

[9] Hacein-Bey-Abina S, von Kalle C, Schmidt M, et al. A serious adverse event after successful gene therapy for X-linked severe combined immunodeficiency. N Engl J Med 2003;348:255–6.

[10] Hacein-Bey-Abina S, Von Kalle C, Schmidt M, et al. LMO2-associated clonal T cell proliferation in two patients after gene therapy for SCID-X1. Science 2003;302:415–9.

[11] Kohn DB, Sadelain M, Dunbar C, et al. American Society of Gene Therapy (ASGT) ad hoc subcommittee on retroviral-mediated gene transfer to hematopoietic stem cells. Mol Ther 2003;8:180–7.

[12] Naldini L, Blomer U, Gage FH, et al. Efficient transfer, integration, and sustained long-term expression of the transgene in adult rat brains injected with a lentiviral vector. Proc Natl Acad Sci USA 1996;93:11382–8.

[13] Naldini L, Blomer U, Gallay P, et al. In vivo gene delivery and stable transduction of non-dividing cells by a lentiviral vector. Science 1996;272:263–7.

[14] Park F, Ohashi K, Chiu W, et al. Efficient lentiviral transduction of liver requires cell cycling in vivo. Nat Genet 2000;24:49–52.

[15] Kumar M, Keller B, Makalou N, et al. Systematic determination of the packaging limit of lentiviral vectors. Hum Gene Ther 2001;12:1893–905.

[16] Kang Y, Stein CS, Heth JA, et al. In vivo gene transfer using a nonprimate lentiviral vector pseudotyped with Ross River Virus glycoproteins. J Virol 2002;76:9378–88.

[17] Park F. Correction of bleeding diathesis without liver toxicity using arenaviral-pseudotyped HIV-1-based vectors in hemophilia A mice. Hum Gene Ther 2003;14:1489–94.

[18] Qian Z, Haessler M, Lemos JA, et al. Targeting vascular injury using hantavirus-pseudo-typed lentiviral vectors. Mol Ther, in press.

[19] Sinn PL, Penisten AK, Burnight ER, et al. Gene transfer to respiratory epithelia with lentivirus pseudotyped with Jaagsiekte sheep retrovirus envelope glycoprotein. Hum Gene Ther 2005;16:479–88.

[20] Miyoshi H, Blomer U, Takahashi M, et al. Development of a self-inactivating lentivirus vector. J Virol 1998;72:8150–7.

[21] De Palma M, Montini E, de Sio FR, et al. Promoter trapping reveals significant differences in integration site selection between MLV and HIV vectors in primary hematopoietic cells. Blood 2005;105:2307–15.

[22] Ohashi K, Park F, Kay MA. Role of hepatocyte direct hyperplasia in lentivirus-mediated liver transduction in vivo. Hum Gene Ther 2002;13:653–63.

[23] Park F, Ohashi K, Kay MA. Therapeutic levels of human factor VIII and IX using HIV-1-based lentiviral vectors in mouse liver. Blood 2000;96:1173–6.

[24] Tsui LV, Kelly M, Zayek N, et al. Production of human clotting Factor IX without toxicity in mice after vascular delivery of a lentiviral vector. Nat Biotechnol 2002;20:53–7.

[25] Park F, Ohashi K, Kay MA. The effect of age on hepatic gene transfer with self-inactivating lentiviral vectors in vivo. Mol Ther 2003;8:314–23.

[26] VandenDriessche T, Thorrez L, Naldini L, et al. Lentiviral vectors containing the human immunodeficiency virus type-1 central polypurine tract can efficiently transduce nondividing hepatocytes and antigen-presenting cells in vivo. Blood 2002;100:813–22.

[27] Case SS, Price MA, Jordan CT, et al. Stable transduction of quiescent CD34(+)CD38(-) human hematopoietic cells by HIV-1-based lentiviral vectors. Proc Natl Acad Sci USA 1999;96: 2988–93.

[28] Mostoslavsky G, Kotton DN, Fabian AJ, et al. Efficiency of transduction of highly purified murine hematopoietic stem cells by lentiviral and oncoretroviral vectors under conditions of minimal in vitro manipulation. Mol Ther 2005;11:932–40.

[29] Humeau LM, Binder GK, Lu X, et al. Efficient lentiviral vector-mediated control of HIV-1 replication in CD4 lymphocytes from diverse HIV + infected patients grouped according to CD4 count and viral load. Mol Ther 2004;9:902–13.

[30] Manilla P, Rebello T, Afable C, et al. Regulatory considerations for novel gene therapy products: a review of the process leading to the first clinical lentiviral vector. Hum Gene Ther 2005;16:17–25.

[31] Bank A, Dorazio R, Leboulch PA. Phase I/II clinical trial of β-globin gene therapy for β-thalassemia. Ann N Y Acad Sci 2005;1054:308–16.

[32] Bergelson JM, Krithivas A, Celi L, et al. The murine CAR homolog is a receptor for coxsackie B viruses and adenoviruses. J Virol 1998;72:415–9.

[33] Lozier JN, Csako G, Mondoro TH, et al. Toxicity of a first-generation adenoviral vector in rhesus macaques. Hum Gene Ther 2002;13:113–24.

[34] Lozier JN, Metzger ME, Donahue RE, et al. Adenovirus-mediated expression of human co-agulation factor IX in the rhesus macaque is associated with dose-limiting toxicity. Blood 1999;94:3968–75.

[35] Raper SE, Chirmule N, Lee FS, et al. Fatal systemic inflammatory response syndrome in a ornithine transcarbamylase deficient patient following adenoviral gene transfer. Mol Genet Metab 2003;80:148–58.

[36] Delatte SJ, Hazen-Martin DJ, Re GG, et al. Restoration of p53 function in anaplastic Wilms' tumor. J Pediatr Surg 2001;36:43–50.

[37] Borovjagin AV, Krendelchtchikov A, Ramesh N, et al. Complex mosaicism is a novel approach to infectivity enhancement of adenovirus type 5-based vectors. Cancer Gene Ther 2005;12:475–86.

[38] Douglas JT, Rogers BE, Rosenfeld ME, et al. Targeted gene delivery by tropism-modified adenoviral vectors. Nat Biotechnol 1996;14:1574–8.

[39] Haviv YS, Blackwell JL, Kanerva A, et al. Adenoviral gene therapy for renal cancer requires retargeting to alternative cellular receptors. Cancer Res 2002;62:4273–81.

[40] Ehrhardt A, Kay MA. A new adenoviral helper-dependent vector results in long-term therapeutic levels of human coagulation factor IX at low doses in vivo. Blood 2002;99:3923–30.

[41] Ehrhardt A, Xu H, Dillow AM, et al. A gene-deleted adenoviral vector results in phenotypic correction of canine hemophilia B without liver toxicity or thrombocytopenia. Blood 2003; 102:2403–11.

[42] DelloRusso C, Scott JM, Hartigan-O'Connor D, et al. Functional correction of adult mdx mouse muscle using gutted adenoviral vectors expressing full-length dystrophin. Proc Natl Acad Sci USA 2002;99:12979–84.

[43] Miao CH, Snyder RO, Schowalter DB, et al. The kinetics of rAAV integration in the liver. Nat Genet 1998;19:13–5.

[44] Snyder RO, Miao CH, Patijn GA, et al. Persistent and therapeutic concentrations of human factor IX in mice after hepatic gene transfer of recombinant AAV vectors. Nat Genet 1997;16:270–6.

[45] Nakai H, Yant SR, Storm TA, et al. Extrachromosomal recombinant adeno-associated virus vector genomes are primarily responsible for stable liver transduction in vivo. J Virol 2001; 75:6969–76.

[46] Couto LB. Preclinical gene therapy studies for hemophilia using adeno-associated virus (AAV) vectors. Semin Thromb Hemost 2004;30:161–71.

[47] Miao CH, Nakai H, Thompson AR, et al. Nonrandom transduction of recombinant adeno-associated virus vectors in mouse hepatocytes in vivo: cell cycling does not influence hepatocyte transduction. J Virol 2000;74:3793–803.

[48] Nakai H, Thomas CE, Storm TA, et al. A limited number of transducible hepatocytes restricts a wide-range linear vector dose response in recombinant adeno-associated virus-mediated liver transduction. J Virol 2002;76:11343–9.

[49] Kay MA, Manno CS, Ragni MV, et al. Evidence for gene transfer and expression of factor IX in haemophilia B patients treated with an AAV vector. Nat Genet 2000;24:257–61.

[50] Manno CS, Chew AJ, Hutchison S, et al. AAV-mediated factor IX gene transfer to skeletal muscle in patients with severe hemophilia B. Blood 2003;101:2963–72.

[51] Kaiser J. Gene therapy. Side effects sideline hemophilia trial. Science 2004;304:1423–5.

[52] Gao G, Lu Y, Calcedo R, et al. Biology of AAV serotype vectors in liver-directed gene transfer to nonhuman primates. Mol Ther 2006;13:77–87.

[53] Gao G, Vandenberghe LH, Wilson JM. New recombinant serotypes of AAV vectors. Curr Gene Ther 2005;5:285–97.

[54] Grimm D, Zhou S, Nakai H, et al. Preclinical in vivo evaluation of pseudotyped adeno-associated virus vectors for liver gene therapy. Blood 2003;102:2412–9.

[55] Nakai H, Fuess S, Storm TA, et al. Unrestricted hepatocyte transduction with adeno-associated virus serotype 8 vectors in mice. J Virol 2005;79:214–24.

[56] Gao GP, Alvira MR, Wang L, et al. Novel adeno-associated viruses from rhesus monkeys as vectors for human gene therapy. Proc Natl Acad Sci USA 2002;99:11854–9.

[57] Shankar P, Manjunath N, Lieberman J. The prospect of silencing disease using RNA interference. JAMA 2005;293:1367–73.

[58] Sangkhathat S, Kusafuka T, Miao J, et al. In vitro RNA interference against beta-catenin inhibits the proliferation of pediatric hepatic tumors. Int J Oncol 2006;28:715–22.

[59] Damm-Welk C, Fuchs U, Wossmann W, et al. Targeting oncogenic fusion genes in leukemias and lymphomas by RNA interference. Semin Cancer Biol 2003;13:283–92.

[60] Bauer G, Selander D, Engel B, et al. Gene therapy for pediatric AIDS. Ann N Y Acad Sci 2000;918:318–29.

[61] Kohn DB, Bauer G, Rice CR, et al. A clinical trial of retroviral-mediated transfer of a rev-responsive element decoy gene into CD34(+) cells from the bone marrow of human immunodeficiency virus-1-infected children. Blood 1999;94:368–71.

[62] Morris KV, Rossi JJ. Lentiviral-mediated delivery of siRNAs for antiviral therapy. Gene Ther 2006;13(6):553–8.

[63] Sullenger BA. Targeted genetic repair: an emerging approach to genetic therapy. J Clin Invest 2003;112:310–1.

[64] Yang Y, Walsh CE. Spliceosome-mediated RNA trans-splicing. Mol Ther 2005;12:1006–12.

[65] Chao H, Mansfield SG, Bartel RC, et al. Phenotype correction of hemophilia A mice by spliceosome-mediated RNA trans-splicing. Nat Med 2003;9:1015–9.

[66] Lai Y, Yue Y, Liu M, et al. Efficient in vivo gene expression by trans-splicing adeno-associated viral vectors. Nat Biotechnol 2005;23:1435–9.

[67] Liu X, Luo M, Zhang LN, et al. Spliceosome-mediated RNA trans-splicing with recombinant adeno-associated virus partially restores cystic fibrosis transmembrane conductance regulator function to polarized human cystic fibrosis airway epithelial cells. Hum Gene Ther 2005;16:1116–23.

[68] Lipshutz GS, Gruber CA, Cao Y, et al. In utero delivery of adeno-associated viral vectors: intraperitoneal gene transfer produces long-term expression. Mol Ther 2001;3:284–92.

[69] Lipshutz GS, Sarkar R, Flebbe-Rehwaldt L, et al. Short-term correction of factor VIII deficiency in a murine model of hemophilia A after delivery of adenovirus murine factor VIII in utero. Proc Natl Acad Sci USA 1999;96:13324–9.

[70] Waddington SN, Mitrophanous KA, Ellard FM, et al. Long-term transgene expression by administration of a lentivirus-based vector to the fetal circulation of immuno-competent mice. Gene Ther 2003;10:1234–40.

[71] Waddington SN, Nivsarkar MS, Mistry AR, et al. Permanent phenotypic correction of hemophilia B in immunocompetent mice by prenatal gene therapy. Blood 2004;104:2714–21.

[72] Follenzi A, Battaglia M, Lombardo A, et al. Targeting lentiviral vector expression to hepatocytes limits transgene-specific immune response and establishes long-term expression of human antihemophilic factor IX in mice. Blood 2004;103:3700–9.

[73] American Academy of Pediatrics Committee on Genetics. Molecular genetic testing in pediatric practice: A subject review. Pediatrics 2000;106:1494–7.

[74] Jooss K, Ertl HC, Wilson JM. Cytotoxic T-lymphocyte target proteins and their major histocompatibility complex class I restriction in response to adenovirus vectors delivered to mouse liver. J Virol 1998;72:2945–54.

[75] Wang L, Cao O, Swalm B, et al. Major role of local immune responses in antibody formation to factor IX in AAV gene transfer. Gene Ther 2005;12:1453–64.

[76] Mingozzi F, Liu YL, Dobrzynski E, et al. Induction of immune tolerance to coagulation factor IX antigen by in vivo hepatic gene transfer. J Clin Invest 2003;111:1347–56.

[77] Kay MA, Holterman AX, Meuse L, et al. Long-term hepatic adenovirus-mediated gene expression in mice following CTLA4Ig administration. Nat Genet 1995;11:191–7.

[78] Halbert CL, Standaert TA, Wilson CB, et al. Successful readministration of adeno-associated virus vectors to the mouse lung requires transient immunosuppression during the initial exposure. J Virol 1998;72:9795–805.

[79] Feili-Hariri M, Dong X, Alber SM, et al. Immunotherapy of NOD mice with bone marrow-derived dendritic cells. Diabetes 1999;48:2300–8.

[80] Xiao BG, Duan RS, Link H, et al. Induction of peripheral tolerance to experimental autoimmune myasthenia gravis by acetylcholine receptor-pulsed dendritic cells. Cell Immunol 2003;223:63–9.

[81] Zhao P, Park F, Cui Y. Engineering hematopoietic stem cells to modulate immune response. In: LaRussa VF, editor. Stem cell: research tools and transplantation (methods in molecular biology). New Jersey: Humana Press; in press.

[82] Seshidhar Reddy P, Ganesh S, Limbach MP, et al. Development of adenovirus serotype 35 as a gene transfer vector. Virology 2003;311:384–93.

[83] Franco LM, Sun B, Yang X, et al. Evasion of immune responses to introduced human acid alpha-glucosidase by liver-restricted expression in glycogen storage disease type II. Mol Ther 2005;12:876–84.

[84] Liu YL, Mingozzi F, Rodriguez-Colon SM, et al. Therapeutic levels of factor IX expression using a muscle-specific promoter and adeno-associated virus serotype 1 vector. Hum Gene Ther 2004;15:783–92.

[85] Zaiss AK, Son S, Chang LJ. RNA 3′ readthrough of oncoretrovirus and lentivirus: implications for vector safety and efficacy. J Virol 2002;76:7209–19.

[86] Germano IM, Fable J, Gultekin SH, et al. Adenovirus/herpes simplex-thymidine kinase/ganciclovir complex: preliminary results of a phase I trial in patients with recurrent malignant gliomas. J Neurooncol 2003;65:279–89.

[87] Wiewrodt R, Amin K, Kiefer M, et al. Adenovirus-mediated gene transfer of enhanced Herpes simplex virus thymidine kinase mutants improves prodrug-mediated tumor cell killing. Cancer Gene Ther 2003;10:353–64.

[88] Painter RG, Lanson NA Jr, Jin Z, et al. Conditional expression of a suicide gene by the telomere reverse transcriptase promoter for potential post-therapeutic deletion of tumorigenesis. Cancer Sci 2005;96:607–13.

[89] Boucher PD, Shewach DS. In vitro and in vivo enhancement of ganciclovir-mediated bystander cytotoxicity with gemcitabine. Mol Ther 2005;12:1064–71.

[90] Ginsburg DS, Calos MP. Site-specific integration with phiC31 integrase for prolonged expression of therapeutic genes. Adv Genet 2005;54:179–87.

[91] Bertoni C, Jarrahian S, Wheeler TM, et al. Enhancement of plasmid-mediated gene therapy for muscular dystrophy by directed plasmid integration. Proc Natl Acad Sci USA 2006;103:419–24.

[92] Held PK, Olivares EC, Aguilar CP, et al. In vivo correction of murine hereditary tyrosinemia type I by phiC31 integrase-mediated gene delivery. Mol Ther 2005;11:399–408.

[93] Olivares EC, Hollis RP, Chalberg TW, et al. Site-specific genomic integration produces therapeutic Factor IX levels in mice. Nat Biotechnol 2002;20:1124–8.

[94] Tan W, Zhu K, Segal DJ, et al. Fusion proteins consisting of human immunodeficiency virus type 1 integrase and the designed polydactyl zinc finger protein E2C direct integration of viral DNA into specific sites. J Virol 2004;78:1301–13.

PEDIATRIC CLINICS
OF NORTH AMERICA

ELSEVIER
SAUNDERS

Pediatr Clin N Am 53 (2006) 639–648

Pediatric Ethics in the Age of Molecular Medicine

Raymond C. Barfield, MD, PhD[a,*], Eric Kodish, MD[b]

[a]Division of Stem Cell Transplantation, St. Jude Children's Research Hospital,
332 North Lauderdale Street, Memphis, TN 38104, USA
[b]Department of Bioethics, Cleveland Clinic Foundation, Lerner College of Medicine at Case,
9500 Euclid Avenue (JJ-6), Cleveland, OH 44195, USA

The diagnosis and treatment of childhood disorders is being revolutionized through research into their environmental and genetic bases and through the application of new technologies for therapy [1]. With these technological and scientific advances, it is reasonable to expect new ethical issues to arise. Lessons learned from past ethical challenges can shed light on new issues and, through analogy, can reveal aspects common to both the novel and the familiar [2]. In approaching the challenges raised by molecular medicine, it can be enormously helpful to understand some of the history of ethical thought. The ethics endeavor also is made easier in many ways because each of the areas of molecular medicine pursues a common goal—to improve the diagnosis and treatment of diseases afflicting children.

Starting points for ethical thought in the age of molecular medicine

The fundamental challenge to developing a coherent approach to complex bioethical questions is the diversity of experience with which participants from various political, religious, philosophical, and vocational backgrounds enter the discussion. This pluralism can reveal new and interesting perspectives, but it also can lead to impasse, especially regarding fundamental assumptions. Population-based genetic research has led the World Health Organization to question "whether the individual can remain of paramount importance in this context" [3]. Embryo selection based on genetic profiles tests how far parents and physicians can go in choosing a child's

---

* Corresponding author.
E-mail address: raymond.barfield@stjude.org (R.C. Barfield).

characteristics. Cognitive neuroscience raises profound questions about the way we think of ourselves as persons and as moral agents [3,4]. Each of these examples—and there are many more—challenges some important aspect of our concept of the human subject. This is a vital point, because it was reports of human subject abuse in, for example, the Nuremberg trials, the US Public Health Service–sponsored Tuskegee syphilis study, and President Clinton's advisory committee on human radiation experiments that prompted repeated attempts to explicate ethical principles that are comprehensive, broadly applicable, and flexible enough to meet new challenges [5].

The most recent attempt to develop a widely (internationally) applicable bioethics code is the adoption of the *Universal Declaration of Bioethics and Human Rights* in October 2005 by the United Nations Educational, Scientific, and Cultural Organizations. But whose interests are affected by genomics? Will pharmacogenomics make new therapies available for diseases, such as malaria and influenza, that may threaten millions, or will it deepen the so-called "10/90" gap in which less than 10% of global health care expenditure is devoted to 90% of the world's disease burden [6]? Will pharmacogenomics make possible a paternalistic distribution of potential therapies to populations because of economic or political expediency, without the safeguard of the personal physician–patient relationship? Some questions may seem better suited to science fiction until one considers the implications of widespread access to information coupled with the reality of profoundly detailed "information" that plumbs one's very molecular structure.

This preface sets the tone for a discussion of technical innovations that promise unprecedented advances in the care of children with a wide range of disorders but also hold the potential for abuses that undermine the struggle for good health and longevity.

Bioinformatics, genomics, and proteomics

Bioinformatics attempts to organize and understand biological information on a large scale. The available information to be organized includes genomic data, nucleic acid and protein structures, gene and protein expression data, and molecular interactions [7]. Genomics is revolutionizing the diagnosis and treatment of disease by elucidating its molecular foundations [8]. Microarrays can profile the expression patterns of tens of thousands of genes simultaneously [9]. Despite the promise offered by such information, however, several questions remain. For example, if a disease gene or disease susceptibility gene profile is discovered, should a subject be notified? Should the subject's family be informed also? Would informing family members be a breach of the patient's confidentiality? If there has been a time lapse between the tissue sampling and the genomic study and the donor has died, should the relatives be contacted [10]? These questions have not yet been answered, but they point to a theme that will be recurrent in the age of molecular medicine: the technology and information gathering is already under way; as ethical thought catches up, what will be the practical outcome and what can be done if ethical consensus conflicts with current practice or technical capability?

Another way to phrase the question is to ask which enterprise leads: the inquiry into what is scientifically and technically possible or the inquiry into what is good to achieve? Does the fact that something is scientifically or technically possible make it good? There are many cases that challenge the assumption that what is possible is also good. But if the answer is no, then from what quarter do such answers come, if not from the arenas of science and technology? The answer is not simple, and any pragmatic solution must include the ethical and technological realms, demonstrating a checks-and-balances effect—both efforts striving for the goal of good for all children.

In the case of genomics, although much has been accomplished technically, the human genome is enormously varied, and much remains to be learned about determining when medical intervention is necessary [11]. This fact calls for advancement of the technology and, given the available time, reflection on the meaning and moral import of advancing the technology.

The American Society of Clinical Oncology (ASCO) has recommended that genetic testing for cancer predisposition be offered when (1) the individual has a personal or family history or features suggestive of a genetic cancer susceptibility, (2) the test can be adequately interpreted, and (3) the result will aid in the diagnosis or the medical or surgical management of a patient or family members who have hereditary risk for cancer [12]. ASCO has also recommended that the regulatory oversight of laboratories providing such tests be strengthened and that federal laws be established to prohibit discrimination by health care providers and employers because of such information.

Although some maintain that genetic discrimination will not affect insurance coverage, several surveys have shown that the public fears this possibility [13–15]. What is unique about the concerns regarding genetic information? Only 0.1% of the 3.2 billion bases in the human genome differ between unrelated people [16]. Lin and colleagues pointed out that someone with access to individual data who performs matches to public single nucleotide polymorphisms (SNPs), given that the world population is roughly 10^{10}, can define a single person by specifying DNA sequence at only 30 to 80 statistically independent SNP positions [17]. Other genotypic and phenotypic information also might be accessible through this approach. The obvious moral dilemma is how to maximize potential good through the development of accurate genetic databases while protecting confidentiality. Likewise, the trustworthiness of researchers and governmental agencies that formulate policy or use the data will be an issue.

At the level of the individual, many of the ethical issues in genomics do not differ substantially from other issues of confidentiality, in light of modern handling of medical records and demographic databases. One unique problem is that a person's genetic information is applicable to family members. If one person gives consent for release of his or her genetic information, therefore, some of that information may apply to others who have not given such consent [18].

Much more work in bioethics, public policy, and human subjects' protection will be required to address the availability of individual genetic information to researchers who seek population-wide facts and the disclosure of genetic information about people other than those who consent. Commentaries have addressed these issues using the concepts of citizenship, commonality, and universality [19]. From each of these perspectives, the central issue is not one of individual autonomy but the benefit of the larger community and the common good of humanity [20,21]. Resistance to such values often is based on the fear of eugenics, which was widely endorsed during the early twentieth century and has some well-intended potential support today, as discussed later.

In pediatrics, a new level of complexity is added. Decisions that may affect the subject's future employability, insurability, privacy, and other interests are made by surrogates (usually parents). When the intervention is clearly understood and the risks and benefits are transparent, consensus and precedent support permission-giving in the best interest of the child. But in the age of molecular medicine, as interventions and technology become increasingly complex, it also becomes more difficult for surrogates to understand the intervention and its possible consequences. Consider the application of pharmacogenomics to the dosing of medications or the application of nanotechnology to infectious disease and transplantation. Even the patient's primary care physician might find such information-dense technology challenging. How much can be expected of the average parent? And to what extent will a signed consent document serve more to reassure and protect the researchers and their institutions than to attest to a truly informed decision?

On the other hand, another question concerns the necessity of a full understanding of the treatment and the character of the understanding that is necessary for informed consent. When we board an airplane with our children, we have no idea what most of the gadgets in the cockpit do. Furthermore, there are crashes that kill hundreds of people despite federal and international regulations and flight standards, yet we continue to board jets to distant destinations. Are we approaching a comparable situation in medicine? This question is meant not to provide an answer but to provoke a discussion about what can be expected realistically in the process of informing parents and patients in the age of molecular medicine, and how much a lack of real understanding could or should affect the conduct of clinical trials.

One study in adults had the interesting hypothesis "[that] in the context of a potentially life-saving procedure without any viable treatment alternatives for a potential cure, 'informed consent' has little significance to the patient in his or her autonomous decision to proceed with treatment and that other factors influence the patient's decision-making process" [22]. The authors assessed the importance of four factors in the patient's decision-making process: (1) a full understanding of treatment, (2) trust in the physician, (3) trust in the treatment team, and (4) best chance for a good outcome. Interestingly, the most important factor was "best chance for a good outcome," and the least important factor was "a full understanding of the treatment." In the past, the caregiver has customarily been trusted to make treatment decisions without the necessity for understanding by the patient. In the future, will such a custom again become a matter of practical necessity? If so, the power and impact of oaths to advance the best interest of patients take on a renewed significance.

Although the study described above has not been replicated in the pediatric setting, it suggests that in a high-tech, complex, and potentially high-risk endeavor, beneficence may be the most important principle in making decisions. Trust in the physician-investigator, the health care team, and the regulatory agencies takes on greater significance. What are the limits of this line of thought?

Pharmacogenomics

A category of genomic research known as pharmacogenomics that has enormous potential for benefit to children illustrates how far-reaching bioethics issues may be in the age of molecular medicine. Here, in addition to the potential for benefit, we also see the potential for national and international financial impact, social and economic discrimination, and the abuse of the information in genomic databases.

Pharmacogenomics combines pharmacogenetics and human genomics to study the role of inheritance in an individual's response to a drug [23]. Its goal has been touted as selection of "the right medicine, for the right patient, at the right dose" [24]. Anyone who has witnessed the undertreatment or overtreatment of a patient knows the power of this idea. But what questions should be considered more closely?

First, some ethical questions regarding pharmacogenomics are related to questions about pharmacoeconomics. Pharmacogenomics could decrease the cost of drug development by ensuring that only those patients who are likely to benefit from a medicine are enrolled on a trial of that medicine. But might pharmacogenomic criteria eventually become regulatory requirements for the development and testing of all medicines [25]? What would be the cost in real terms and in terms of exclusion of subgroups of people from studies? The pharmaceutical industry, functioning on a business model, is unlikely to develop medicines that will benefit only a small, narrowly defined group of patients. Orphan drugs may become more common. How are economic risks to be weighed against the potential clinical benefit for a small group of patients? This question is familiar to all pediatricians.

A second question is the corollary to the first: if a child has disease X for which drug Z is indicated, but pharmacogenomic analysis suggests that the child is less likely than others to benefit from the drug, will that child be denied the therapy? To what extent would the child have to be less likely to respond to be excluded? Ten percent? Thirty percent? The question of insurance coverage for specific therapies arises here: if a patient is less likely to benefit from a drug, is the insurance company still obligated to pay for it? If not, will this create a further divide between the rich, who can pay for a drug even if the chance for benefit is modest, and others [26]?

The third issue that has arisen in pharmacogenomics is race. According to the Institute of Medicine, nonwhite populations tend to receive lower quality health care than whites, even when insurance status, income, age, and severity of condition are controlled [27,28]. This is a complex issue, because pathophysiological factors are not associated with race-related superficial physical features. The concept of race itself is complex and controversial. Even multi-locus genotyping of populations shows only moderate correlation with genetically determined population clusters and even less with ethnicity. And despite the genetic variation within purported racial groups, if genetic variance peculiar to a racial or ethnic group is found, what are the implications? Might medicines be developed or not developed for certain populations because of political or economic motivation [24]?

Each of these questions spawns many others. The point here is to consider the impact of these technical advances and to stimulate further inquiry, debate, and discussion.

Neuroethics

"Ethics in the age of molecular medicine" can sound like science fiction, because it looks at what actually has been accomplished in medicine and science and asks, "What is possible?" Neuroethics is a field in which advances can lead to unexpected consequences, not all of which are met with enthusiasm. Some neuroscience breakthroughs have the potential to challenge our views of freedom, personal responsibility, and personality by reducing mental states to brain states or by providing the means to directly manipulate brain states to alter mental capacity.

The philosophical issue of the relation of mental events to physical events in the brain and the contribution of molecular science to the debate is a vital and fascinating discussion but one that is too large for this essay. The alteration of brain states is an issue that is of immediate relevance to the pediatrician in everyday practice, however.

Enhancement of brain function through medication has led to the widespread use of psychoactive drugs by people who would not have been considered ill two decades ago [4]. Part of this trend is based on real benefit and part is based on aggressive marketing of psychiatric medications (a profound ethical issue of its own). Enhancement drugs include those that affect mood, sleep, eating, libido, depression, anxiety, and memory (whereas most are intended to enhance memory, some hold the fascinating possibility of doing the opposite—preventing the retention of memories) [29]. What is the relevance of psychopharmacology to the pediatrician? In some schools, one third of boys are on methylphenidate (Ritalin) or a related compound [30]. If medicated children begin to perform better than others, how do we assess the motivation for medicating a child? And if a family cannot afford a medicine that enhances function, what are the larger implications for people in lower socioeconomic groups? Congress has taken on the issue of steroid use in sports. What do we do when the spelling bee is won by a medicated fifth grader?

Another, somewhat surprising, neuroethics issue that is directly relevant to pediatric practitioners regards advances in understanding of the critical periods of brain development. What effect do events during different periods of brain development have on the growth of language ability? Is the development of such skills affected by physical activity or by the use of video games, cell phones, and other electronics during different periods of brain development [31]? Tools such as functional MRI can demonstrate changes associated with learning a new language [32]. Illes and colleagues, discussing Japanese progress in the study of the biology of neural plasticity, point out a report documenting the synchronized, photic seizures induced in almost 1000 Japanese children by an episode of *Pokemon* [31,33]. When more is understood about neural development, the next logical step in neural research will be genetic modification to relieve known disorders and enhance mental capacity. The scope of neuroethics comprises a wide range of considerations as pragmatic as assigning legal responsibility for behavior and as fundamental as the nature of human identity.

Stem cell therapy and selection of embryo donors

On the subject of stem cell therapy using adult and embryonic stem cells, one of the pioneers in stem cell research wrote that "these interventions require physicians and physician-scientists to determine for themselves whether patient welfare or personal ethics will dominate in their practices" [34]. The desire to heal and to exploit all means available to benefit patients is profoundly admirable. Identification of a benefit, however profound, does not automatically justify the end of obtaining that benefit at any cost. For example, one effective answer to the shortage of liver and kidney transplants might be to round up all people with brown hair and remove their livers and kidneys. The objection to this solution is based not on science but on ethics—both personal and public. The debate about the use of embryonic stem cells will no doubt take its place in history, as did the cases of Galileo and Scopes. But all of these cases point to the fundamental question of who we are as humans, and this sort of question is not amenable to scientific investigation.

The importance of this point is that technology often progresses irrespective of ethical thought. This fact is not surprising, for scientific and technical advancement are limited only by the ideas of scientists and physicians and the reluctance of nature to yield its secrets. In contrast, ethics must take into account many competing issues, such as the just distribution of resources and the principles of beneficence and respect for persons.

We make these statements in the context of transplantation and embryonic selection because these issues are common, complex, and contentious. Many stem cell transplant physicians have faced the issue of a sibling who is conceived to serve as the source of a matched hematopoietic stem cell transplant. This topic is not new. What is relatively new is the practice of preimplantation genetic diagnosis (PGD) of embryos to determine whether they carry known genetic diseases. Currently, more than 100 different genetic diseases are putative indications for PGD [35]. When this procedure is used, "sick" embryos often are discarded. More recently, PGD has been used for human leukocyte antigen (HLA) testing to obtain a matched sibling for donation in the context of nongenetic diseases [36,37]. With this procedure, embryos are rejected not because of a burdensome disease but because they do not have the desired HLA type. This practice is more permissive, and it raises the question whether this approach to generating new humans shows adequate respect for the human potential of each embryo [38].

As with other issues in the age of molecular medicine, embryo selection based on genetic profiling also raises important questions about the delivery of a level of medical care based on a family's financial assets. The cost of each clinical cycle of in vitro fertilization and PGD is $15,000 to $20,000. Multiple cycles often are required for success, and because insurance rarely pays for such interventions, only the wealthy can afford them.

Other issues arise, mentioned briefly here. There are currently no polices in place regarding adoption of a child after stem cell donation to ensure that the donor child is adequately cared for and to prevent the family from putting it up for adoption without adequate oversight. In the midst of questions about the status of an unborn fetus, what of the use of PGD to select a disease-free embryo with the intent to abort the fetus and collect stem cells? Why should this practice be illegal, when it is legal to abort the same fetus for reasons of convenience? Finally, there are already more than 400,000 frozen embryos in the United States alone. What is the import and impact of this growing number?

Summary

It is only lack of space, not lack of questions or content, that limits this discussion. Other issues that might be fruitfully addressed include (1) the medical uses of nanotechnology; (2) the redesign of clinical trials, such as the "first time in human" studies, to match advances in technology; (3) the role of individual choice, risk–benefit ratios, and international priorities in vaccine development; and (4) international bioethics and the just distribution of resources (eg, to what extent is it ethical to develop and deliver therapies for small populations at great expense, when large populations might benefit from current therapies produced in larger amounts at less cost?).

In the end, bioethics in the age of molecular medicine is not different from bioethics in any other age. We ask what we value. We ask who "we" are. We attend to the issues of justice, suffering, and inequality. And we do the best we can. We also must keep in mind that science cannot tell us what we ought to do with the knowledge generated by science. This question requires a different marvel of human endeavor: the quest for wisdom.

Acknowledgments

We thank Sharon Naron for her helpful criticism and editorial assistance.

References

[1] Feigin RD. Prospects for the future of child health through research. JAMA 2005;294: 1373–9.

[2] Smith B. Analogy in moral deliberation: the role of imagination and theory in ethics. J Med Ethics 2002;28:244–8.

[3] World Health Organization. Genetic databases: assessing the benefits and the impact on human and patient rights. Geneva: World Health Organization; 2003.

[4] Farah MJ. Neuroethics: the practical and the philosophical. Trends Cogn Sci 2005;9:34–40.

[5] Kodish E. Informed consent for pediatric research: is it really possible? J Pediatr 2003;142: 89–90.

[6] Global Forum for Health Research. The 10/90 report on health research 2000. Geneva: Global Forum for Health Research; 2000.

[7] Hocquette JF. Where are we in genomics? J Physiol Pharmacol 2005;56(Suppl 3):37–70.

[8] Segal E, Friedman N, Kaminski N, et al. From signatures to models: understanding cancer using microarrays. Nat Genet 2005;37(Suppl):S38–45.

[9] Joos L, Eryuksel E, Brutsche MH. Functional genomics and gene microarrays: the use in research and clinical medicine. Swiss Med Wkly 2003;133:31–8.

[10] D'Ambrosio C, Gatta L, Bonini S. The future of microarray technology: networking the genome search. Allergy 2005;60:1219–26.

[11] Kuehn BM. Genetic information: how much can patients handle? JAMA 2005;294:295–6.

[12] American Society of Clinical Oncology. Policy statement update: genetic testing for cancer susceptibility. J Clin Oncol 2003;21:2397–406.

[13] Thomas SM. Society and ethics: the genetics of disease. Curr Opin Genet Dev 2004;14: 287–91.

[14] Nowlan W. Human genetics. A rational view of insurance and genetic discrimination. Science 2002;297:195–6.

[15] Rothenberg KH, Terry SF. Human genetics. Before it's too late: addressing fear of genetic information. Science 2002;297:196–7.

[16] Li WH, Sadler LA. Low nucleotide diversity in man. Genetics 1991;129:513–23.

[17] Lin Z, Owen AB, Altman RB. Genetics. Genomic research and human subject privacy. Science 2004;305:183.

[18] Claerhout B, DeMoor GJ. Privacy protection for clinical and genomic data. The use of privacy-enhancing techniques in medicine. Int J Med Inform 2005;74:257–65.

[19] Knoppers BM, Chadwick R. Human genetic research: emerging trends in ethics. Nat Rev Genet 2005;6:75–9.

[20] UNESCO. Universal declaration on the human genome and human rights. J Med Philos 1998;23:334–41.

[21] Knoppers BM, Hirtle M, Glass KC. Policy forum: genetic technologies. Commercialization of genetic research and public policy. Science 1999;286:2277–8.

[22] Jacoby LH, Maloy B, Cirenza E, et al. The basis of informed consent for BMT patients. Bone Marrow Transplant 1999;23:711–7.

[23] Weinshilboum R, Wang L. Pharmacogenomics: bench to bedside. Nat Rev Drug Discov 2004;3:739–48.

[24] Lipton P. Pharmacogenetics: the ethical issues. Pharmacogenomics J 2003;3:14–6.

[25] Breckenridge A, Lindpaintner K, Lipton P, et al. Pharmacogenetics: ethical problems and solutions. Nat Rev Genet 2004;5:676–80.

[26] Service RF. Genetics and medicine. Recruiting genes, proteins for a revolution in diagnostics. Science 2003;300:236–9.

[27] Nelson A. Unequal treatment: confronting racial and ethnic disparities in health care. J Natl Med Assoc 2002;94:666–8.

[28] Wilson JF, Weale ME, Smith AC, et al. Population genetic structure of variable drug response. Nat Genet 2001;29:265–9.

[29] Pitman RK, Sanders KM, Zusman RM, et al. Pilot study of secondary prevention of post-traumatic stress disorder with propranolol. Biol Psychiatry 2002;51:189–92.

[30] Diller LH. The run on Ritalin. Attention deficit disorder and stimulant treatment in the 1990s. Hastings Cent Rep 1996;26:12–8.

[31] Illes J, Blakemore C, Hansson MG, et al. Science and society: international perspectives on engaging the public in neuroethics. Nat Rev Neurosci 2005;6:977–82.

[32] Tatsuno Y, Sakai KL. Language-related activations in the left prefrontal regions are differentially modulated by age, proficiency, and task demands. J Neurosci 2005;25:1637–44.

[33] Takahashi T, Tsukahara Y. Pocket Monster incident and low luminance visual stimuli: special reference to deep red flicker stimulation. Acta Paediatr Jpn 1998;40:631–7.

[34] Weissman I. Stem cell research: paths to cancer therapies and regenerative medicine. JAMA 2005;294:1359–66.

[35] Grewal SS, Kahn JP, MacMillan ML, et al. Successful hematopoietic stem cell transplantation for Fanconi anemia from an unaffected HLA-genotype-identical sibling selected using preimplantation genetic diagnosis. Blood 2004;103:1147–51.

[36] Verlinsky Y. Designing babies: what the future holds. Reprod Biomed Online 2005; 10(Suppl 1):24–6.

[37] Verlinsky Y, Rechitsky S, Sharapova T, et al. Preimplantation HLA testing. JAMA 2004; 291:2079–85.

[38] Burgio GR, Locatelli F. Ethics of creating programmed stem-cell donors. Lancet 2000;356: 1868–9.

PEDIATRIC CLINICS
OF NORTH AMERICA

Pediatr Clin N Am 53 (2006) 649–684

Cellular and Genetic Basis of Primary Immune Deficiencies

James W. Verbsky, MD, PhD[a],
William J. Grossman, MD, PhD[b],*

[a]Division of Rheumatology, Department of Pediatrics, Medical College of Wisconsin,
8701 Watertown Plank Road, Milwaukee, WI 53226, USA
[b]Division of Hematology/Oncology/Blood & Marrow Transplantation,
Department of Pediatrics, Medical College of Wisconsin, 8701 Watertown Plank Road,
Milwaukee, WI 53226, USA

Although primary immune deficiencies (PIDs) are thought to be rare, it is estimated that there are over 500,000 cases in the United States [1]. Approximately 50,000 new cases are diagnosed yearly and are present in up to 1 in 2000 live births [2–5]. Possible reasons for this increase in new diagnoses are a better awareness and recognition of PIDs by physicians, the development of sophisticated diagnostic testing, and improved intensive care allowing prolonged survival of these patients until they are properly diagnosed.

There are currently more than 120 PIDs with known genetic causes [6], compared with the approximately 66 classified PIDs in 1989 [7]. The recent sudden increase in classified PIDs has been facilitated by the completion of the Human Genome Project in April of 2003 [8]. This article attempts to help the general pediatrician gain a grasp of the rapidly expanding field of immunodeficiencies [9–12], with specific emphasis on developing clinical approaches to recognizing immune deficiencies, clinical evaluations for suspected deficiencies, and understanding the genetic and cellular basis of congenital immunodeficiency syndromes.

Recognizing immune deficiencies

The majority of PIDs are diagnosed in infancy, when there is a 5:1 predominance of males over females because of the X-linked inherited PIDs. Although most PIDs are recognized in infancy or childhood, a large fraction

* Corresponding author.
E-mail address: wgrossma@mcw.edu (W.J. Grossman).

0031-3955/06/$ - see front matter © 2006 Elsevier Inc. All rights reserved.
doi:10.1016/j.pcl.2006.05.005   *pediatric.theclinics.com*

($\sim$ 40%) of PIDs are not diagnosed until adolescence or early adulthood, when the distribution between males and females is nearly equal [3,13]. Part of the delay in these latter diagnoses is thought to result from the masking of symptoms [3,14], and hence their diagnosis, by the frequent use of antibiotics and better intensive care. Thus it is important to know the clinical presentation of PIDs at all ages.

The recognition of these PIDs can be a daunting task for the pediatrician. A basic strategy for recognizing possible immune defects is accomplished by an understanding of what is considered abnormal rather than normal in the clinical presentation and history of the patient. A list of warning signs has been developed by the Jeffrey Model Foundation/Immune Deficiency Foundation and serves as an excellent basic tool in helping physicians determine what should be considered abnormal, leading to further immunologic evaluation [15]. A modified list of these warning signs includes the following: eight or more otitis media infections per year; two or more serious sinus infections per year; two or more pneumonias per year; recurrent deep infections or infections in unusual areas (eg, muscle, liver); the need for intravenous antibiotics to clear infections; infection with an opportunistic organism (eg, *Pneumocystis carinii, Giardia*); and persistent thrush in patients older than 1 year of age. In addition, a family history of primary immune deficiencies, early childhood deaths, and consanguinity should prompt the physician to consider further immunologic evaluations for an underlying PID [15].

In addition to the previously mentioned warning signs, there are a multitude of physical examination and clinical findings that should raise suspicion of an underlying PID. The sinopulmonary system, gastrointestinal tract, and the skin are the principal sites of environment–host interactions, and consequently these organs are associated with many of the initial presenting symptoms associated with PIDs, including failure to thrive and recurrent/persistent infections. Gastrointestinal complications are found in the majority of PID patients and include infections with opportunistic organisms (eg, *Giardia, Cryptococcus, Cryptosporidium, Clostridium difficile* [*C difficile*]), malabsorption/protein-losing enteropathy, and severe food allergies [12,16–18]. Other physical examination findings include absent or abnormally enlarged lymph node tissue, skin/hair findings (severe eczema, alopecia, erythrodermia, silvery hair, albinism), ataxia, mucocutaneous candidiasis, dystrophic nails, hepatosplenomegaly, early childhood polyendocrinopathies, recurrent oral ulcers, and a variety of facial features (eg, microcephaly, midline defects, coarse facial features) [2,5,12,19,20].

In addition to recognition of these clinical presentations and physical examination findings, a basic understanding of the immune system is instrumental in deciding how to evaluate patients for possible immune defects. The immune system is historically divided into two basic arms, the innate and the adaptive arms of the immune system. The innate immune system is comprised of neutrophils, macrophages, natural killer (NK) cells, and complement proteins. This arm responds rapidly to infections in a manner that is relatively nonspecific to any particular infection. The adaptive immune system is composed primarily of T and B cells and typically responds to infections more slowly than the innate immune system. The adaptive immune system, however, is much more specific to particular infections than the innate immune system, a response known as "memory." This memory response by the adaptive immune system has evolved primarily through the ability to arrange and mutate receptors of T cells (T-cell receptors, TCRs) and B cells (immunoglobulins, also known as B-cell receptors, BCRs) randomly into billions of different combinations. This diversification in turn allows the adaptive immune system to recognize billions of different epitopes of infectious organisms. Through the preferential expansion and survival of T and B cells that better recognize certain organisms, the immune system enriches itself for those T and B cells that are the most efficacious at clearing certain organisms. This process subsequently allows a larger starting fraction of lymphocytes that can respond more quickly and better to future infections with the same organisms, creating what is called "immunologic memory" [1,20,21].

The adaptive immune system has been defined further into the humoral and cellular immune arms. The humoral immune system historically has been restricted to B cells and their production of immunoglobulins, whereas the cellular immune system classically has been limited to T cells and their ability to produce various cytokines, and in the case of cytotoxic T lymphocytes, the killing of cells infected with intracellular organisms. What has become clear during the past several years is that the humoral and cellular immune arms are functionally dependent on each other in mounting effective immune responses. For instance, B cells are reliant on certain cytokines produced by different helper T cells to produce different types of immunoglobulins (ie, IgG versus IgE). Likewise, cytotoxic T lymphocytes also rely on specific immunoglobulin responses by B cells to clear viral infections effectively by binding and destroying cell-free virus particles and preventing their spread to other cellular targets [1,20,21].

Similar to the functional dependence between the humoral and cellular immune arms, the innate and adaptive immune arms are intimately dependent on each other for optimal immune responses. Examples of this dependence are the need for certain T-cell–derived cytokines to activate macrophages to destroy intracellular organisms such as *Listeria monocytogenes*, and the increased ability of neutrophils to destroy bacteria coated with specific antibodies produced by B cells [1,21]. These close relationships between the different arms of the immune system demonstrate how disruption of any part can result in severe immune deficiencies and life-threatening consequences.

Evaluations for suspected immune deficiencies

As suggested previously, the approach to diagnosing possible immune defects in patients relies on understanding the contribution of the different arms of the immune system in responding to various infections. Understanding the roles of the different immune cells in clearing different types of infections allows the physician to focus on specific clinical tests that will help in determining if the patient has an immune deficiency. A suggested approach to evaluating patients is discussed here and is summarized in Fig. 1.

	Suspect T cell or Combined Immune Defect
Presentation:	Failure to thrive, chronic diarrhea, opportunistic infections, polyendocrinopathies, persistent thrush (>1 year of age)
Infections:	Opportunistic (Mycobacterium, Pneumocystis carnii, Candida, EBV, CMV, disseminated varicella)

Clinical Evaluations:	1. CBC with differential + Lymphocyte subsets (flow cytometry)
	  - Note: Normal CBC does not rule out a lymphocyte subset deficiency
	2. Vaccine titers (tetanus, diphtheria, pneumococcal)
	  - If non-protective titers: re-vaccinate and check titer levels in 3-4 weeks
	2. Quantitative Immunoglobulin levels: IgA, IgE, IgM, IgG
	  - Note: can have normal levels but defective specific responses
	3. T cell proliferation assay (mitogens, PMA/ionomycin, CD3 ligation)

	4. Consider: Skin testing (candida, PPD; need to consider exposure history)
	5. Advanced: a. NK cell cytotoxicity (suspect NK cell defect; i.e., HLH)
	         b. Cytokine receptor expression (flow cytometry)
	         c. Cytokine production

	Suspect Humoral Defect
Presentation:	Recurrent sinopulmonary infections, poor growth, autoimmunity, GI malabsorption
Infections:	Encapsulated bacteria, viruses (enteroviruses)

Clinical Evaluations:	1. Vaccine titers (tetanus, diphtheria, pneumococcal)
	  - If non-protective titers: re-vaccinate and check titer levels in 3-4 weeks
	2. Quantitative Immunoglobulin levels: IgA, IgE, IgM, IgG
	  - Note: can have normal levels but defective specific responses

	3. Consider: Sweat test for CF, evaluation of sinus/chest anatomy with CT scan
	4. Advanced: a. B cell subset evaluation (flow cytometry) for memory development
	         b. IgG subclass determination (rare/controversial deficiencies)
	         c. B cell proliferation assay
	         d. Ciliary evaluation (Kartagener's, etc.)

	Suspect Neutrophil Defect
Presentation:	Abscesses, deep-seeded infections, oral ulcers, pneumonias, poor wound healing, delayed umbilical cord separation
Infections:	Catalase positive bacteria (Staph. aureus, Pseudomonas, Serratia, Klebsiella), Candida, Nocardia, Aspergillus
Clinical Evaluations:	1. CBC with manual differential: 2. Nitroblue tetrazolium (NBT) test: tests oxidative burst (evaluates for CGD)
	3. Consider: Flow cytometry (DHR) - more quantitative than NBT (female carriers), test for MRSA carrier status 4. Advanced: chemotaxis assay, phagocytosis assay

	Suspect Complement Defect
Presentation:	Rheumatoid disorders (lupus, scleroderma), recurrent infections (pyogenic, Neisseria), angioedema
Clinical Evaluations:	1. Total hemolytic complement assay (CH50) - measures classical and alternative pathways - If abnormal: quantitation of individual complement components 2. C3, C4 levels 3. Angioedema: measure level of C1 inhibitor
	4. Advanced: serum opsonic and chemotactic assays

Fig. 1. Laboratory evaluations for suspected primary immunodeficiencies. Suggested work-up for T cell or combined immune defects, humoral defects, neutrophil defects, and complement defects. Typical presentations and infectious complications for each immune defect are listed. Front-line clinical evaluations for the different suspected immune defects are listed along with follow-up evaluations for abnormal results. Tests to consider for suspected defects, as well as advanced clinical evaluations, are separated from front-line evaluations by a solid line. CBC, complete blood cell count; CF, cystic fibrosis; CGD, chronic granulomatous disease; CMV, cytomegalovirus; DHR, dihydrorhodamine; EBV, Epstein-Barr virus; GI, gastrointestinal; HLH, hemophagocytic lymphohistiocytosis; MRSA, methicillin-resistant Staphylococcus aureus; NBT, nitroblue tetrazolium; NK, natural killer; PMA, phorbol myristyl acetate.

Determining defects in cellular immune responses

Cellular immune defects typically are classified as T-cell defects. Because T cells are critical in the killing of intracellular organisms, patients who has T-cell defects often presents with opportunistic infections and disseminated viral infections. These infections include *Pneumocystis carinii, Cryptococcus, Mycobacteria* spp, *Candida* spp, and a variety of viruses (eg, cytomegalovirus, Epstein-Barr virus, adenovirus, varicella). Because of the typical chronicity of these infections, patients who have T-cell defects commonly present with failure to thrive, refractory diarrhea, and persistent thrush after 1 year of age [2,5,12,19,22,23]. In severely T-cell deficient patients, infants are occasionally born with evidence of severe graft-versus-host disease (ie, severe skin rash at birth, liver dysfunction, enteropathy, and reactive pulmonary disease). This complication is caused by the transfer through the placenta of maternal lymphocytes that subsequently recognize the infant's organs as foreign and begin to attack and destroy them [24]. This condition occurs in T-cell–deficient patients because they lack a normal immune system that would recognize these maternal lymphocytes as nonself and destroy them. In addition, patients who have T-cell defects can present with a variety of different autoimmune syndromes (eg, type 1 diabetes in infancy, hypothyroidism, Addison's disease) caused by their own immune cells [25–31]. The reasons for these clinical complications are unclear, but they may be caused by the lack of T-regulatory cells, a subset of T cells that are essential in controlling autoimmune T and B cells [26].

Although patients who have T-cell deficiencies typically present before 6 months of age secondary to the life-threatening complications associated with opportunistic infections and viruses, many patients are not diagnosed until much later [3]. For this reason it is important for the pediatrician to monitor the growth of children carefully using standard growth charts. A pediatrician should suspect a cellular immune deficiency if the child demonstrates a significant decrease in weight/height velocity without a clear cause, often defined as a decrease in more than two isobars.

As noted previously, B cells are functionally dependent on T-cell help for proper immunoglobulin responses, and hence T-cell defects often present with a combined T- and B-cell clinical deficiency phenotype. If a T-cell or combined T- and B-cell immune deficiency is suspected, the first line of laboratory evaluations should include (1) lymphocyte subset enumeration by flow cytometry, (2) quantitative immunoglobulin levels (IgA, IgE, IgM, and IgG), (3) vaccine titer levels (tetanus, diphtheria, pneumococcus, and hepatitis B), and (4) determining T-cell proliferative responses to mitogens (phytohemaglutinin [PHA], Concanavalin A [ConA]) and phorbol myristyl acetate [PMA]/ionomycin) (see Fig. 1) [2,20,32].

It is important for the pediatrician to consider lymphopenia in neonates and infants as a probable immune deficiency until proven otherwise. This level of suspicion is critical to diagnose severe combined immune deficiencies before life-threatening infections occur and to prevent the administration of live attenuated virus vaccines (eg, measles, mumps, rubella, varicella, bacille Calmette-Guérin) that could be lethal in such individuals [33–36]. On the other hand, it is also vital for physicians to understand that a complete blood cell count (CBC) does not rule out a lymphocyte subset defect. Patients who have specific lymphocyte subset defects often have a normal absolute lymphocyte count, which is why subset enumeration by flow cytometry is required. If a lymphocyte subset deficiency is found, these patients should be referred immediately to an immunologist for further evaluation.

Because B cells require proper help from T cells for specific immunoglobulin production, low quantitative IgM and IgG are often helpful in suggesting a defect in the ability of T cells to stimulate B-cell immunoglobulin production properly. Normal quantitative immunoglobulins do not rule out the possibility of a defect in T-cell–B-cell interactions, however, and patients who have such defects often may have normal immunoglobulin levels. For this reason, it is more informative to demonstrate functional T-cell–B-cell interactions as determined by vaccine titer levels. The presence of protective vaccine titers suggests a basic level of T-cell–B-cell interactions and would make a severe T-cell defect much less likely [2,19,20,32]. Patients shown to have nonprotective vaccine titers should be rechallenged with those respective vaccines (no live-virus vaccinations) to determine if they are able to make functional immunoglobulin responses (typically retested 3–4 weeks after vaccination). If they are able to make appropriate vaccine titer levels upon revaccination, a severe T-cell defect is unlikely. Conversely, a patient's inability to make protective vaccine titer levels suggests a B- or T-cell defect. Additional information that needs to be considered when evaluating vaccine titer levels is the age of patient (maternal transfer of IgG), vaccination history, and potential drugs (steroids) that may interfere with vaccine responses.

Skin testing is another important tool in determining functional defects in T cells. The immunologic response to skin testing is often referred to as a "delayed-type hypersensitivity response." Such testing is functionally informative because it determines the ability of T cells to respond to foreign antigen presented on professional antigen-presenting cells, producing skin induration and erythema. Typical protein adjuncts used to test this response include purified protein derivative from heat-killed mycobacterium and Candida protein. The age of the patient, likelihood of prior exposure, vaccination history (bacille Calmette-Guérin), and drug treatments (eg, steroids) need to be considered in determining true anergic responders [2,19,20,32].

T-cell proliferation assays are often performed in individuals suspected of having a T-cell defect. These proliferative assays should employ agents that cross-link the TCR (PHA, ConA, anti-CD3 antibody) to stimulate T-cell proliferation as well as agents that can stimulate T-cell division by bypassing the TCR signaling complex (PMA/ionomycin). Using this combination of agents allows the determination of proximal TCR signaling defects (PHA, ConA, anti-CD3) versus more downstream signaling defects (PMA/ionomycin) [2,19,20,32].

Finally, more advanced laboratory testing such as cytokine production, cytokine receptor detection, signaling molecule detection, gene sequencing, and NK-cell cytotoxicity assays may also be important in the diagnosis of certain cellular immunodeficiencies. For example, infants that have primary hemophagocytic lymphohistiocytosis (HLH) typically have defects in the ability of NK cells to kill target cells (ie, decreased cytotoxicity). Consultation with an immunologist is recommended before performing these more advanced immunology tests [20,37–39].

Determining defects in humoral immune responses

Humoral immune deficiencies typically are caused by defects in the ability of B cells to produce functional immunoglobulins. Patients who have such defects often present with recurrent sinopulmonary infections, diarrhea, poor growth, and autoimmunity. The types of infections in humoral defects characteristically involve encapsulated bacteria (eg, *Haemophilus influenza*, *Pneumococcus* spp, *Streptococci* spp, among others), but humoral defects also can present with difficulties in controlling parasitic infections such as *Giardia* as well as certain viruses such as enteroviruses and papillomaviruses. Humoral defects also can present with chronic autoimmune complications such as autoimmune hemolytic anemia, immune thrombocytopenia, and autoimmune neutropenia, all caused by the inappropriate production of self-reactive immunoglobulins by B cells.

The primary immunologic tests to determine whether a patient has a humoral defect include (1) quantitative immunoglobulins (IgA, IgE, IgM and IgG) and (2) vaccine titer levels (see Fig. 1). As noted previously, although low immunoglobulin levels can indicate an underlying humoral defect, normal levels do not rule out a B-cell defect. Therefore it is important to determine the functional abilities of B cells to make protective vaccine titers. Patients who have low vaccine titer levels should be revaccinated and tested for vaccine titer levels approximately 3 to 4 weeks after vaccination [2,19,20,32].

Other laboratory tests that should be considered in patients who have recurrent sinopulmonary infections include a sweat test to rule out cystic fibrosis, sinus/chest CT scans to evaluate patients for anatomic abnormalities, and sinopulmonary biopsy with evaluation by electron microscopic for ciliary defects. Finally, more advanced testing for B-cell defects includes flow cytometry evaluation of B-cell subsets (ie, naive and memory B-cell subsets), B-cell proliferation assay, and IgG subclass determination [2,19,20,32].

Determining defects in phagocyte function

Phagocytes (neutrophils and monocytes) are part of the innate immune system and are critical in initiating immune responses to bacterial infections quickly. Patients who have neutrophil defects present with a history of recurrent abscesses, abscesses in unusual areas (eg, liver, muscle, abdominal cavity), recurrent oral ulcers, severe pneumonias, poor wound healing, or delayed umbilical cord separation. Patients who have chronic granulomatous disease (CGD) have difficulty clearing catalase positive organisms (eg, *Staphylococcus aureus, Serratia, Klebsiella*) because of the lack of oxygen radical production by the NADPH oxidative system. Patients who have CGD and other neutrophil defects also have a high incidence of infections with other organisms such as *Candida, Nocardia*, and *Aspergillus* [20,40,41].

The initial clinical evaluation for patients suspected of having a neutrophil defect is the CBC with a manual differential (see Fig. 1). Although the presence of a normal absolute neutrophil count is encouraging, it does not rule out a functional defect in the neutrophils. In fact, a persistently elevated absolute neutrophil count (typically $> 20,000/\mu L$) is associated with certain defects affecting the neutrophil's ability to migrate from the vasculature (ie, leukocyte adhesion deficiency, LAD). If the patient has few or no detectable neutrophils, a quick determination is required to evaluate that patient for congenital neutropenia, also known as Kostmann's syndrome. Frequently, multiple CBCs with manual differentials are needed to establish the level of neutropenia and to help distinguish other possible causes, such as cyclic neutropenia. In addition to being evaluated for intrinsic causes of their neutropenia, neutropenic patients also should be evaluated for possible extrinsic causes. Such extrinsic causes include a variety of drugs, malignancy, isoimmune/autoimmune disorders, and hypersplenism [20,40,41].

In addition to CBC evaluations for neutrophil defects, patients should have their neutrophils evaluated for possible deficiencies in the NADPH oxidative system. The primary functional test for this system is the nitroblue tetrazolium (NBT) test. The NBT test determines the ability of activated neutrophils to produce oxygen radicals that reduce NBT to an insoluble blue dye that can be seen microscopically in neutrophils. A similar flow-based assay is used by many reference laboratories and is based on the ability of stimulated neutrophils to reduce a nonfluorescent molecule, dihydrorhodamine, to a fluorescent molecule by oxygen radicals. If a male patient is found to have CGD, it should be considered mandatory to evaluate the patient's biologic mother as a potential carrier status of the X-linked form of CGD. The flow-based dihydrorhodamine test typically is much more quantitative and sensitive than the NBT test in determining the percentage of affected neutrophils in females carriers of the X-linked form of CGD, which is caused by random X chromosome inactivation (ie, lyonization) [42,43]. This analysis is crucial in female carriers of X-linked CGD, as it is in all X-linked diseases, because a small fraction of such female patients can be clinically symptomatic because of skewing toward the mutant X chromosome. Other more advanced testing for possible neutrophil defects includes examination for chemotaxis and phagocytosis defects. Such deficiencies are quite rare, and their evaluations are primarily research based [40].

Determining defects in the complement immune system

Defects in the complement system are rare compared with other immune system defects and account for less than 2% of the known patients who have PIDs. Some of the most common clinical presentations for individuals who have complement system defects include recurrent infections with pyogenic bacteria and *Neisseria* spp, as well as an increased prevalence of auto-immune disorders (eg, lupus and scleroderma).

Screening for most complement defects is accomplished by performing a total hemolytic complement (CH_{50}) assay. The CH_{50} assay measures the amount of complement in serum required to lyse 50% of red blood cell targets. This test measures both the classic and alternative complement pathways because it relies on properly formed C9 complement pores to lyse red blood cell targets, which are the end products of both pathways. C3 and C4 levels should also be measured if the CH_{50} assay is abnormal, because levels of these proteins can help define the pathway in which the complement defect is located. Patients with the clinical presentation of angioedema should be suspected of having a defect in the C1 inhibitor, and quantitative measurements of this protein and its function are required [44,45]. More advanced tests, such as serum opsonic and chemotactic assays, are primarily research based [32,46–48].

Categorization of primary immune deficiencies

An expert international committee sponsored by the International Union of Immunological Societies and the Jeffrey Model Foundation currently classifies all PIDs [6]. This committee meets approximately every 2 to 3 years and is responsible for updating and refining the current classification of PIDs based on their known molecular causes. The reader is referred to these published reports for updated summaries of PIDs [6]. Given the interrelated and interdependent components of the innate and adaptive immune systems, the current classification of PIDs is somewhat artificial. Nonetheless, the grouping of PIDs based on these immunologic definitions is essential to understand their genetic etiologies, cellular consequences, and, ultimately, their clinical implications.

Severe combined immune deficiencies (SCIDs) are disorders that can affect both T and B cells and usually are further classified according to the presence or absence of lymphocyte subsets. For instance, classifying a patient as $T^-B^+NK^-$ SCID indicates that both the T-cell and NK-cell numbers are markedly reduced in the peripheral blood and thus would most likely carry a mutation in one of the known genes that can cause $T^-B^+NK^-$ SCID (eg, γ_c or JAK3 deficiency) [6]. This type of classification of patients who have SCIDs is helpful when attempting to determine the underlying genetic mutation, but a full understanding of this type of classification system requires a considerable understanding of the genetic and cellular requirements for lymphocyte development and function.

Further complicating the classification of PIDs, especially SCID phenotypes, is the recent understanding of the different clinical phenotypes that can occur with hypomorphic gene mutations. In comparison with null mutations, in which there is a complete absence of gene product expression and function, hypomorphic mutations result in reduced gene product expression or function. These mutations can result in reduced, but not absent, peripheral lymphocyte subsets. In addition, hypomorphic mutations can result in atypical clinical presentations of PID caused by the presence of dysregulated lymphocyte subsets, including increased end-organ (skin, lung, intestines, liver) damage and severe autoimmunity [49–53]. A prototypical example of these hypomorphic mutations is Omenn's syndrome ($T^+B^-NK^+$ SCID) caused by missense mutations in either the recombination-activating genes 1 and 2 (*RAG1* or *RAG2*) [53]. In comparison to other mutations in *RAG1* or *RAG2* that result in absence of both T and B cells ($T^-B^-NK^+$ SCID), patients who have Omenn's syndrome have relatively normal levels of peripheral T cells, but they also have other unusual clinical complications, including erythrodermia, eosinophilia, and organomegaly, that are not typically observed in the more complete Rag1 or Rag2 mutations [6]. Nonetheless, such hypomorphic gene mutations can be just as life threatening as complete null mutations and in some cases cause significantly more clinical morbidity.

Finally, it is important to understand the concept that "genotype does not equal phenotype," meaning that an identical genetic mutation in two different individuals can result in very different clinical phenotypes and presentations. This concept is best exemplified in patients who have 22q11 microdeletion syndrome (also known as DiGeorge syndrome type 1), in which approximately 85% of patients carry the same microdeletion [54]. Despite the identical gene deletion, the clinical presentation in these patients is extremely broad, ranging from absence of heart defects and a normal immune system to severe congenital heart defects and complete absence of T cells. The "genotype does not equal phenotype" concept is understood better by examining family members and monozygotic twins who have identical disease-causing mutations [55–57]. In such instances, there also is a broad clinical presentation of these diseases, indicating the importance of other inherited maternal and paternal genes and also how differences in gene expression patterns can substantially affect clinical presentations (as demonstrated in monozygotic twins carrying identical mutations).

In this review the authors have attempted to help the general pediatrician better understand the PIDs. In grouping PIDs, the general categorization of the international consortium has been observed where possible, but the review has emphasized groups of mutations based on the pathophysiology of the different genetic deficiencies. Finally, the review has been restricted to known defects that primarily present with immunodeficiency as a significant part of the clinical presentation. For example, the authors have not discussed the recently described group of autoinflammatory disorders (ie, hereditary fever syndromes), because these patients typically do not present with increased susceptibility to infections but rather with unexplained fevers and inflammatory symptoms. For additional information on these conditions, the reader is referred to excellent recent reviews [58–60].

Deficiencies in lymphocyte signaling and growth factors

T cells require proper signaling through receptors to survive and proliferate in response to foreign antigens. Many of the genetic causes that result in a SCID phenotype are the result of defects in lymphocyte signaling or growth factors (Fig. 2) [1,6,20,21]. After recognition of antigen–major histocompatibility (MHC) complexes by the heterodimer α/β TCR, signaling through the physically associated CD3 complex subunits occurs. This complex usually is composed of heterodimer subunits of either CD3γ/ε chains or CD3δ/ε chains and a CD3ζ homodimer [1,6,20,21]. Deficiency in either the CD3δ or CD3ε chain results in decreased circulating T cells and a T$^-$B$^+$NK$^+$ SCID phenotype. The CD3ε chain also seems to be required for $\gamma\delta$ T cell development. A defect in the CD3γ chain results in a milder PID with decreased circulating CD8 T cells but normal numbers of circulating CD4 T cells. The few patients reported with a CD3γ chain defect also seem to have a higher incidence of autoimmunity, including autoimmune hemolytic anemia, enteropathy, and autoimmune thyroid disease [61]. Downstream signaling events of the CD3 complex include activation of the tyrosine kinase molecule Zap70. Patients who have Zap70 defects have been shown to have severely reduced circulating CD8 T cells but normal CD4 T cells [62,63]. In addition to TCR recognition of antigen-MHC complexes, the CD4 and CD8 molecules found on their respective T-cell subsets facilitate T-cell interaction with the antigen-presenting cells by forming adhesive interactions with the MHC class II and class I molecules, respectively. As expected, patients who have a defect in the *CD8* gene have a lack of circulating CD8 T cells [64]. Although there are no reported patients with *CD4* gene defects, a patient who had a reported deficiency in the CD4-associated signaling molecule, Lck, was demonstrated to have a reduction in circulating CD4 T cells [65]. For proper and repetitive signaling to occur through the TCR/CD3 complex, expression of the tyrosine phosphatase CD45 is also required to reset the signaling complex. A patient who had a deficiency in CD45 was shown to have a clinical phenotype of a T$^-$B$^+$NK$^+$ SCID, demonstrating its central role in maintaining normal T-cell signaling, which is required for their survival [66].

Besides the need for proper TCR/CD3 signaling for survival, T cells also require stimulation through the γ_c cytokine receptor complex for their function and survival. The γ_c cytokine receptor family includes interleukin (IL)-2, IL-4, IL-7, IL-9, IL-15, and IL-21, all of which use the γ_c subunit as part of their signaling complex. Besides the γ_c subunit, each individual cytokine also recognizes and binds a separate ligand-specific subunit (eg, IL-4Rα, IL-7Rα, IL-9Rα). In some cases, certain cytokines (eg, IL-2) are

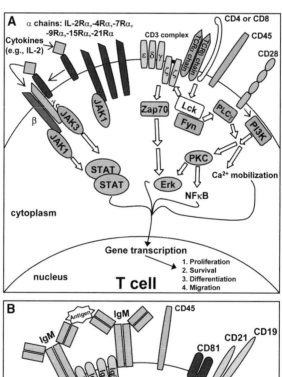

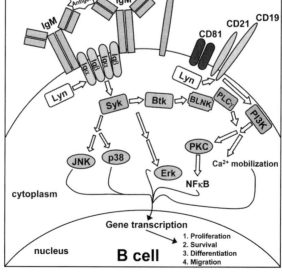

recruited to the signaling subunits through a third unique α chain (eg, IL-2Rα; also known as CD25). Both the γ_c and ligand-specific subunits are associated with Janus kinase (JAK) signaling molecules (eg, JAK3 and JAK1) that become activated upon cytokine binding and phosphorylate the receptor subunits. These phosphorylated receptor subunits then recruit signal transducer and activator of transcription (STAT) molecules. The STAT molecules are subsequently phosphorylated by the JAKs, leading to their dimerization and translocation to the nucleus where they regulate gene transcription [67–69]. Defects in the IL-7Rα chain produces a $T^-B^+NK^+$ SCID phenotype, establishing IL-7 as a key developmental cytokine [6,70,71]. Defects in the γ_c subunit and Jak3 result in a $T^-B^+NK^-$ SCID phenotype [9,72–80], demonstrating their role in T-cell signaling and also their role in NK-cell signaling and survival. Finally, a deficiency in the IL-2Rα chain (also known as CD25) has been described in two individuals [81], resulting in a PID that includes T-cell lymphopenia and several auto-immune features (eg, enteropathy, diabetes, eczema). This autoimmunity is most likely caused by a reduction in the number or function of T-regulatory cells, which have been demonstrated to be essential in preventing autoimmunity (Verbsky, unpublished observations).

For B cells, signaling occurs by antigen-induced aggregation of surface immunoglobulins (BCRs) and their associated signaling heterodimer complex composed of Igα and Igβ. The BCR signaling complex subsequently delivers signals through a number of molecules, including src-family kinases (eg, Lyn, Fyn, Blk) and tyrosine kinases (eg, Bruton's tyrosine kinase, Btk), which also rely on adapter molecules such as B-cell linker protein (BLNK) [82–85]. Deficiencies in the μ (mu heavy-chain; IgM), Igα, Btk and BLNK all result in profoundly decreased levels of circulating B cells, along with decreases in serum immunoglobulins [6,86–91].

◄────────────────────

Fig. 2. Deficiencies in human lymphocyte signaling and growth factors. Simplified signaling cascades for T cells and B cells are illustrated. (A) Primary T cell signaling occurs through the TCR-associated CD3 complex via Zap70, as well as well as cytokine signaling through the γ_c receptor complex and the JAK–STAT pathway. Proximal signaling occurs through Lck, Fyn, PLCγ, and ERK. Downstream effector molecules, including dimerized STAT molecules and nuclear factor κB, translocate to the nucleus, where they affect gene transcription that controls T cell proliferation, survival, differentiation, and migration. The known human signaling defects resulting in primary immune deficiencies are as follows: (1) γ_c receptor complex: (a) gamma common chain receptor (γ_c), (b) IL-2Rα chain (CD25), (c) IL-7Rα chain; (2) CD3 signaling complex: (a) CD3ε, (b) CD3δ, (c) CD3γ; (3) Zap70; (4) Lck; (5) CD8; (6) CD45. See text for clinical presentation of each defect. (B) Primary B cell signaling occurs through the BCR (IgM)-associated signaling molecules Igα/β, as well as the costimulatory molecules CD21 and CD19. Proximal signaling occurs through Syk, Btk, BLNK, Lyn, PLCγ, and PKC. Downstream effector molecules include nuclear factor κB and NFAT that translocate to the nucleus where they affect gene transcription that controls B cell proliferation, survival, differentiation, and migration. The known human signaling defects resulting in primary immune deficiencies are as follows: (1) μ gene (IgM); (2) Igα; (3) BLNK; (4) Btk. See text for clinical presentation of each defect.

Deficiencies in development and survival

Similar to the previously described genetic mutations that cause deficiencies of T- and B-cell signaling, several other known genetic defects result in the failure of T- and B-cell development or their subsequent survival. A summary of these other known genetic defects is illustrated in Fig. 3.

Both B- and T-cell receptors require somatic gene recombination, a process commonly referred to as "V-(D)-J recombination," to produce diverse combinations of immunoglobulins or TCRs. Two of the genes central to this process in both B and T cells are *RAG1* and *RAG2*. Defects in either *RAG1* or *RAG2* genes result in the inability of developing B and T cells to produce

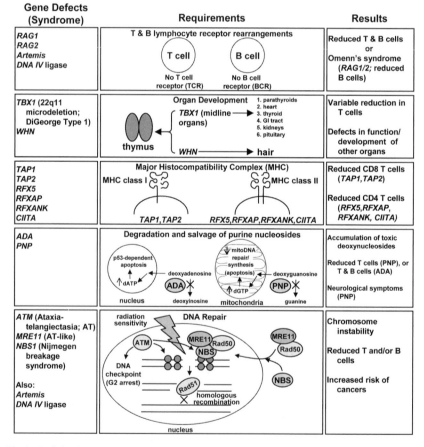

Fig. 3. Deficiencies in human lymphocyte development and survival. Genes and their associated syndromes (*left column*), mechanisms of action associated with the genes (*center column*), and clinical result of gene defects (*right column*) are depicted. Deficiencies are grouped according to the mechanisms of action of genes and include T and B lymphocyte receptor rearrangements, organ development, major histocompatibility complex expression, degradation and salvage of purine nucleosides, and DNA repair.

functional receptors required for survival signals during their development [92–94]. Both Rag1 and Rag2 deficiencies result in $T^-B^-NK^+$ SCID phenotype, with the exceptions of certain hypomorphic mutations, as noted previously, that can result in Omenn's syndrome ($T^+B^-NK^+$ SCID) characterized by erythrodermia, eosinophilia, organomegaly, alopecia, and lack of peripheral B cells [6,92,93,95–98]. It should be noted, however, that the T cells in Omenn's patients are often dysfunctional T-cell clones that are thought to be responsible for much of the observed secondary end-organ damage in these patients. Two additional genes, termed *Artemis* and *DNA IV ligase*, also have been shown to play critical roles in both V-(D)-J recombination and DNA repair. Similar to Rag1 and Rag2 deficiencies, defects in either Artemis or DNA IV ligase produce a $T^-B^-NK^+$ SCID clinical phenotype [6,49,80,99–103]. In contrast to Rag1 and Rag2, however, Artemis and DNA IV ligase are also involved in other types of DNA repair; thus defects in these genes also demonstrate radiation sensitivity in both lymphoid and nonlymphoid organs. For these reasons, defects in Artemis and DNA IV ligase often are referred to as "radiation-sensitive SCIDs."

Not only is there a need for T cells to develop functional TCRs; these TCRs also need to interact subsequently with antigen-MHC complexes in the thymus to receive a survival signal during their development. Several genes have been discovered that are required for normal expression of MHC class I and class II. For MHC class I to be expressed properly on the cell surface, a heterodimer transporter associated with antigen-processing polypeptides (TAP1 or TAP2) loads peptides from the cytosol into awaiting MHC class I in the endoplasmic reticulum [1,20]. Defects in either Tap1 or Tap2 result in absent MHC class I expression and subsequent lack of circulating CD8 T cells that require MHC class I for their thymic development, resulting in the syndrome called "bare lymphocyte syndrome, type I" [6,104,105]. In a similar fashion, development of CD4 T cells in the thymus requires their TCR to interact with antigen-MHC class II complexes. Defects in a number of genes for DNA-binding proteins (*RFX5*, *RFXAP*, *RFXANK*, *CIITA*) that promote expression of MHC class II result in the lack of circulating CD4 T cells [106–109]. The lack of MHC class II commonly is referred to as "bare lymphocyte syndrome, type II" and can be associated with several other clinical features besides lack of CD4 T cells, including multiple types of autoimmune disorders (eg, rheumatoid arthritis, multiple sclerosis).

For T cells to develop normally, they require a normal thymus that contributes thymic epithelial cells that are an essential component of T-cell development through a process called "positive selection." Defects in two genes, *Tbx1* and *WHN*, lead to abnormal thymic epithelial development and consequently decreased levels of circulating T cells. Haploinsufficiency in the *Tbx1* gene occurs in the 22q11.2 microdeletion syndrome, commonly referred to as "DiGeorge syndrome type 1" [110–113]. Tbx1 is a transcription factor that is required for the normal migration of neural crest cells during development of the brachial apparatus and cardiac outflow tract. Insufficiency of this transcription factor can lead to the abnormal growth of many midline structures and organs, including the central nervous system, pituitary gland, heart, parathyroid, thyroid, thymus, skeletal system, gastrointestinal tract, and kidneys [114–118]. Although 85% of patients who have 22q11.2 microdeletion syndrome carry the same 3-mega base pairs (Mbp) deletion, the immunodeficiency spectrum observed in these patients is quite diverse, ranging from completely normal T-cell numbers to complete absence of T cells [54]. This clinical spectrum demonstrates that Tbx1 is a dosage-sensitive transcription factor and that genotype does not equal phenotype. WHN is a transcription factor that also is required for normal development of thymic epithelium and hair follicles. Patients who have gene mutations in *WHN* display a severe decrease in circulating T cells and also present with congenital alopecia and nail dystrophy, a clinical presentation commonly referred to as a "nude" phenotype [119].

A number of genes have been shown to be important in normal DNA repair that allows cells to survive after encountering DNA-damaging agents. When eukaryotic cells are exposed to ionizing/gamma radiation, they halt their progression through the cell cycle by a process called "radiation-induced S-phase checkpoint" to repair damaged DNA. Defects in the ataxia telangiectasia mutated (*ATM*), meiotic recombination 11 homologue (*MRE11*), or nibrin (*NBN*) genes lead to failure in this checkpoint and to continued DNA synthesis in the face of DNA damage [103,120,121] resulting in either cell death or acquisitions of gene mutations that can ultimately lead to the development of cancer. Given the high mitotic rate of lymphoid cells, defects in the *ATM*, *MRE11*, or *NBN* DNA repair genes can lead to reduced numbers of circulating T cells or, in the case of defects in the *Artemis* or *DNA IV ligase* genes (as discussed previously), significantly reduced levels of both T and B cells [122,123]. As predicted, defects in all these DNA repair genes also carry a significantly increased risk of various cancers as well as a variety of other gene-specific clinical associations such as microcephaly (*NBN*) and ataxia (*ATM*, *MRE11*) [102].

Finally, because lymphoid cells are highly proliferative during their development and peripheral responses, they use high amounts of nucleotides for DNA synthesis. Defects in two genes involved in the purine catabolic pathway, adenosine deaminase (*ADA*) and purine nucleoside phosphorylase (*PNP*), result in a buildup of toxic nucleosides that can lead to lymphocyte cell death [124–128]. In ADA deficiency, there is a buildup of the enzyme's precursor deoxyadenosine that ultimately leads to a toxic increase of nuclear deoxyadenosine triphosphate and p53-dependent cell death. *ADA* deficiency results in a progressive $T^-B^-NK^-$ SCID clinical phenotype. Similarly, PNP deficiency results in an increase in the enzyme's precursor deoxyguanosine that results in the toxic buildup of deoxyguanosine triphosphate in cellular mitochondria. *PNP* deficiency results in a progressive decrease in circulating T cells (B cells are usually spared) as well as the development of neurologic symptoms and various autoimmune complications (eg, autoimmune hemolytic anemia).

Deficiencies in T- and B-cell interactions

As noted previously, B cells are functionally dependent on T cells to make proper functional immunoglobulin responses. It is not surprising, therefore, to find that several PIDs are caused by defects in genes that mediate these cellular interactions between T and B cells and their downstream signals (Fig. 4).

Defects in two genes, *CD40L* and *CD40*, result in a similar clinical syndrome termed "hyper-IgM syndrome" [129–135]. *CD40L* is an X-linked gene that is expressed on activated T cells, whereas hyper-IgM syndrome

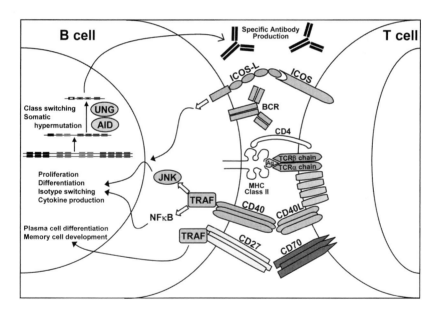

Fig. 4. Deficiencies in human T and B lymphocyte interactions. Simplified illustration of key proteins expressed on T cells and their cognate B cell proteins that are required for proper B cell costimulation. Proper B cell costimulation through CD40 and ICOS-L results in proximal signaling through TRAF. Downstream effector molecules include nuclear factor κB, which translocates to the nucleus and controls B cell proliferation, differentiation, isotype switching, and cytokine production. Additional signaling through the TRAF pathway promotes development of plasma cell and memory B cell differentiation. Similar secondary B cell costimulation results in class switching and somatic hypermutation through UNG and AID. The known human defects in T–B cell interaction are: (1) CD40L (X-linked hyper-IgM), whose cellular consequences include defective B cell signaling and defective dendritic cell signaling; (2) CD40 (AR hyper-IgM), whose cellular consequences include defective B cell signaling and defective dendritic cell signaling; (3) ICOS, whose cellular consequences include decreased B cells; (4) UNG, whose cellular consequences include impaired B cell differentiation and lack of somatic hypermutation; and (5) AID, whose cellular consequences include impaired B cell differentiation and lack of somatic hypermutation.

caused by defective expression of CD40 on B cells is inherited in an autosomal recessive manner. The term "hyper-IgM" is somewhat of a misnomer, because the majority of patients who have defects in either *CD40* or *CD40L* genes have normal serum levels of IgM. Interaction between CD40 and CD40L is required for proper B-cell costimulation and production of functional antibodies. As such, defects in either gene result in the inability to produce functional antibodies but still allow normal levels of circulating T and B cells in most patients. CD40–CD40L contacts are also important in dendritic cell–T-cell interactions, and defects in either gene result an increased rate of opportunistic infections such as *Pneumocystis carinii* and *Cryptococcus* spp [130,136,137]. Similarly, the costimulatory molecules ICOS and ICOS-L expressed on T and B cells, respectively, have also been shown to be important in producing critical costimulatory signals that are required for B cells to produce functional immunoglobulin responses. A defect in the inducible T-cell costimulator (*ICOS*) gene on T cells inhibits functional immunoglobulin responses and also results in a significant decrease in circulating B cells and has been shown to be the genetic cause in a small fraction of patients who have common variable immune deficiency [138,139].

As noted previously immunoglobulin diversity is produced primary through V-(D)-J recombination. In addition, B cells are able to undergo somatic hypermutation of recombined immunoglobulin genes that can produce additional diversity and potentially higher-affinity immunoglobulins. This somatic hypermutation requires proper B-cell–T-cell interaction and signaling, which ultimately leads to the activity of two genes involved in this somatic hypermutation process, uracil-DNA glycosylase (*UNG*) and activation-induced cytidine deaminase (*AID*) [140,141]. Defects in either gene result in decreased production and somatic mutations in plasma B-cell immunoglobulins (IgA and IgG). In addition, both are associated clinically with significant lymphadenopathy. Defects in the *AID* gene are commonly grouped in the autosomal recessive form of hyper-IgM along with CD40 but are not associated with increased opportunistic infections.

Phagocyte defects

Phagocytes include polymorphonuclear leukocytes and monocytes, which are components of the innate immune system and are the first line of defense against microbes. Polymorphonuclear leukocytes and monocytes exist briefly in the circulation (for 7 hours and 2–4 days, respectively) and are recruited to tissues responding to microbial invasion (Fig. 5). The release of inflammatory cytokines (eg, tumor necrosis factor α, IL-1) from these tissues in response to infections activates vessel endothelium to express adhesion molecules, resulting in the margination of phagocytes on the vessels near the site of infection. Chemokines (eg, IL-8) released by tissues binds to chemokine receptors on the marginated phagocytes resulting in their activation

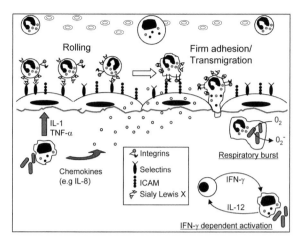

Fig. 5. Phagocyte defects. Phagocyte defects can be divided into defects in production, defects in recruitment, and defects in bactericidal activity. Once produced in the bone marrow, phagocytes are recruited to tissues in a multistep process. First, selectin molecules on endothelium bind to fucose resides expressed on phagocytes resulting in their rolling along the vessel wall. Chemokines released by tissues bind to chemokine receptors of the rolling phagocytes, resulting in activation and integrin-dependent adhesion of the phagocytes. Finally, phagocytes migrate through the endothelial monolayer toward the infected area in response to a chemokine gradient. Upon phagocytosis of pathogens, the NADPH-dependent respiratory burst produces reactive oxygen species that are toxic to microbes. In cases of resistant organisms, IFN-γ production from T cells is required to activate the phagocyte and kill the organism. The known defects in generation or recruitment of phagocytes include: (1) severe congenital neutropenia (elastase, GFI1); (2) Cyclic neutropenia (elastase); (3) LAD I (β2 integrin); (4) LAD II (fucosylation); (5) LAD III (Rap-1 activation). The known defects in phagocyte activation/killing include: (1) chronic granulomatous disease (X-linked [gp91phox], AR [p22-, p47-, p67-phox]); (2) IL-12Rβ1 deficiency; (3) IL-12p40 deficiency; (4) IFN-γR1; (5) IFN-γR2; (6) Stat1; (7) MPO; (8) G-6-PD.

and expression of integrins that mediate adhesion of these rolling phagocytes to the vessel endothelium. Finally the adherent cells disperse through the vessel wall toward the chemokine gradient into the infected area. Phagocytes then recognize these pathogens by direct recognition of bacterial components (eg, mannose), by attached antibodies, or by complement components, resulting in phagocytosis of the offending organism. Once in the phagocyte, granules fuse with the phagosomes, resulting in activation of cytotoxic mechanisms that eventually kill the pathogens. Immunodeficiency can result from defects in any step along this pathway.

The first phagocyte defects to consider are defects in phagocyte number. Severe congenital neutropenia, also known as "Kostmann's syndrome," is a group of disorders characterized by neutropenia, granulocyte maturational arrest, and increased susceptibility to myeloid leukemias. Defects in neutrophil elastase (*Ela2*) have been described in most patients who have congenital neutropenia [142,143]. Recent work has shown that mutations in neutrophil elastase result in the abnormal cellular localization of this protein and enhanced apoptosis of the myeloid precursors [144]. The progression to myeloid dysplasia or myeloid leukemia in these patients can be associated with mutations in the granulocyte colony-stimulating factor receptor, possibly explaining initial reports that granulocyte colony-stimulating factor receptor mutations were also a cause of congenital neutropenia [145–147]. Severe congenital neutropenia also can be caused by mutations in the proto-oncogene *Gfi1*, possibly because it controls the expression of neutrophil elastase, thus linking these two syndromes [148]. Finally, a related disorder, cyclic neutropenia, also is caused by mutations in neutrophil elastase [143,149]. This disorder is characterized by recurrent episodes of neutropenia associated with periodic fevers and recurrent bacterial infections. Why the episodes of neutropenia are cyclical is unknown, but it has been suggested that episodes are associated with normal bursts of polymorphonuclear (PMN) leukocyte; in addition, in patients who have cyclic neutropenia, the mutations of neutrophil elastase group in a different area of the Ela2 protein than do the mutations found in patients who have severe congenital neutropenia [150].

The inflammatory cascade is a three-step process resulting in phagocyte recruitment to a site of infection. First, phagocytes express glycosylated receptors for selectin molecules (eg, Sialyl Lewis X) on the cell surface that interact with selectins on the surface of endothelium resulting in their rolling along the vessel walls, a process known as margination. Firm adhesion of the leukocytes to endothelium is mediated subsequently by integrins and their receptors, a process that is increased by a G protein–mediated activation of leukocytes in response to chemokines binding to their receptors. Finally, the leukocyte migrates through endothelium monolayer into tissues in response to a chemokine gradient (reviewed in [151]). Leukocyte adhesion deficiency type I (LAD I) is a defect in the expression of the $\beta2$-integrin subunit CD18 [152,153]. Phagocytes with deficits in CD18 expression are not able to adhere firmly to the endothelium monolayer and thus cannot migrate into tissues. This lack of adhesion results in a relative increase in circulating neutrophils, because neutrophils that normally would be marginated to endothelium remain in circulation. Leukocyte adhesion deficiency type II (LAD II) is a defect in the fucosylation, or the modification of proteins such as selectin ligands with fucose [154,155]. LAD II seems to be caused by a defect in the uptake of fucose into the Golgi apparatus by a fucose-specific transporter. This rare disease has been described in five patients of Arab decent and results in neutrophilia similar to LAD I but is associated also with severe metal retardation. Finally, a third LAD has been described in a single patient who suffered delayed cord separation, neutrophilia, cellulitis, and excessive bleeding caused by defective platelet function [156]. This condition has been labeled "leukocyte adhesion deficiency III" and seems to be caused by the defective activation of Rap-1, a Ras-related GTP-ase that is critical to integrin activation in response to chemokines. Because these cells cannot be activated at the endothelial surface in response to che-mokines, firm adhesion and transmigration are prevented. Regulation of ac-tin cytoskeleton (Rac2) deficiency has also been described in one patient who had delayed umbilical cord separation, invasive bacterial infections, and neutrophilia [157,158]. Rac2 seems to be important to several aspects of neutrophil function following activation, including chemotaxis and super-oxide generation.

Once phagocytes have entered tissues and encountered pathogens, they must be phagocytosed and eradicated. One mechanism of eradication of mi-crobes is through the generation of superoxide derivatives (hydrogen perox-ide and hydroxyl radical) through the NADPH oxidase complex, a process known as the "respiratory burst." Activation of this pathway seems to re-quire Rac2, described previously, and once activated ultimately transfers electrons from NADPH to oxygen using a multi-subunit complex composed of the proteins p67phox (NCF2), p47phox (NCF1), p22phox (CYBA), or gp91phox (CYBB). Mutations in any of these subunits has been linked to CGD, a disease characterized by infections with catalase-positive bacteria and fungi [159–166]. The CYBB gene is X-linked, whereas the other three genes are autosomal recessive in their inheritance. Glucose-6-phosphate de-hydrogenase deficiency (G6PD) is usually associated with hemolytic anemia, but with complete deficiency defective respiratory burst and susceptibility to infections can also be seen [167–169]. G6PD is required to produce NADPH through the hexose monophosphate shunt pathway. Myeloperoxidase (MPO) is produced by neutrophil and monocyte granules, and deficiency can lead to susceptibility to candidal infections [170–173]. MPO is involved in the conversion of hydrogen peroxide to hypohalous acid, thus enhancing the toxicity of superoxide molecules.

Some microorganisms, such as mycobacteria, are resistant to the phago-cyte-killing mechanism. Responses to these organisms require monocyte/macrophage activation by helper T cells. When macrophages engulf these organisms, IL-12 is produced, which acts on helper T cells to become Th type 1 cells characterized by high levels of interferon (IFN)-γ production. IFN-γ then leads to the activation of macrophages and efficient killing of the engulfed mycobacteria or other resistant organisms. Defects in receptors for IFNγ or its signal transduction components (Stat1) and defects in the production of IL-12 or IL-12 receptor result in increased sensitivity to my-cobacterial infections, salmonella, and certain viruses [174–177]. Most defi-ciencies in IFN-γ receptor subunits (IFN-γR1 and IFN-γR2) are inherited in an autosomal recessive manner, whereas certain IFN-γR1 mutations re-sult in autosomal dominant disease transmission from receptor subunits that act in a dominant negative manner [178,179]. Stat1 mutations are auto-somal recessive, but dominant negative mutations have been reported also [178,180]. Deficiency in either the p40 subunit of IL-12 or the IL-12 receptor β1 chain results in increased susceptibility to mycobacterial infections and exhibits autosomal recessive inheritance [174,181,182].

Complement defects

The complement system consists of a group of heat-labile serum proteins that interact with antibodies and lead to the destruction of microorganisms, either through their direct lysis or by enhancement of phagocytosis (opsonization). Complement deficiencies result in increased sensitivity to pyogenic infections with encapsulated organisms (eg, *pneumococcus, Haemophilus Influenza*) as well as neisserial infections (meningococcus and gonococcus) [20]. Complement deficiencies can result in immune deficiencies and also in autoimmunity, particularly systemic lupus erythematosus (SLE) [183]. This observation can be explained by the involvement of complement in the dissolution of immune complexes and the targeting of apoptotic cells for their clearance from the circulation [184,185]. The inability to clear these complexes can lead to the persistence of self-antigens in the body and the development autoimmunity. The complement cascade can be initiated in three ways: (1) activation by antibodies (IgG and IgM) in what is known as the "classic pathway"; (2) through mannose-binding lectin, known as the "lectin pathway"; and (3) through the spontaneous activation of complement on foreign organisms, known as the "alternative pathway" (Fig. 6) [1]. These pathways converge by the activation of a protein complex known as the C3 convertase, which deposits C3b on the surface of microorganisms. Deposited C3b can act as an opsonin that enhances phagocytosis, or the pathway can lead to the activation of the terminal complement components (C5b–C9) and the generation of the pore-forming membrane attack complex that causes direct lysis of the organism. In addition, the deposition of C3b activates the alternative pathway, leading to the generation of more C3b and the amplification of the response. Finally, the proteolysis of complement components results in the production of peptide fragments that initiate inflammation (C3a, C5a) [1].

The classic pathway is activated when antibody binds to its target and the associated C1q protein leads to the activation of the serine proteases C1r and then C1s. Similarly, binding of the mannose-binding protein (MBP) to mannose residues on bacteria result in the activation of MBP-associated serine protease 1 and 2. Activation of these complexes results in the cleavage of C4 and the deposition of C4b on the surface of the target organism. C2 then is cleaved into C2b, which binds to deposited C4b on the cell surface, resulting in the formation of the C3 convertase (C4b2b). This complex can deposit hundreds of C3b molecules on the bacterial surface that can bind to C3b forming the C5 convertase, or the deposited C3b can bind to factor B to initiate the alternative pathway and amplify the response (see later discussion). Defects in the early components of the classic pathway are predominantly associated with the development of SLE and other autoimmune diseases, although infections do occur [20]. C1q is made up of three homologous genes, *C1QA, C1QB*, and *C1QC*, located on the long arm of chromosome 1. Mutations in any of these subunits can lead to clinically significant

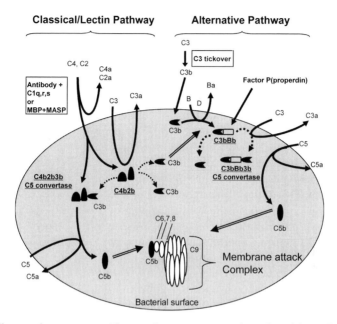

Fig. 6. The complement system. The complement system can be activated by antibodies and associated C1q,r,s proteins (classical pathway), mannose-binding protein (MBP) and MBP-associated serine protease (MASP) (lectin pathway), or spontaneously on foreign surfaces (alternative pathway). The activation of these complement pathways on foreign surfaces results in the formation of the C3 convertase (C4b2b or C3bBb) that deposits many C3b molecules on the surface. C3b can then feed into the alternative pathway to amplify the response. C3b can also bind to the C3 convertases to form the C5 convertases (C3bBb3b or C4b2b3b) that can activate the membrane attack complex (C5-9), resulting in the lysis of the organsism. Complement defects presenting with pyogenic infections or autoimmune disease: C1q, C1s, C1r, C2, C3, C4, factor I, factor D, MBP, MASP. Complement defects presenting with Neiserrial infections: C5, C6, C7, C8, C9, factor I.

C1q deficiency [186,187]. Ninety-three percent of patients who have C1q deficiency develop SLE; approximately 30% suffer significant bacterial infections, with 10% succumbing to sepsis [188,189]. C1s and C1r deficiency results in SLE or other autoimmune processes including glomerulonephritis, although bacterial infections are also common [188,189]. C2 deficiency is the most common inherited complement deficiency (1:10,000 whites). The gene is located within the MHC on chromosome 6 and is associated with SLE and a variety of autoimmune diseases as well as susceptibility to infections by encapsulated organisms [188,189]. C3 deficiency most commonly presents with increased susceptibility to infections, but SLE and other autoimmune phenomenon can also be seen [188,189]. The increased susceptibility to infections and the relatively decreased likelihood of autoimmune disease probably reflects the location of C3 at the convergence of the alternative and classic pathways. Thus C3 defects may have a more severe phenotype than do defects in other complement components. Complete C4 deficiency is very rare, because

C4 comprises two linked genes, and all four alleles of C4 must be deleted for complete C4 deficiency [188,189]. C4 deficiency presents with early-onset SLE, although bacterial infections are common and can be severe. The two C4 alleles are termed "*C4A*" and "*C4B*." It is estimated that up to 14% of whites carry a null C4A allele, and 1% are homozygous deficient for C4A. Approximately 15% to 16% of whites carry a null *C4B* allele; 1% to 3% are completely deficient in C4B [20,190]. Homozygous deficiencies in either C4A or C4B increase the risk for the development of autoimmune diseases such as SLE, Henoch-Schönlein purpura, immune thrombocytopenia, and celiac disease [188,189].

The alternative complement pathway is activated when C3b is deposited on a cell surface. This deposition can occur spontaneously in a process known as "C3 tickover" or can occur by activation of the C3 convertase by the classic pathway or the lectin pathway (see previous discussion) [1]. Once C3b is deposited, factor B binds to C3b and is cleaved by factor D resulting in the alternative pathway C3 convertase (C3bBb). The serum protein factor P, also known as properdin, stabilizes this interaction. Properdin deficiency is one of the strongest risk factors for meningococcal infections, with up to 50% of affected individuals suffering meningococcal infections [188,189]. In addition, patients who have properdin deficiency have much higher mortality when infected with Meningococcus. The stabilized C3 convertase (C3Bb) can lead to more C3 deposition and more C3 convertase generation, resulting in amplification of both the classic and alternative pathways. Finally, C3 can bind to the C3Bb complex, forming the C5 convertase (C3bBb3b).

Once the C5 convertase is generated from either the classic/lectin or alternative pathways (C3bBb3b or C4b2b3b, respectively), C5 binds and is cleaved into C5a, a mediator of inflammation, and C5b, which initiates the membrane attack complex. C5b binds to C6 and C7; then C8 is inserted into the membrane of the target organism and recruits C9, which polymerizes to form a pore in the organism leading to its lysis [1]. Defects in the terminal components of complement (C5–C9) are associated with increased susceptibility to certain gram-negative bacteria, in particular *Neisseria* [188,189]. C5 deficiency, C6 deficiency, C7 deficiency, C8 deficiency, and C9 deficiency all show autosomal recessive inheritance and usually present with neisserial infections, usually Meningococcus but also gonococcal infections [20]. Rarely, SLE or other autoimmune illnesses have been reported in these patients.

The complement system can be destructive if activated on self-tissues, and therefore a system of complement inhibitors works together to prevent such inappropriate activation. The serum proteins C1 inhibitor, factor I, factor H, membrane cofactor protein (MCP), decay accelerating factor (DAF), and CD59 all work together to inhibit complement activation either by the dissociation of activated complement components or by their cleavage and inactivation. Factor I deficiency results in the excessive activation of the alternative pathway and secondary consumption of C3 and in an increased susceptibility to infections with encapsulated organisms [20]. CD59 and

DAF deficiencies do not seem to cause clinically apparent disease on their own, but combined defects of these components occur in the disease paroxysma nocturnal hemoglobinuria (PNH) [191]. A clonal expansion of red blood cells that lack glycosylphosphatidylinositol (GPI)-linked proteins results in DAF and CD59 deficiency, because these are GPI-linked proteins. Red blood cells in patients who have PNH are susceptible to complement-mediated lysis, and thus these patients exhibit episodes of red blood cell hemolysis and hemoglobinuria. Factor H deficiency is reported to result in the spontaneous activation of the alternative pathway and the secondary consumption of C3, resulting in recurrent pyogenic infections [192]. Factor H deficiency and MCP deficiency cause hemolytic uremic syndrome (HUS) that can be familial in nature and occurs without the preceding diarrheal illnesses classically seen in patients who have nonfamilial HUS [193–195]. C1 inhibitor deficiency results in the clinical presentation of hereditary angioedema and presents with attacks of submucosal or subcutaneous edema [20].

Disorders of immune regulation

CD8 T cells and NK cells contain cytotoxic granules containing perforin and granzyme molecules that are important for the killing of virally infected cells and tumor cells [196–198]. Recently, a variety of genetic defects in the granule exocytosis pathway (Fig. 7) have been described that result in difficulty clearing virus and, more importantly, in immune dysregulation. When a cytotoxic lymphocyte recognizes a target cell, an activation signal is transduced that is dependent on signaling lymphocyte activation marker–associated protein (SAP). This transduction leads to the activation and movement of cytotoxic granules toward the target cell, which requires a Ras-like GTPase, Rab27. The granules fuse with the plasma membrane to release their contents into the immunologic synapse formed by the cytotoxic cell and the target cell. The fusion of cytotoxic granules with the plasma membrane requires the protein Munc 13-4 as well as the protein Lyst. Finally, perforin inserts into the target cell plasma membrane and allows entry of the granzyme proteins into the target cell and resultant apoptosis [199,200].

Deficiencies in proteins involved in granule exocytosis can result in HLH. This disorder is characterized by excessive immune activation following viral infections, most notably herpes virus infections (cytomegalovirus, Epstein-Barr virus), followed by macrophage activation and eventual death of the affected individuals if not properly treated. Perforin and Munc 13-4 deficiencies are the most common cause of HLH [201–204]. SAP deficiency results in X-linked lymphoproliferative disorder, which usually is seen after Epstein-Barr virus infections in affected individuals [205]. Lyst deficiency results in Chediak Higashi syndrome characterized by partial albinism, bleeding tendencies, neurologic abnormalities, poor NK- and T-cell cytotoxicity, frequent pyogenic infections, and abnormally large lysosomes [206,207]. Rab27 deficiency results in Griscelli syndrome type II, which presents

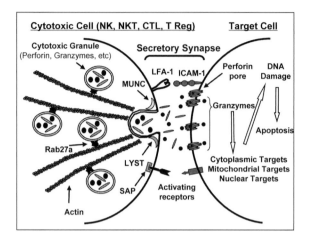

Fig. 7. Disorders of immune regulation. The perforin/granzyme cytotoxic pathway is involved in the killing of virally infected cells and tumor cells. Once a cytotoxic cell recognizes a target through specific receptors, an activation signal is transduced that involves signaling lymphocyte activation marker–associated protein/SH2D1A (SAP). This results in the movement of cyto- toxic granule along actin via Rab27. The granules fuse with the plasma membrane in a process that appears to require MUNC-13 and Lyst proteins. Perforin and granzymes are released into the immunologic synapse formed between the cytotoxic cell and its target. Perforin inserts into the target membrane forming a pore, and granzymes enter, causing apoptosis of the target cell. Genes and their associated human diseases are as follows: (1) perforin, HLH; (2) SH2D1A (SAP), XLP/Duncan's disease; (3) UNC13D (MUNC13-4), HLH; (4) RAB27A, Griscelli syn- drome; (5) CHS1 (LYST), Chediak-Higasi syndrome.

with partial albinism, and low NK cell cytotoxicity [208]. All these syn- dromes are autosomal recessively inherited with the exception of X-linked lymphoproliferative disease.

The pathophysiology of HLH is not clear but probably is multifactorial. Patients who have defects in the granule exocytosis pathway exhibit the in- ability to clear virally infected cells, but this inability does not explain all the features of the disease [209]. Recent studies have shown that this pathway also is involved in terminating an immune response. The authors have shown that human T-regulatory cells also express perforin and granzymes upon activation and kill autologous target cells [210,211]. T-regulatory cells are critical regulators of the immune response, and the finding that these cells can use the granule exocytosis pathway to kill autologous target is an attractive hypothesis to explain the dysregulated immune response seen in HLH [209].

Summary

PIDs are a diverse group of genetic disorders that result in a variety of disease phenotypes. Most PIDs are classified on the basis of which arm of the immune system is affected. As more is learned more about immunodeficiencies, however, it becomes clear that multiple aspects of the immune response are perturbed with each genetic mutation. In addition, such genetic defects show that the immune system is a carefully balanced system, and often symptoms of autoimmunity are observed with PIDs. The future study of these patients and further delineation of mutations that affect the immune response will provide further insight into the function of the immune system and also will provide valuable insights into autoimmunity, allergic responses, and tumorigenesis.

References

[1] Abbas AK, Lichtman AH. Cellular and molecular immunology. 5th edition. Philadelphia: W.B. Saunders; 2004.

[2] Cooper MA, Pommering TL, Koranyi K. Primary immunodeficiencies [see comment]. Am Fam Physician 2003;68(10):2001–8.

[3] Primary immune deficiency diseases in America: the first national survey of patients and specialists. Available at: http://www.primaryimmune.org/pid/survey.htm. Accessed May 1, 2006.

[4] Chapel H, Geha R, Rosen F, for the IPC committee. Primary immunodeficiency diseases: an update [see comment]. Clin Exp Immunol 2003;132(1):9–15.

[5] Bonilla FA, Geha RS. 2. Update on primary immunodeficiency diseases. J Allergy Clin Immunol 2006;117(2 Suppl Mini-Primer):S435–41.

[6] Notarangelo L, Casanova JL, Fischer A, et al. Primary immunodeficiency diseases: an update. J Allergy Clin Immunol 2004;114(3):677–87.

[7] Stiehm ER. New and old immunodeficiencies. Pediatr Res 1993;33(1 Suppl):S2–7.

[8] International consortium completes human genome project. Available at: http://www.genome.gov/11006929. Accessed May 1, 2006.

[9] Buckley RH, Schiff RI, Schiff SE, et al. Human severe combined immunodeficiency: genetic, phenotypic, and functional diversity in one hundred eight infants [see comment]. J Pediatr 1997;130(3):378–87.

[10] Fischer A. Human primary immunodeficiency diseases: a perspective. Nat Immunol 2004; 5(1):23–30.

[11] Fischer A, Cavazzana-Calvo M, De Saint Basile G, et al. Naturally occurring primary deficiencies of the immune system. Annu Rev Immunol 1997;15:93–124.

[12] Simonte SJ, Cunningham-Rundles C. Update on primary immunodeficiency: defects of lymphocytes. Clin Immunol 2003;109(2):109–18.

[13] Rosen FS, Cooper MD, Wedgwood RJ. The primary immunodeficiencies. N Engl J Med 1995;333(7):431–40.

[14] Riminton DS, Limaye S. Primary immunodeficiency diseases in adulthood. Intern Med J 2004;34(6):348–54.

[15] The Jeffrey Modell Foundation Medical Advisory Board. 10 warning signs of primary immunodeficiency. Available at: http://www.info4pi.org/patienttopatient/index.cfm?section=patienttopatient&content=warningsigns&TrkId=15&CFID=16613484&CFTOKEN=94038628. Accessed May 1, 2006.

[16] Mulholland MW, Delaney JP, Foker J, et al. Gastrointestinal complications of congenital immunodeficiency states. The surgeon's role. Ann Surg 1983;198(6):673–80.

[17] Lai Ping So A, Mayer L. Gastrointestinal manifestations of primary immunodeficiency disorders. Semin Gastrointest Dis 1997;8(1):22–32.

[18] Katz AJ, Rosen FS. Gastrointestinal complications of immunodeficiency syndromes. Ciba Found Symp 1977;46:243–61.

[19] Bonilla FA, Geha RS. 12. Primary immunodeficiency diseases [erratum appears in J Allergy Clin Immunol 2003;112(2):267]. J Allergy Clin Immunol 2003;111(2 Suppl):S571–81.

[20] Stiehm ER, Ochs HD, Winkelstein JA, et al. Immunologic disorders in infants and children. 5th edition. Philadelphia: W.B. Saunders; 2004.

[21] Paul WE. Fundamental immunology. 5th edition. Philadelphia: Lippincott Williams & Wilkins; 2003.

[22] Fischer A. Primary T-lymphocyte immunodeficiencies. Clin Rev Allergy Immunol 2001; 20(1):3–26.

[23] Fischer A, Le Deist F, Hacein-Bey-Abina S, et al. Severe combined immunodeficiency. A model disease for molecular immunology and therapy. Immunol Rev 2005;203:98–109.

[24] Le Deist F, Raffoux C, Griscelli C, et al. Graft vs graft reaction resulting in the elimination of maternal cells in a SCID patient with maternofetal GVHd after an HLA identical bone marrow transplantation. J Immunol 1987;138(2):423–7.

[25] Rosen FS. Autoimmunity and immunodeficiency disease. Ciba Found Symp 1987;129: 135–48.

[26] Reinherz EL, Rubinstein A, Geha RS, et al. Abnormalities of immunoregulatory T cells in disorders of immune function. N Engl J Med 1979;301(19):1018–22.

[27] Gennery AR, Barge D, O'Sullivan JJ, et al. Antibody deficiency and autoimmunity in 22q11.2 deletion syndrome. Arch Dis Child 2002;86(6):422–5.

[28] Davies JK, Telfer P, Cavenagh JD, et al. Autoimmune cytopenias in the 22q11.2 deletion syndrome. Clin Lab Haematol 2003;25(3):195–7.

[29] Cunningham-Rundles C. Hematologic complications of primary immune deficiencies. Blood Rev 2002;16(1):61–4.

[30] Choi JH, Shin YL, Kim GH, et al. Endocrine manifestations of chromosome 22q11.2 microdeletion syndrome. Horm Res 2005;63(6):294–9.

[31] Cavadini P, Vermi W, Facchetti F, et al. AIRE deficiency in thymus of 2 patients with Omenn syndrome. J Clin Invest 2005;115(3):728–32.

[32] Noroski LM, Shearer WT. Screening for primary immunodeficiencies in the clinical immunology laboratory. Clin Immunol Immunopathol 1998;86(3):237–45.

[33] Stiehm ER, Chin TW, Haas A, et al. Infectious complications of the primary immunodeficiencies. Clin Immunol Immunopathol 1986;40(1):69–86.

[34] Stephan JL, Vlekova V, Le Deist F, et al. Severe combined immunodeficiency: a retrospective single-center study of clinical presentation and outcome in 117 patients. J Pediatr 1993; 123(4):564–72.

[35] Levy O, Orange JS, Hibberd P, et al. Disseminated varicella infection due to the vaccine strain of varicella-zoster virus, in a patient with a novel deficiency in natural killer T cells [see comment]. J Infect Dis 2003;188(7):948–53.

[36] Jouanguy E, Altare F, Lamhamedi S, et al. Interferon-gamma-receptor deficiency in an infant with fatal bacille Calmette-Guerin infection. N Engl J Med 1996;335(26): 1956–61.

[37] Pacheco SE, Shearer WT. Laboratory aspects of immunology. Pediatr Clin North Am 1994;41(4):623–55.

[38] De Vries JE, Noordzij JG, Kuijpers TW, et al. Flow cytometric immunophenotyping in the diagnosis and follow-up of immunodeficient children. Eur J Pediatr 2001;160:583–91.

[39] Grossman WJ, Radhi M, Schauer D, et al. Development of hemophagocytic lymphohistiocytosis in triplets infected with HHV-8. Blood 2005;106(4):1203–6.

[40] Rosenzweig SD, Holland SM. Phagocyte immunodeficiencies and their infections. J Allergy Clin Immunol 2004;113(4):620–6.

[41] Lakshman R, Finn A. Neutrophil disorders and their management. J Clin Pathol 2001; 54(1):7–19.

[42] Jirapongsananuruk O, Malech HL, Kuhns DB, et al. Diagnostic paradigm for evaluation of male patients with chronic granulomatous disease, based on the dihydrorhodamine 123 assay. J Allergy Clin Immunol 2003;111(2):374–9.

[43] Vowells SJ, Sekhsaria S, Malech HL, et al. Flow cytometric analysis of the granulocyte respiratory burst: a comparison study of fluorescent probes. J Immunol Methods 1995; 178(1):89–97.

[44] Johnson AM, Alper CA, Rosen FS, et al. C1 inhibitor: evidence for decreased hepatic synthesis in hereditary angioneurotic edema. Science 1971;173(996):553–4.

[45] Bissler JJ, Aulak KS, Donaldson VH, et al. Molecular defects in hereditary angioneurotic edema. Proc Assoc Am Physicians 1997;109(2):164–73.

[46] Tangsinmankong N, Bahna SL, Good RA. The immunologic workup of the child suspected of immunodeficiency. Ann Allergy Asthma Immunol 2001;87(5):362–9.

[47] Chinen J, Shearer WT. Basic and clinical immunology. J Allergy Clin Immunol 2005; 116(2):411–8.

[48] Colten HR, Rosen FS. Complement deficiencies. Annu Rev Immunol 1992;10:809–34.

[49] Buck D, Moshous D, de Chasseval R, et al. Severe combined immunodeficiency and microcephaly in siblings with hypomorphic mutations in DNA ligase IV. Eur J Immunol 2006; 36(1):224–35.

[50] de Villartay JP, Lim A, Al-Mousa H, et al. A novel immunodeficiency associated with hypomorphic RAG1 mutations and CMV infection [see comment]. J Clin Invest 2005;115(11): 3291–9.

[51] Blaeser F, Kelly M, Siegrist K, et al. Critical function of the CD40 pathway in parvovirus B19 infection revealed by a hypomorphic CD40 ligand mutation. Clin Immunol 2005; 117(3):231–7.

[52] Moshous D, Pannetier C, Chasseval RD R, et al. Partial T and B lymphocyte immunodeficiency and predisposition to lymphoma in patients with hypomorphic mutations in Artemis. J Clin Invest 2003;111(3):381–7.

[53] de Saint-Basile G, Le Deist F, de Villartay JP, et al. Restricted heterogeneity of T lymphocytes in combined immunodeficiency with hypereosinophilia (Omenn's syndrome). J Clin Invest 1991;87(4):1352–9.

[54] Saitta SC, Harris SE, Gaeth AP, et al. Aberrant interchromosomal exchanges are the predominant cause of the 22q11.2 deletion. Hum Mol Genet 2004;13(4):417–28.

[55] Lu JH, Chung MY, Hwang B, et al. Monozygotic twins with chromosome 22q11 microdeletion and discordant phenotypes in cardiovascular patterning. Pediatr Cardiol 2001;22(3): 260–3.

[56] Yamagishi H, Ishii C, Maeda J, et al. Phenotypic discordance in monozygotic twins with 22q11.2 deletion. Am J Med Genet 1998;78(4):319–21.

[57] Goodship J, Cross I, Scambler P, et al. Monozygotic twins with chromosome 22q11 deletion and discordant phenotype [see comment]. J Med Genet 1995;32(9):746–8.

[58] Centola M, Aksentijevich I, Kastner DL. The hereditary periodic fever syndromes: molecular analysis of a new family of inflammatory diseases. Hum Mol Genet 1998;7(10):1581–8.

[59] Kobayashi S. Hereditary periodic fever syndromes: autoinflammatory diseases [comment]. Intern Med 2005;44(7):694–5.

[60] Padeh S. Periodic fever syndromes. Pediatr Clin North Am 2005;52(2):577–609.

[61] Fischer A, de Saint Basile G, Le Deist F. CD3 deficiencies. Curr Opin Allergy Clin Immunol 2005;5(6):491–5.

[62] Elder ME. SCID due to ZAP-70 deficiency. J Pediatr Hematol Oncol 1997;19(6):546–50.

[63] Elder ME. ZAP-70 and defects of T-cell receptor signaling. Semin Hematol 1998;35(4): 310–20.

[64] de la Calle-Martin O, Hernandez M, Ordi J, et al. Familial CD8 deficiency due to a mutation in the CD8 alpha gene. J Clin Invest 2001;108(1):117–23.

[65] Goldman FD, Ballas ZK, Schutte BC, et al. Defective expression of p56lck in an infant with severe combined immunodeficiency. J Clin Invest 1998;102(2):421–9.

[66] Kung C, Pingel JT, Heikinheimo M, et al. Mutations in the tyrosine phosphatase CD45 gene in a child with severe combined immunodeficiency disease. Nat Med 2000; 6(3):343–5.

[67] O'Shea JJ, Park H, Pesu M, et al. New strategies for immunosuppression: interfering with cytokines by targeting the Jak/Stat pathway. Curr Opin Rheumatol 2005;17(3):305–11.

[68] Johnston JA, Bacon CM, Riedy MC, et al. Signaling by IL-2 and related cytokines: JAKs, STATs, and relationship to immunodeficiency. J Leukoc Biol 1996;60(4):441–52.

[69] Leonard WJ, O'Shea JJ. Jaks and STATs: biological implications. Annu Rev Immunol 1998;16:293–322.

[70] Giliani S, Mori L, de Saint Basile G, et al. Interleukin-7 receptor alpha (IL-7Ralpha) deficiency: cellular and molecular bases. Analysis of clinical, immunological, and molecular features in 16 novel patients. Immunol Rev 2005;203:110–26.

[71] Puel A, Ziegler SF, Buckley RH, et al. Defective IL7R expression in T(-)B(+)NK(+) severe combined immunodeficiency. Nat Genet 1998;20(4):394–7.

[72] Candotti F, Oakes SA, Johnston JA, et al. Structural and functional basis for JAK3-deficient severe combined immunodeficiency. Blood 1997;90(10):3996–4003.

[73] Leonard WJ. Dysfunctional cytokine receptor signaling in severe combined immunodeficiency. J Investig Med 1996;44(6):304–11.

[74] Notarangelo LD, Giliani S, Mella P, et al. Combined immunodeficiencies due to defects in signal transduction: defects of the gammac-JAK3 signaling pathway as a model. Immunobiology 2000;202(2):106–19.

[75] Notarangelo LD, Mella P, Jones A, et al. Mutations in severe combined immune deficiency (SCID) due to JAK3 deficiency. Hum Mutat 2001;18(4):255–63.

[76] Russell SM, Tayebi N, Nakajima H, et al. Mutation of Jak3 in a patient with SCID: essential role of Jak3 in lymphoid development. Science 1995;270(5237):797–800.

[77] Macchi P, Villa A, Giliani S, et al. Mutations of Jak-3 gene in patients with autosomal severe combined immune deficiency (SCID). Nature 1995;377(6544):65–8.

[78] Rosen FS, Janeway CA. The gamma globulins. 3. The antibody deficiency syndromes. N Engl J Med 1966;275(14):769–75.

[79] Noguchi M, Yi H, Rosenblatt HM, et al. Interleukin-2 receptor gamma chain mutation results in X-linked severe combined immunodeficiency in humans. Cell 1993;73(1):147–57.

[80] Buckley RH. Molecular defects in human severe combined immunodeficiency and approaches to immune reconstitution. Annu Rev Immunol 2004;22:625–55.

[81] Roifman CM. Human IL-2 receptor alpha chain deficiency. Pediatr Res 2000;48(1):6–11.

[82] Dal Porto JM, Gauld SB, Merrell KT, et al. B cell antigen receptor signaling 101. Mol Immunol 2004;41(6–7):599–613.

[83] Gauld SB, Cambier JC. Src-family kinases in B-cell development and signaling. Oncogene 2004;23(48):8001–6.

[84] Kurosaki T. Functional dissection of BCR signaling pathways. Curr Opin Immunol 2000; 12(3):276–81.

[85] Kurosaki T. Regulation of B cell fates by BCR signaling components. Curr Opin Immunol 2002;14(3):341–7.

[86] Yel L, Minegishi Y, Coustan-Smith E, et al. Mutations in the mu heavy-chain gene in patients with agammaglobulinemia [see comment]. N Engl J Med 1996;335(20):1486–93.

[87] Minegishi Y, Rohrer J, Coustan-Smith E, et al. An essential role for BLNK in human B cell development. Science 1999;286(5446):1954–7.

[88] Milili M, Antunes H, Blanco-Betancourt C, et al. A new case of autosomal recessive agammaglobulinaemia with impaired pre-B cell differentiation due to a large deletion of the IGH locus. Eur J Pediatr 2002;161(9):479–84.

[89] Hagemann TL, Rosen FS, Kwan SP. Characterization of germline mutations of the gene encoding Bruton's tyrosine kinase in families with X-linked agammaglobulinemia. Hum Mutat 1995;5(4):296–302.

[90] Tsukada S, Saffran DC, Rawlings DJ, et al. Deficient expression of a B cell cytoplasmic tyrosine kinase in human X-linked agammaglobulinemia. Cell 1993;72(2):279–90.

[91] Vetrie D. Isolation of the defective gene in X linked agammaglobulinaemia. J Med Genet 1993;30(6):452–3.

[92] Villa A, Sobacchi C, Vezzoni P. Recombination activating gene and its defects. Curr Opin Allergy Clin Immunol 2001;1(6):491–5.

[93] Villa A, Sobacchi C, Notarangelo LD, et al. V(D)J recombination defects in lymphocytes due to RAG mutations: severe immunodeficiency with a spectrum of clinical presentations. Blood 2001;97(1):81–8.

[94] Corneo B, Moshous D, Gungor T, et al. Identical mutations in RAG1 or RAG2 genes leading to defective V(D)J recombinase activity can cause either T-B-severe combined immune deficiency or Omenn syndrome. Blood 2001;97(9):2772–6.

[95] Santagata S, Villa A, Sobacchi C, et al. The genetic and biochemical basis of Omenn syndrome. Immunol Rev 2000;178:64–74.

[96] Villa A, Santagata S, Bozzi F, et al. Omenn syndrome: a disorder of Rag1 and Rag2 genes. J Clin Immunol 1999;19(2):87–97.

[97] Villa A, Santagata S, Bozzi F, et al. Partial V(D)J recombination activity leads to Omenn syndrome. Cell 1998;93(5):885–96.

[98] Schwarz K, Gauss GH, Ludwig L, et al. RAG mutations in human B cell-negative SCID. Science 1996;274(5284):97–9.

[99] Ege M, Ma Y, Manfras B, et al. Omenn syndrome due to ARTEMIS mutations. Blood 2005;105(11):4179–86.

[100] Kalman L, Lindegren ML, Kobrynski L, et al. Mutations in genes required for T-cell development: IL7R, CD45, IL2RG, JAK3, RAG1, RAG2, ARTEMIS, and ADA and severe combined immunodeficiency: HuGE review. Genet Med 2004;6(1):16–26.

[101] Moshous D, Callebaut I, de Chasseval R, et al. Artemis, a novel DNA double-strand break repair/V(D)J recombination protein, is mutated in human severe combined immune deficiency. Cell 2001;105(2):177–86.

[102] O'Driscoll M, Cerosaletti KM, Girard PM, et al. DNA ligase IV mutations identified in patients exhibiting developmental delay and immunodeficiency. Mol Cell 2001;8(6):1175–85.

[103] O'Driscoll M, Jeggo P. Immunological disorders and DNA repair. Mutat Res 2002; 509(1–2):109–26.

[104] Furukawa H, Murata S, Yabe T, et al. Splice acceptor site mutation of the transporter associated with antigen processing-1 gene in human bare lymphocyte syndrome. J Clin Invest 1999;103(5):755–8.

[105] de la Salle H, Hanau D, Fricker D, et al. Homozygous human TAP peptide transporter mutation in HLA class I deficiency [erratum appears in Science 1994;266(5190):1464]. Science 1994;265(5169):237–41.

[106] Dziembowska M, Fondaneche MC, Vedrenne J, et al. Three novel mutations of the CIITA gene in MHC class II-deficient patients with a severe immunodeficiency. Immunogenetics 2002;53(10–11):821–9.

[107] Masternak K, Muhlethaler-Mottet A, Villard J, et al. Molecular genetics of the bare lymphocyte syndrome. Rev Immunogenet 2000;2(2):267–82.

[108] Villard J, Lisowska-Grospierre B, van den Elsen P, et al. Mutation of RFXAP, a regulator of MHC class II genes, in primary MHC class II deficiency [see comment]. N Engl J Med 1997;337(11):748–53.

[109] Wiszniewski W, Fondaneche MC, Lambert N, et al. Founder effect for a 26-bp deletion in the RFXANK gene in North African major histocompatibility complex class II-deficient patients belonging to complementation group B. Immunogenetics 2000;51(4–5): 261–7.

[110] Gong W, Gottlieb S, Collins J, et al. Mutation analysis of TBX1 in non-deleted patients with features of DGS/VCFS or isolated cardiovascular defects. J Med Genet 2001; 38(12):e45.

[111] Baldini A. Dissecting contiguous gene defects: TBX1. Curr Opin Genet Dev 2005;15(3): 279–84.

[112] Merscher S, Funke B, Epstein JA, et al. TBX1 is responsible for cardiovascular defects in velo-cardio-facial/DiGeorge syndrome. Cell 2001;104(4):619–29.

[113] Chieffo C, Garvey N, Gong W, et al. Isolation and characterization of a gene from the Di-George chromosomal region homologous to the mouse Tbx1 gene. Genomics 1997;43(3): 267–77.

[114] Yagi H, Furutani Y, Hamada H, et al. Role of TBX1 in human del22q11.2 syndrome [see comment]. Lancet 2003;362(9393):1366–73.

[115] Perez E, Sullivan KE. Chromosome 22q11.2 deletion syndrome (DiGeorge and velocardio-facial syndromes). Curr Opin Pediatr 2002;14(6):678–83.

[116] Weinzimer SA. Endocrine aspects of the 22q11.2 deletion syndrome. Genet Med 2001;3(1): 19–22.

[117] Antshel KM, Kates WR, Roizen N, et al. 22q11.2 deletion syndrome: genetics, neuroanatomy and cognitive/behavioral features keywords. Child Neuropsychol 2005;11(1):5–19.

[118] Sullivan KE. DiGeorge syndrome/chromosome 22q11.2 deletion syndrome. Curr Allergy Asthma Rep 2001;1(5):438–44.

[119] Frank J, Pignata C, Panteleyev AA, et al. Exposing the human nude phenotype. Nature 1999;398(6727):473–4.

[120] Carney JP. Chromosomal breakage syndromes. Curr Opin Immunol 1999;11(4):443–7.

[121] Tauchi H. Positional cloning and functional analysis of the gene responsible for Nijmegen breakage syndrome, NBS1. J Radiat Res (Tokyo) 2000;41(1):9–17.

[122] Michalkiewicz J, Barth C, Chrzanowska K, et al. Abnormalities in the T and NK lymphocyte phenotype in patients with Nijmegen breakage syndrome [see comment]. Clin Exp Immunol 2003;134(3):482–90.

[123] Chrzanowska KH, Kleijer WJ, Krajewska-Walasek M, et al. Eleven Polish patients with microcephaly, immunodeficiency, and chromosomal instability: the Nijmegen breakage syndrome. Am J Med Genet 1995;57(3):462–71.

[124] Hershfield MS. Adenosine deaminase deficiency: clinical expression, molecular basis, and therapy. Semin Hematol 1998;35(4):291–8.

[125] Markert ML. Molecular basis of adenosine deaminase deficiency. Immunodeficiency 1994; 5(2):141–57.

[126] Arpaia E, Benveniste P, Di Cristofano A, et al. Mitochondrial basis for immune deficiency. Evidence from purine nucleoside phosphorylase-deficient mice. J Exp Med 2000;191(12): 2197–208.

[127] Agarwal RP, Crabtree GW, Parks RE Jr, et al. Purine nucleoside metabolism in the erythrocytes of patients with adenosine deaminase deficiency and severe combined immunodeficiency. J Clin Invest 1976;57(4):1025–35.

[128] Markert ML. Purine nucleoside phosphorylase deficiency. Immunodefic Rev 1991;3(1): 45–81.

[129] Ferrari S, Plebani A. Cross-talk between CD40 and CD40L: lessons from primary immune deficiencies. Curr Opin Allergy Clin Immunol 2002;2(6):489–94.

[130] Fontana S, Moratto D, Mangal S, et al. Functional defects of dendritic cells in patients with CD40 deficiency. Blood 2003;102(12):4099–106.

[131] Ferrari S, Giliani S, Insalaco A, et al. Mutations of CD40 gene cause an autosomal recessive form of immunodeficiency with hyper IgM. Proc Natl Acad Sci U S A 2001;98(22):12614–9.

[132] Levy J, Espanol-Boren T, Thomas C, et al. Clinical spectrum of X-linked hyper-IgM syndrome [see comment]. J Pediatr 1997;131(1 Pt 1):47–54.

[133] Korthauer U, Graf D, Mages HW, et al. Defective expression of T-cell CD40 ligand causes X-linked immunodeficiency with hyper-IgM [see comment]. Nature 1993;361(6412): 539–41.

[134] DiSanto JP, Bonnefoy JY, Gauchat JF, et al. CD40 ligand mutations in x–linked immunodeficiency with hyper-IgM [see comment]. Nature 1993;361(6412):541–3.

[135] Allen RC, Armitage RJ, Conley ME, et al. CD40 ligand gene defects responsible for X-linked hyper-IgM syndrome [see comment]. Science 1993;259(5097):990–3.

[136] Winkelstein JA, Marino MC, Ochs H, et al. The X-linked hyper-IgM syndrome: clinical and immunologic features of 79 patients. Medicine 2003;82(6):373–84.

[137] Lee WI, Torgerson TR, Schumacher MJ, et al. Molecular analysis of a large cohort of patients with the hyper immunoglobulin M (IgM) syndrome. Blood 2005;105(5):1881–90.

[138] Grimbacher B, Hutloff A, Schlesier M, et al. Homozygous loss of ICOS is associated with adult-onset common variable immunodeficiency. Nat Immunol 2003;4(3):261–8.

[139] Salzer U, Maul-Pavicic A, Cunningham-Rundles C, et al. ICOS deficiency in patients with common variable immunodeficiency. Clin Immunol 2004;113(3):234–40.

[140] Minegishi Y, Lavoie A, Cunningham-Rundles C, et al. Mutations in activation-induced cytidine deaminase in patients with hyper IgM syndrome [see comment]. Clin Immunol 2000; 97(3):203–10.

[141] Imai K, Slupphaug G, Lee WI, et al. Human uracil-DNA glycosylase deficiency associated with profoundly impaired immunoglobulin class-switch recombination [see comment]. Nat Immunol 2003;4(10):1023–8.

[142] Ancliff PJ, Gale RE, Liesner R, et al. Mutations in the ELA2 gene encoding neutrophil elastase are present in most patients with sporadic severe congenital neutropenia but only in some patients with the familial form of the disease. Blood 2001;98(9):2645–50.

[143] Dale DC, Person RE, Bolyard AA, et al. Mutations in the gene encoding neutrophil elastase in congenital and cyclic neutropenia. Blood 2000;96(7):2317–22.

[144] Aprikyan AA, Liles WC, Boxer LA, et al. Mutant elastase in pathogenesis of cyclic and severe congenital neutropenia. J Pediatr Hematol Oncol 2002;24(9):784–6.

[145] Dong F, Hoefsloot LH, Schelen AM, et al. Identification of a nonsense mutation in the granulocyte-colony-stimulating factor receptor in severe congenital neutropenia. Proc Natl Acad Sci U S A 1994;91(10):4480–4.

[146] Dong F, Brynes RK, Tidow N, et al. Mutations in the gene for the granulocyte colony-stimulating-factor receptor in patients with acute myeloid leukemia preceded by severe congenital neutropenia. N Engl J Med 1995;333(8):487–93.

[147] Carlsson G, Aprikyan AA, Goransdotter EK, et al. Neutrophil elastase and granulocyte colony-stimulating factor receptor mutation analyses and leukemia evolution in severe congenital neutropenia patients belonging to the original Kostmann family in northern Sweden. Haematologica 2006;91:589–95.

[148] Person RE, Li FQ, Duan Z, et al. Mutations in proto-oncogene GFI1 cause human neutropenia and target ELA2. Nat Genet 2003;34(3):308–12.

[149] Horwitz M, Benson KF, Person RE, et al. Mutations in ELA2, encoding neutrophil elastase, define a 21-day biological clock in cyclic haematopoiesis. Nat Genet 1999;23(4):433–6.

[150] Aprikyan AA, Dale DC. Mutations in the neutrophil elastase gene in cyclic and congenital neutropenia. Curr Opin Immunol 2001;13(5):535–8.

[151] Simon SI, Green CE. Molecular mechanics and dynamics of leukocyte recruitment during inflammation. Annu Rev Biomed Eng 2005;7:151–85.

[152] Kishimoto TK, Hollander N, Roberts TM, et al. Heterogeneous mutations in the beta subunit common to the LFA-1, Mac-1, and p150, 95 glycoproteins cause leukocyte adhesion deficiency. Cell 1987;50(2):193–202.

[153] Dana N, Todd RF, Pitt J, Springer TA, et al. Deficiency of a surface membrane glycoprotein (Mo1) in man. J Clin Invest 1984;73(1):153–9.

[154] Luhn K, Wild MK, Eckhardt M, et al. The gene defective in leukocyte adhesion deficiency II encodes a putative GDP-fucose transporter. Nat Genet 2001;28(1):69–72.

[155] Etzioni A, Harlan JM, Pollack S, et al. Leukocyte adhesion deficiency (LAD) II: a new adhesion defect due to absence of sialyl Lewis X, the ligand for selectins. Immunodeficiency 1993;4(1–4):307–8.

[156] Kinashi T, Aker M, Sokolovsky-Eisenberg M, et al. LAD-III, a leukocyte adhesion deficiency syndrome associated with defective Rap1 activation and impaired stabilization of integrin bonds. Blood 2004;103(3):1033–6.

[157] Ambruso DR, Knall C, Abell AN, et al. Human neutrophil immunodeficiency syndrome is associated with an inhibitory Rac2 mutation. Proc Natl Acad Sci U S A 2000;97(9):4654–9.

[158] Williams DA, Tao W, Yang F, et al. Dominant negative mutation of the hematopoietic-specific Rho GTPase, Rac2, is associated with a human phagocyte immunodeficiency. Blood 2000;96(5):1646–54.

[159] Ariga T, Sakiyama Y, Furuta H, et al. Molecular genetic studies of two families with X-linked chronic granulomatous disease: mutation analysis and definitive determination of carrier status in patients' sisters. Eur J Haematol 1994;52(2):99–102.

[160] Ariga T, Furuta H, Cho K, et al. Genetic analysis of 13 families with X-linked chronic granulomatous disease reveals a low proportion of sporadic patients and a high proportion of sporadic carriers. Pediatr Res 1998;44(1):85–92.

[161] Roos D, de Boer M, Kuribayashi F, et al. Mutations in the X-linked and autosomal recessive forms of chronic granulomatous disease. Blood 1996;87(5):1663–81.

[162] Roos D. The genetic basis of chronic granulomatous disease. Immunol Rev 1994;138: 121–57.

[163] Bolscher BG, de Boer M, de Klein A, et al. Point mutations in the beta-subunit of cytochrome b558 leading to X-linked chronic granulomatous disease. Blood 1991;77(11): 2482–7.

[164] Rae J, Newburger PE, Dinauer MC, et al. X-linked chronic granulomatous disease: mutations in the CYBB gene encoding the gp91-phox component of respiratory-burst oxidase. Am J Hum Genet 1998;62(6):1320–31.

[165] Rae J, Noack D, Heyworth PG, et al. Molecular analysis of 9 new families with chronic granulomatous disease caused by mutations in CYBA, the gene encoding p22(phox). Blood 2000;96(3):1106–12.

[166] Heyworth PG, Cross AR, Curnutte JT. Chronic granulomatous disease. Curr Opin Immunol 2003;15(5):578–84.

[167] Gray GR, Stamatoyannopoulos G, Naiman SC, et al. Neutrophil dysfunction, chronic granulomatous disease, and non-spherocytic haemolytic anaemia caused by complete deficiency of glucose-6-phosphate dehydrogenase. Lancet 1973;2(7828):530–4.

[168] Ardati KO, Bajakian KM, Tabbara KS. Effect of glucose-6-phosphate dehydrogenase deficiency on neutrophil function. Acta Haematol 1997;97(4):211–5.

[169] Roos D, van Zwieten R, Wijnen JT, et al. Molecular basis and enzymatic properties of glucose 6-phosphate dehydrogenase volendam, leading to chronic nonspherocytic anemia, granulocyte dysfunction, and increased susceptibility to infections. Blood 1999;94(9): 2955–62.

[170] Kitahara M, Eyre HJ, Simonian Y, et al. Hereditary myeloperoxidase deficiency. Blood 1981;57(5):888–93.

[171] Nauseef WM, Root RK, Malech HL. Biochemical and immunologic analysis of hereditary myeloperoxidase deficiency. J Clin Invest 1983;71(5):1297–307.

[172] Nauseef WM. Myeloperoxidase deficiency. Hematol Oncol Clin North Am 1988;2(1): 135–58.

[173] Parry MF, Root RK, Metcalf JA, et al. Myeloperoxidase deficiency: prevalence and clinical significance. Ann Intern Med 1981;95(3):293–301.

[174] Altare F, Jouanguy E, Lamhamedi S, et al. Mendelian susceptibility to mycobacterial infection in man. Curr Opin Immunol 1998;10(4):413–7.

[175] Altare F, Durandy A, Lammas D, et al. Impairment of mycobacterial immunity in human interleukin-12 receptor deficiency. Science 1998;280(5368):1432–5.

[176] Altare F, Lammas D, Revy P, et al. Inherited interleukin 12 deficiency in a child with bacille Calmette-Guerin and Salmonella enteritidis disseminated infection. J Clin Invest 1998; 102(12):2035–40.

[177] Picard C, Fieschi C, Altare F, et al. Inherited interleukin-12 deficiency: IL12B genotype and clinical phenotype of 13 patients from six kindreds. Am J Hum Genet 2002;70(2): 336–48.

[178] Dorman SE, Picard C, Lammas D, et al. Clinical features of dominant and recessive interferon gamma receptor 1 deficiencies. Lancet 2004;364(9451):2113–21.

[179] Jouanguy E, Lamhamedi-Cherradi S, Lammas D, et al. A human IFNGR1 small deletion hotspot associated with dominant susceptibility to mycobacterial infection [see comment]. Nat Genet 1999;21(4):370–8.

[180] Dupuis S, Doffinger R, Picard C, et al. Human interferon-gamma-mediated immunity is a genetically controlled continuous trait that determines the outcome of mycobacterial invasion. Immunol Rev 2000;178:129–37.

[181] Fieschi C, Casanova JL. The role of interleukin-12 in human infectious diseases: only a faint signature. Eur J Immunol 2003;33(6):1461–4.

[182] de Jong R, Altare F, Haagen IA, et al. Severe mycobacterial and Salmonella infections in interleukin-12 receptor-deficient patients. Science 1998;280(5368):1435–8.

[183] Manderson AP, Botto M, Walport MJ. The role of complement in the development of systemic lupus erythematosus. Annu Rev Immunol 2004;22:431–56.

[184] Botto M, Dell'Agnola C, Bygrave AE, et al. Homozygous C1q deficiency causes glomerulonephritis associated with multiple apoptotic bodies. Nat Genet 1998;19(1):56–9.

[185] Botto M. Links between complement deficiency and apoptosis. Arthritis Res 2001;3(4):207–10.

[186] Berkel AI, Birben E, Oner C, et al. Molecular, genetic and epidemiologic studies on selective complete C1q deficiency in Turkey. Immunobiology 2000;201(3–4):347–55.

[187] Bowness P, Davies KA, Norsworthy PJ, et al. Hereditary C1q deficiency and systemic lupus erythematosus. QJM 1994;87(8):455–64.

[188] Figueroa JE, Densen P. Infectious diseases associated with complement deficiencies. Clin Microbiol Rev 1991;4(3):359–95.

[189] Ross SC, Densen P. Complement deficiency states and infection: epidemiology, pathogenesis and consequences of neisserial and other infections in an immune deficiency. Medicine (Baltimore) 1984;63(5):243–73.

[190] Awdeh ZL, Alper CA. Inherited structural polymorphism of the fourth component of human complement. Proc Natl Acad Sci U S A 1980;77(6):3576–80.

[191] Shichishima T, Saitoh Y, Terasawa T, et al. Complement sensitivity of erythrocytes in a patient with inherited complete deficiency of CD59 or with the Inab phenotype. Br J Haematol 1999;104(2):303–6.

[192] Ault BH, Schmidt BZ, Fowler NL, et al. Human factor H deficiency. Mutations in framework cysteine residues and block in H protein secretion and intracellular catabolism. J Biol Chem 1997;272(40):25168–75.

[193] Pichette V, Querin S, Schurch W, et al. Familial hemolytic-uremic syndrome and homozygous factor H deficiency. Am J Kidney Dis 1994;24(6):936–41.

[194] Noris M, Brioschi S, Caprioli J, et al. Familial haemolytic uraemic syndrome and an MCP mutation. Lancet 2003;362(9395):1542–7.

[195] Atkinson JP, Liszewski MK, Richards A, et al. Hemolytic uremic syndrome: an example of insufficient complement regulation on self-tissue. Ann N Y Acad Sci 2005;1056:144–52.

[196] Lieberman J. The ABCs of granule-mediated cytotoxicity: new weapons in the arsenal. Nat Rev Immunol 2003;3(5):361–70.

[197] Catalfamo M, Henkart PA. Perforin and the granule exocytosis cytotoxicity pathway. Curr Opin Immunol 2003;15(5):522–7.

[198] Raja SM, Metkar SS, Froelich CJ. Cytotoxic granule-mediated apoptosis: unraveling the complex mechanism. Curr Opin Immunol 2003;15(5):528–32.

[199] Russell JH, Ley TJ. Lymphocyte-mediated cytotoxicity. Annu Rev Immunol 2002;20:323–70.

[200] Grossman WJ, Revell PA, Lu ZH, et al. The orphan granzymes of humans and mice [erratum appears in Curr Opin Immunol 2003;15(6):731]. Curr Opin Immunol 2003;15(5):544–52.

[201] Kogawa K, Lee SM, Villanueva J, et al. Perforin expression in cytotoxic lymphocytes from patients with hemophagocytic lymphohistiocytosis and their family members. Blood 2002;99(1):61–6.

[202] Ueda I, Morimoto A, Inaba T, et al. Characteristic perforin gene mutations of haemophagocytic lymphohistiocytosis patients in Japan. Br J Haematol 2003;121(3):503–10.

[203] Feldmann J, Callebaut I, Raposo G, et al. Munc13–c14 is essential for cytolytic granules fusion and is mutated in a form of familial hemophagocytic lymphohistiocytosis (FHL3). Cell 2003;115(4):461–73.

[204] Ishii E, Ohga S, Tanimura M, et al. Clinical and epidemiologic studies of familial hemophagocytic lymphohistiocytosis in Japan. Japan LCH Study Group. Med Pediatr Oncol 1998; 30(5):276–83.

[205] Arico M, Imashuku S, Clementi R, et al. Hemophagocytic lymphohistiocytosis due to germline mutations in SH2D1A, the X-linked lymphoproliferative disease gene. Blood 2001;97(4):1131–3.

[206] Stinchcombe J, Bossi G, Griffiths GM. Linking albinism and immunity: the secrets of secretory lysosomes. Science 2004;305(5680):55–9.

[207] Kumar M, Sackey K, Schmalstieg F, et al. Griscelli syndrome: rare neonatal syndrome of recurrent hemophagocytosis. J Pediatr Hematol Oncol 2001;23(7):464–8.

[208] Menasche G, Pastural E, Feldmann J, et al. Mutations in RAB27A cause Griscelli syndrome associated with haemophagocytic syndrome. Nat Genet 2000;25(2):173–6.

[209] Verbsky JW, Grossman WJ. Hemophagocytic lymphohistiocytosis: diagnosis, pathophysiology, treatment, and future perspectives. Ann Med 2006;38(1):20–31.

[210] Grossman WJ, Verbsky JW, Barchet W, et al. Human T regulatory cells can use the perforin pathway to cause autologous target cell death. Immunity 2004;21(4):589–601.

[211] Grossman WJ, Verbsky JW, Tollefsen BL, et al. Differential expression of granzymes A and B in human cytotoxic lymphocyte subsets and T regulatory cells. Blood 2004;104(9): 2840–8.

PEDIATRIC CLINICS
OF NORTH AMERICA

ELSEVIER
SAUNDERS

Pediatr Clin N Am 53 (2006) 685–698

Recent Molecular and Cellular Advances in Pediatric Bone Marrow Transplantation

Julie-An M. Talano, MD*, David A. Margolis, MD

*Division of Pediatric Hematology and Oncology, Medical College of Wisconsin,
8701 Watertown Plank Road, Milwaukee, WI 53226, USA*

Hematopoietic cell transplantation (HCT) has evolved as a treatment for a variety of congenital and acquired malignant and nonmalignant disorders. The first successful human bone marrow transplant occurred in pediatrics for severe combined immunodeficiency. Reported in 1968, the patient received marrow from an HLA-matched sibling [1]. Presently, in adults and children, the majority of allogeneic transplants are performed for the treatment of malignant disorders such as leukemias and lymphomas, although the field continues to expand to include autoimmune disorders, metabolic diseases, and hemoglobinopathies. Since its inception, the field of pediatric HCT has made vast improvements in morbidity and mortality related to transplantation, but there still are many hurdles that must be overcome. The major barriers that still contribute significantly to the morbidity and mortality of allogeneic transplantation are relapse of disease, infection, and graft-versus-host disease (GVHD). This article summarizes the recent molecular and cellular advances in the field of allogeneic HCT. The topics reviewed are

1. Induction of an antitumor/antileukemia response using adoptive immunotherapy with donor leukocyte infusions (DLI), activated DLI, natural killer (NK) cells, gamma delta T cells, and cytotoxic T cells (CTL) against minor HLA antigens
2. Prevention of infections caused by Epstein-Barr virus (EBV), cytomegalovirus (CMV), and adenovirus using cellular therapy

---

* Corresponding author.
  E-mail address: jtalano@mail.mcw.edu (J.M. Talano).

0031-3955/06/$ - see front matter
doi:10.1016/j.pcl.2006.05.007
pediatric.theclinics.com

Induction of antitumor/antileukemia response

Donor leukocyte infusions

DLI entails obtaining leukocytes from a normal donor with the intent of enhancing a specific immunologic effect. Most often the desired effect is a graft-versus-malignancy (GVM) effect or a graft-versus-malignancy effect. DLI is performed at a time after the hematopoietic progenitor cell transplantation. Historically the major limiting side effect with DLI is GVHD, when the donor T cells see the host as foreign and attack the host. Also, DLI has made a significant impact in only one disease, chronic myelogenous leukemia (CML).

Kolb and colleagues [2] reported on the first successful DLI infusions in patients who had CML. Three patients who had hematologic relapse after bone marrow transplantation for CML were treated with DLI and interferon alpha. All had a complete hematologic remission. In two patients, GVHD developed and was treated by immunosuppression. Since that time multiple studies have confirmed that DLI is effective in treating CML that has relapsed after bone marrow transplantation. In 1995 Kolb and colleagues [3] reported the effects of DLI on acute and chronic leukemia in relapse after bone marrow transplantation. Complete remissions were induced by DLI in 54 patients who had CML (73%) and in five patients (29%) who had acute myelogenous leukemia (AML). In contrast, acute lymphoblastic leukemia (ALL) did not respond to the DLI. Remissions were durable in patients treated for CML in the chronic phase (87% probability of remission at 3 years). The remissions for AML or advanced-phase CML were not long lasting. Fifty-two patients (41%) developed GVHD of grade 2 or more, and 41 patients (34%) showed signs of myelosuppression.

Collins and colleagues [4] reported on the use of DLI in 25 North American bone marrow transplant programs. One hundred forty patients were available for analysis. Complete responses were observed in 60% of patients who had CML; response rates were greater in patients who had cytogenetic and chronic-phase relapse (75.7%) than in patients who had accelerated-phase (33.3%) or blast-phase (16.7%) relapse. The actuarial probability of remaining in complete remission at 2 years was 89.6%. Complete remission rates in AML (n = 39) and ALL (n = 11) in patients who had not received pre-DLI chemotherapy were 15.4% and 18.2%, respectively. Complications of DLI included acute GVHD (60%), chronic GVHD (60.7%), and pancytopenia (18.6%).

To minimize the complications associated with DLI, studies have examined the optimal initial starting dose of lymphocytes. Response of disease to DLI is not always associated with the development of GVHD, suggesting that there may be a GVL effect independent of the development of GVHD. Guglielmi and colleagues [5] analyzed the effect of initial cell dose of DLI on patient outcomes in 298 patients at 51 centers in Europe.

The results of the analysis showed that the lower initial cell dose was associated with less GVHD, less myelosuppression, same response rate, better survival, better failure-free survival, and less DLI-related mortality. The results suggested that the first DLI dose should not exceed 0.2×10^8 mononuclear cells/kg.

Advances in the treatment of CML provide an example of combining different translational approaches to the same disease. Imatinib mesylate is a tyrosine kinase inhibitor that has had a major impact on the treatment of CML [6]. Imatinib mesylate can place patients in a complete cytogenetic remission, and sometimes molecular remission as well, without the risk of GVHD that is associated with transplantation or DLI. Because advanced-phase posttransplantation relapse CML responds poorly to DLI, Savani and colleagues [7] combined imatinib with DLI and observed a more rapid molecular remission with the combination, and a superior disease-free survival after treatment, compared with DLI or imatinib alone. The synergy may occur because imatinib can reduce the burden of disease below the level of detection, followed by a low dose of DLI that creates a GVL effect to eradicate CML progenitors so that imatinib can be stopped safely. Also, with a lower dose of DLI, one can reduce the incidence of GVHD. The combination of imatinib and DLI will need to be studied further in future prospective trials. As innovative molecularly targeted anticancer agents are developed, combining them with immunotherapy may improve outcomes for diseases that relapse after transplantation (such as AML and ALL) that traditionally have not responded to DLI alone. This approach has recently been used in Philadelphia-chromosome ALL in a case report. Savani and colleagues [8] reported on two patients who were given imatinib combined with DLI as salvage treatment for advanced-phase Philadelphia-chromosome–positive ALL after nonmyeloablative allogeneic HCT. The authors also have had a similar success with a pediatric patient with Philadelphia-chromosome ALL who had a molecular relapse after an HLA-matched unrelated transplant. The patient was given DLI at a dose of 1×10^7 T cells/kg, and treatment with imatinib was restarted. With such therapy he has been in a molecular remission for more than 1 year. These preliminary observations provide the hope that the combination of targeted pharmacotherapy with adoptive immunotherapy may be feasible.

Donor leukocyte infusions: separating graft-versus-leukemia effect from graft-versus-host disease

Manipulating the T cell

A major challenge exists in augmenting the GVL effect and separating it from GVHD. After an allogeneic transplant, T cells mount a response against minor histocompatibility antigens of the recipient (HLA-matched transplantation) and against minor and major histocompatibility antigens (HLA-mismatched transplantations). Michalek and colleagues [9] have demonstrated that GVL and GVHD are mediated by different clones of T cells. They identified two types of T cells based on their T-cell receptor (TCR) sequences in nine donor/recipient pairs. Their results suggested that allodepleted T-cell transplants should exert a GVL effect but only rarely cause GVHD. Also, their study suggested that the expansion and reinfusion of the GVL-specific CD4+ T cells may be useful for immunotherapy. Andre-Schmutz and colleagues [10] reported a phase I/II study in which they sought to infuse T cells selectively depleted of allogeneic T cells that cause GVHD by using an ex vivo procedure designed to eliminate alloactivated donor T cells. They removed alloactivated T cells using an immunotoxin that reacts with the interleukin (IL)-2 receptor (CD25). 1 to 8×10^{5} allodepleted T cells/kg were infused into 15 pediatric patients between days 15 and 47 after allogeneic transplant. No cases of severe (> grade 2) GVHD arose. Evidence for early T-cell expansion was shown in three patients. Because variability in depletion of alloreactivity was documented, the investigators modified their method of depletion using anti-CD25 and magnetic beads. A phase I/II trial has been initiated for 25 pediatric patients who had inherited disorders of the immune system [11].

In an effort to augment the GVL/tumor effect of DLI, Porter and colleagues [12] investigated ex vivo activation of the DLI. They hypothesized that failure of DLI to mediate an antitumor effect in most diseases was caused by inappropriate activation of donor T cells in vivo to induce an antitumor response. Activation of T cells requires two signals, engagement of the TCR and a second costimulatory signal. The second signal, when combined with primary antigen-dependent stimulation of the TCR, is required for the T cell to synthesize maximally and secrete cytokines and then divide in response to antigen. The major positive costimulatory receptor on a T cell is CD28 and its ligands, the B7 family of molecules CD80 and CD86, which are abundantly expressed on activated antigen-presenting cells. T-cell costimulation is critical for induction of full T-cell effector function and therefore represents an attractive immunotherapeutic approach for the treatment of cancer. Suboptimal T-cell activation may occur because of a lack of costimulatory ligands on tumor cells, failure to present antigens to T cells, direct suppression of cytotoxic effector cells by suppressor T cells or cytokines, failure to stimulate CD4+ cells, or quantitative lack of sufficient cytotoxic effector cells. Porter and colleagues [12] activated donor T cells by costimulation and expansion after exposure to magnetic beads coated with anti-CD3 (OKT3) and anti-CD28. Eighteen patients participated in a phase I dose-escalation trial. Patients who had aggressive malignancies received induction chemotherapy, and all patients received conventional DLI followed 12 days later by activated DLI. Activated DLI was dose escalated from 1×10^{6} to 1×10^{8} CD3 cells/kg in five levels. Seven patients developed GVHD (grade 1–2, n = 5; grade 3, n = 2). Four developed chronic GVHD. Eight patients achieved a complete remission, including four of seven who had ALL, two of four who had AML, one who had CLL, and one of two who had non-Hodgkin lymphoma. Overall 10 of 18 remain alive 11 to 53 months after receiving activated DLI. Therefore, one can conclude that adoptive transfer of costimulated activated allogeneic T cells is feasible, does not result in excessive GVHD, and may contribute to durable remissions in diseases in which conventional DLI has been disappointing.

Another approach toward modifying DLI to promote immune reconstitution, augment GVL, and minimize GVHD uses L-leucyl-L-leucine methyl ester (LLME). LLME is a lysosomotropic agent that is taken up by cells and converted to pro-apoptotic metabolites by the action of intracellular dipeptidyl peptidase I. It therefore depletes cells containing cytotoxic granules and perforin, leaving an enriched population of CD4+ T cells. Hsieh and colleagues [13] showed in a murine model that animals that received doses of LLME-treated DLI survived indefinitely without evidence of GVHD compared with the lethal GVHD induced by untreated DLI. Most notably, mice given LLME-treated DLI also experienced DLI dose-dependent increases in survival against the challenge with MMD2-8 leukemia. Filicko and colleagues [14] presented their preliminary results of a phase I human trial using dose-escalated LLME-treated DLI. They have treated 18 patients with initial starting doses of 1×10^4 T cells/kg (haploidentical, n = 3), 1×10^5 T cells/kg (HLA identical unrelated, n = 6), and 1×10^6 T cell/kg (HLA identical sibling, n = 9). All patients received one to three DLI infusions. After the first DLI, six of eight evaluable matched sibling recipients and two of six matched unrelated donors demonstrated early recovery of donor-derived CD4+ cells. Five patients developed GVHD (grade 1–2, n = 4; grade 3, n = 1). These preliminary results suggest that LLME-treated DLI can accelerate CD4+ reconstitution without causing severe GVHD. The authors are participating in this study with pediatric patients who undergo haploidentical transplantation.

Use of natural killer cells

Another cellular-based therapy with potential antileukemic properties is NK cells. NK cells are a subset of peripheral blood lymphocytes defined by the expression of CD56 or CD16 and the absence of a TCR. NK cells recognize and kill cells in a major histocompatibility (MHC) unrestricted fashion and produce important cytokines. The NK-cell response to a target depends on both the activating and inhibitory receptors involved. For a review of these receptors and their role in the immune response, the reader is referred to Hallet and colleagues [15].

An opportunity to capitalize on NK-cell alloreactivity is the setting of haploidentical transplantation. Nearly every patient has a family member (parent, child, sibling, or other relative) identical for one haplotype (haploidentical) who could serve as a donor for a patient in need of a transplant. In

1994 Aversa and colleagues [16] overcame engraftment barriers by introducing the clinical application of the hematopoietic progenitor cell megadose. Giving patients large numbers of CD34 stem cells would enable patients to engraft despite the degree of HLA mismatch. The grafts are depleted of the majority of T cells to minimize GVHD. This approach has been successful and can augment NK-cell alloreactivity. When NK cells are faced with mismatched allogeneic targets, they sense the missing expression of self-MHC class I molecules and mediate an NK alloreaction that kills the leukemia cell [17]. This effect has been documented in a murine model. This phenomenon explains the clinical observation of decreased relapse of adult patients who have AML when a killer cell inhibitory receptor (KIR) alloreactive haploidentical transplantation is performed.

In vitro studies on human tumor cell lines showed that alloreactive NK cells can kill AML, CML, T-cell ALL, and non-Hodgkin lymphoma [18]. Common ALL was the only target to resist killing. Recently, however, Torelli and colleagues [19] reported the expansion of NK cells with lytic activity against autologous blasts from adult and pediatric patients who had ALL. They found that incubating the NK cells with IL-2 and IL-15 for 24 hours significantly increased the cytotoxic function. This report is the first documentation of increased cytotoxicity against autologous ALL blasts. Perhaps the stimulation with IL-2 and IL-15 induces an increased level of the killer-activating receptors at the NK cell surface relative to the activity of the corresponding inhibitory receptors. Leung and colleagues [20] demonstrated that NK cells mediated an antileukemia effect in both pediatric AML and ALL. Childhood ALL blasts express a high rate of adhesion molecules that are essential for NK target conjugation and activation, including members of the Beta1 integrin family (CD29, CD49d), the Beta2 integrin family leukocyte function associated antigen-1 (LFA-1), and the immunoglobulin superfamily (intercellular adhesion molecule-1, LFA-3) [21]. This increased expression of adhesion molecules may explain why childhood ALL responds to NK killing whereas adult ALL does not.

In addition to in vivo expansion after transplantation, NK cells may be adoptively transferred. Miller and colleagues [22] have tested haploidentical, related-donor NK-cell infusions in a nontransplantation setting to determine safety and in vivo NK-cell expansion. Two low-intensity outpatient immune suppressive regimens were tested to see if they would permit the transfer of these cells: (1) low-dose cyclophosphamide and methylprednisolone and (2) fludarabine. A higher-intensity inpatient regimen of high-dose cyclophosphamide and fludarabine was tested in patients who had poor-prognosis AML. All patients received high-dose IL-2 after infusions. Patients who received the lower-intensity regimens showed transient persistence but no in vivo expansion of donor cells. In contrast, infusions after the more intense cyclophosphamide/fludarabine immunosuppression resulted in a marked rise in endogenous IL-15, expansion of donor NK cells, and induction of a complete remission in 5 of 19 patients who had poor-prognosis

AML. None of these patients developed GVHD. The five patients who had AML and who achieved a morphologic complete response were evaluated. Patients were stratified into those who had KIR ligand mismatch, and three of the four patients who had KIR alloreactivity achieved a complete remission. This experience was in marked contrast to those patients who did not have KIR alloreactivity, of whom only 2 of 15 achieved a remission. In those patients who achieved a complete remission, the number of circulating NK cells was significantly greater than in the nonremission group (51% ± 13% versus 12% ± 6%; $P = .04$).

In pediatrics, Koehl and colleagues [23,24] reported ex vivo expansion of highly purified NK cells for immunotherapy after haploidentical stem cell transplantation. So far, three pediatric patients who had multiply relapsed ALL or AML have been treated with repeated transfusions of KIR alloreactive NK cells after HCT. Although all the patients showed blast persistence at the time of transplantation, they reached complete remission and complete donor chimerism within 1 month after transplantation. NK-cell therapy was well tolerated without GVHD induction or other adverse events, but one patient relapsed, and two others died of infections. A phase I protocol is currently open to pursue NK infusions after transplantation.

Use of gamma delta T cells

Most mature T cells have a TCR consisting of the alpha beta subunit that recognizes processed peptide antigens on MHC molecules by antigen-presenting cells. A small subset of cells that comprises less than 10% of the peripheral T-cell compartment has a different TCR consisting of a gamma delta subunit. The gamma delta T cells do not express CD4 or CD8, which is commonly found on alpha beta T cells. These cells directly recognize and respond to a variety of MHC-like, stress-induced self-antigens expressed by malignant cells. Therefore they can recognize malignant cells without prior antigen exposure or priming [25,26]. This mechanism is not well understood, but it is fundamentally different from both alpha beta T cells and NK cells. There is evidence that gamma delta T cells kill cancer cells, in particular human leukemia cells. Duval and colleagues [27] postulated that nonmalignant T lymphocytes remaining within bone marrow from children who have newly diagnosed ALL could be involved in an antileukemia immune response. T lymphocytes that expressed gamma delta TCR comprised less than 1% of all marrow cells. A preferential outgrowth of gamma delta T cells within the CD3 population was observed when marrow cells were cultured with IL-2 alone or with stimulating feeder cells. These results, obtained in a series of 14 patients who had precursor B-cell ALL, differed significantly from expansions from normal marrow cells. These results suggest a prior activation in vivo of some gamma delta T cells by leukemic cells and provide some evidence on the role of these subsets in the immune response to leukemia. Dolstra and colleagues [28] found that gamma delta cytotoxic T lymphocytes

(CTLs) isolated after HCT from the peripheral blood of a patient who had AML efficiently lysed freshly isolated AML cells and AML cell lines. HLA-matched nonmalignant hematopoietic cells were not killed.

Gamma delta T cells have been implicated in protection against relapse in bone marrow transplantation. Lamb and colleagues [29] reported that patients who received bone marrow grafts depleted of alpha beta T cells developed spontaneous increases in gamma delta T cells. These patients had an improved disease-free survival when compared with patients at similar risk. Ten patients (23.2%) were found to have an increased ($\geq$ 10%) proportion of gamma delta–positive T cells in the peripheral blood at 60 to 270 days after bone marrow transplantation. All these patients remain alive, and nine (90% of patients with $\geq$ 10% gamma delta–positive cells) are free of disease at 2.5 years after bone marrow transplantation. This rate compares with a disease-free survival probability of 31% among patients who have a normal proportion and concentration of gamma delta–positive T cells. No other factor was found to be independently associated with improved survival in these patients. These data suggest an association between an increase in the percentage and number of gamma delta–positive T cells and improved disease-free survival following transplantation from a partially mismatched related donor.

Neuroblastoma is a pediatric cancer that is extremely difficult to treat when it is metastatic. Schilbach and colleagues [30] showed that gamma delta T cells exerted natural and IL-2–induced cytotoxicity to neuroblastoma cells. They found that the cells were easy to propagate and expand. The cells had unimpaired highly cellular cytotoxicity during a period of 30 days in cell culture and did not exert alloreactivity; therefore, they could be used across MHC barriers.

The use of gamma delta T cells as adoptive immunotherapy has been limited because of the low levels of these cells in the peripheral blood. Additionally, ex vivo expansion is labor intensive, may result in microbial contamination, and the ex vivo expanded cells tend to undergo activation-induced cell death. Otto and colleagues [31] recently published their success with an automated cell-purification method for the enrichment of gamma delta T cells from leukapheresis products. The mean percentage of gamma delta T cells in the final product was 91%. The isolated cells were cytotoxic against a neuroblastoma cell line and an erythroleukemic line in vitro. With this process Otto and colleagues [32] combined gamma delta T cells with humoral immunotherapy in a mouse model of disseminated neuroblastoma. Anti-GD2 is a monoclonal antibody that binds to disialoganglioside GD-2, which is expressed by most neuroblastoma cells [33]. It has been used in preliminary trials in patients who have neuroblastoma and has had some promising results. For the treatment to be effective, however, the treated patient must have an intact immune system. This situation is uncommon after intensive chemotherapy or transplantation. IL-7 is a cytokine that supports the survival and activity of human T cells in vitro and in vivo. Otto made a novel fusion cytokine with IL-7, Fc-IL-7, that has a much longer half-life in the serum than IL-7 alone. The mice were infused with the neuroblastoma cells 5 to 6 days before therapy. Then they were given five consecutive weekly infusions of gamma delta T cells or gamma delta T cells with anti-GD2 or gamma delta T cells, anti-GD2, and Fc-IL-7. The investigators found that the natural cytotoxicity of gamma delta T cells to the neuroblastoma cells in vitro was enhanced dramatically by the anti-GD2. Combination therapy with gamma delta T cells and anti-GD2 significantly enhanced survival ($P = .001$), as did treatment with gamma delta T cells, anti-GD2, and Fc-IL-7 ($P = .005$). Such promising outcomes may result in a similar approach being adapted to other malignancies.

Changing the target: use of cytotoxic T cells against minor histocompatibility antigens

Thus far we have described attempts made at altering cells to provoke an anticancer response without GVHD. An exciting new approach is to use T cells that target only cancer cells. In theory, this approach would provide a graft versus tumor (GVT) response without any risk of GVHD. In the field of HLA-matched allogeneic HCT transplantation, the triggers of the alloimmune response are peptides derived from polymorphic proteins that are presented by the HLA molecules of the graft. These proteins, minor histocompatibility antigens (mHag), may be expressed ubiquitously or have limited tissue expression. To separate GVT from GVHD, the target for cellular therapy logically is a minor antigen that is expressed only on the cancerous tissue. In hematopoietic cancers such as leukemia, mHag is expressed only on hematopoietic cells, making it an attractive target for GVL effect [34]. Marjit and colleagues [35] have shown that the GVL response in some patients who have CML and multiple myeloma results from T cells targeting the hematopoietic tissue–specific mHags, HA-1 and HA-2. Additionally, the Leiden group has shown the feasibility of generating donor-derived CTL specific for hematopoietic lineage-restricted mHags HA-1 and HA-2 which would theoretically provide a GVL effect without GVHD [36]. Clinical data using this approach have not been published to date.

Cytotoxic T cells against infectious agents

Cytomegalovirus

After HCT, patients remain immunocompromised for months to years. Common viruses that are ubiquitous in the environment can cause substantial morbidity and mortality. CMV commonly can reactivate in patients and cause significant disease. Prophylactic administration of ganciclovir or foscarnet may reduce the risk and protect these patients from fatal CMV disease, but these prophylactic medications can cause complications such as myelosuppression or nephrotoxicity. Subsequently, these patients are at higher risk of fungal or bacterial infections. Also, increasing numbers of CMV strains are becoming resistant to standard antiviral therapy. Innovative methods to prevent and treat this infection in these patients are needed.

Walter and colleagues [37] made clones for CD8+ CMV CTLs from CMV proteins that were isolated from the blood of bone marrow donors. Fourteen patients each received four infusions of these cells 30 to 40 days after bone marrow transplantation. No toxic effects related to the infusions were observed. CTLs specific for CMV were reconstituted in all patients. The level of activity achieved was similar to that of the donors. CTL activity declined in patients who were deficient in CD4+ helper cells specific for CMV. This finding suggests the importance of CD4+ cells in this process. None of the patients developed CMV reactivation or disease. Other groups have replicated this approach [38,39], but it has not become widely adopted because of the significant technical and financial limitations of ex vivo T-cell cultures.

Cobbold and colleagues [40] have recently developed a method that seems to expedite the process of cell development. CMV-specific CD8+ T cells are found in high frequency in the blood of healthy CMV-seropositive donors and represent 0.5% to 4% of the entire pool of CD8+ T cells. Combining HLA-peptide tetramers with magnetic bead technology allows the selection of these CMV-specific CD8+ cells. This process allows the direct selection of CD8+ T cells from the blood of transplant donors and then direct infusion of these cells into patients without a need for accessory in vitro manipulation. Nine patients were treated with these cells; six patients received cells from HLA-matched sibling donors, and three patients received cells from HLA-matched unrelated donors. CMV CTLs were obtained from 250 mL of peripheral blood or a leukapheresis product from the original donor. The cells were infused into patients within 4 hours of selection. No toxicity was observed related to the infusion. CMV-specific CD8+ T cells became detectable in all patients within 10 days of infusion. CMV viremia was reduced in every patient, and eight patients cleared the virus entirely. This approach has significant potential as antigen-specific T-cell therapy.

Adenovirus

Adenovirus is an extremely common cause of viral infections in the pediatric population. More than 51 different adenovirus serotypes have been identified. Over 80% of children will have developed antibodies to at least one serotype before age 5 years. In children who have normal immune systems the virus can cause self-limited disease consisting of gastroenteritis, keratoconjunctivitis, pharyngitis, and cystitis. In the HCT setting, however, significant morbidity and mortality can occur. Adenovirus can cause hemorrhagic cystitis, hepatitis, and gastroenteritis, with a mortality rate as high as 60%. Cidofovir is an antiviral agent with activity against adenovirus, but it is highly nephrotoxic, and its efficacy is limited without an intact immune system. Alternative strategies for prevention and treatment are desperately needed. Recently Feuchtinger and colleagues [41] described the isolation and expansion of human adenovirus–specific CD4+ and CD8+ T cells for adjuvant immunotherapy. Isolated cells were expanded and showed a specific response to adenovirus antigen with confirmatory testing and specific killing of adenovirus-infected B-cell lines. This method has the potential to generate sufficient numbers of adenovirus-specific T cells for adoptive immunotherapy for future therapeutic trials.

Epstein-Barr virus

Like CMV, EBV is a herpes virus that may cause disease after an HCT. In the absence of competent immune surveillance by CTLs after transplantation, B cells directly transformed by EBV can expand and grow opportunistically. The disease caused by this overgrowth, posttransplantation lymphoproliferative disease (PTLD), has a heterogeneous presentation ranging from an infectious mononucleosis syndrome to aggressive non-Hodgkin's lymphoma. The diagnosis, treatment, and prevention of PTLD provide an example of translational medicine.

Because PTLD is primarily a failure of T cells, the cornerstone of treatment includes decreasing the patient's immune suppression. This approach, however, can lead to GVHD. To augment the immune response to treat PTLD, unirradiated DLI have proven effective in resolving PTLD [42]. Once again, the limiting adverse effect with this strategy is GVHD. To overcome the risks of GVHD, one approach has been the use of antigen-specific T-cell lines. Rooney and colleagues [43] have shown that donor-derived antigen-specific CTLs can treat clinical PTLD and prevent the development of PTLD in high-risk patients without the induction of GVHD. The drawbacks to this approach are the length of time needed to make the CTLs as well as the facilities required for CTL production [44].

The classic method of diagnosing PTLD is tissue diagnosis by biopsy. Based on the success of preemptive treatment of CMV, multiple institutions developed assays for the amplification of EBV DNA from peripheral blood (EBV viral load) to identify patients who had uncontrolled B-cell overgrowth who may be able to receive treatment before the overt development of PTLD. A review of this work has been recently published [45]. In general, an increasing EBV viral load is predictive of the development of PTLD [46,47].

Because investigators have shown that an increasing EBV viral load is predictive of the development of PTLD, the logical next step of such findings has been to try to intervene with treatment to prevent the development of PTLD if an increasing viral load is observed. One strategy is to provide CTLs as discussed previously. Another increasingly common strategy is to use the drug rituximab. Rituximab is a chimeric murine/human monoclonal antibody directed against an antigen, CD20, which is expressed on B cells. Van Esser and colleagues [48] have shown that preemptive treatment with rituximab, based on an increasing viral load, is effective in preventing development of PTLD. This strategy, although adopted in many centers, has not been evaluated prospectively in a controlled manner.

Summary

The field of allogeneic transplantation has made vast improvements since its inception in 1968. Improvements in supportive care have greatly improved survival. Delayed immune reconstitution, GVHD, and relapse of disease still pose great obstacles. This article has highlighted novel strategies for using cellular therapy in conjunction with HCT that potentially may lead to improved clinical outcomes for patients undergoing HCT in the future.

References

[1] Gatti RA, Meuwissen HJ, Allen HD, et al. Immunological reconstitution of sex-linked lymphopenic immunological deficiency. Lancet Oncol 1968;2(7583):1366–9.
[2] Kolb H, Mittermuller J, Clemm C, et al. Donor leukocyte transfusions for treatment of recurrent chronic myelogenous leukemia in marrow transplant patients. Blood 1990;76(12): 2462–5.
[3] Kolb HJ, Schattenberg A, Goldman JM, et al. Graft-versus-leukemia effect of donor lymphocyte transfusions in marrow grafted patients. Blood 1995;86(5):2041–50.
[4] Collins RH Jr, Shpilberg O, Drobyski WR, et al. Donor leukocyte infusions in 140 patients with relapsed malignancy after allogeneic bone marrow transplantation. J Clin Oncol 1997; 15(2):433–44.
[5] Guglielmi C, Arcese W, Dazzi F, et al. Donor lymphocyte infusion for relapsed chronic myelogenous leukemia: prognostic relevance of the initial cell dose. Blood 2002;100(2):397–405.
[6] Druker BJ. Imatinib as a paradigm of targeted therapies. Advances in Cancer Research 2004; 91:1–30.
[7] Savani BN, Montero A, Kurlander R, et al. Imatinib synergizes with donor lymphocyte infusions to achieve rapid molecular remission of CML relapsing after allogeneic stem cell transplantation. Bone Marrow Transplant 2005;36(11):1009–15.
[8] Savani BN, Srinivasan R, Espinoza-Delgado I, et al. Treatment of relapsed blast-phase Philadelphia-chromosome-positive leukaemia after non-myeloablative stem-cell transplantation with donor lymphocytes and imatinib. Lancet Oncol 2005;6(10):809–12.
[9] Michalek J, Collins RH, Durrani HP, et al. Definitive separation of graft-versus-leukemia- and graft-versus-host-specific CD4 + T cells by virtue of their receptor. Proc Natl Acad Sci U S A 2003;100(3):1180–4.
[10] Andre-Schmutz I, Le Deist F, Hacein-Bey-Abina S, et al. Immune reconstitution without graft-versus-host disease after haemopoietic stem-cell transplantation: a phase 1/2 study. Lancet 2002;360(9327):130–7.
[11] Dal Cortivo L, Mahloaoui N, Picard B, et al. Adoptive immunotherapy with donor allodepleted T cells [abstract #479]. Blood 2005;106(11):144a.
[12] Porter DL, Levine BL, Bunin N, et al. A phase I trial of donor lymphocyte infusions expanded and activated ex-vivo via CD3/CD28 co-stimulation. Blood 2006;107(4):1325–31.
[13] Hsieh MH, Varadi G, Flomenberg N, et al. Leucyl-leucine methyl ester-treated haploidentical donor lymphocyte infusions can mediate graft-versus-leukemia activity with minimal graft-versus-host disease risk. Biol Blood Marrow Transplant 2002;8(6):303–15.

[14] Filicko J, Grosso D, Flomenberg P, et al. Accelerated immune recovery following LLME Treated donor lymphocyte infusion. Biol Blood Marrow Transplant 2006;12(2 Suppl 1): 77–8.

[15] Hallett WH, Murphy WJ. Natural killer cells: biology and clinical use in cancer therapy. Cell Mol Immunol 2004;1(1):12–21.

[16] Aversa F, Tabilio A, Terenzi A, et al. Successful engraftment of T-cell-depleted haploidentical "three-loci" incompatible transplants in leukemia patients by addition of recombinant human granulocyte colony-stimulating factor-mobilized peripheral blood progenitor cells to bone marrow inoculum. Blood 1994;84(11):3948–55.

[17] Velardi A, Ruggeri L, Moretta A. NK cells: a lesson from mismatched hematopoietic transplantation. Trends Immunol 2002;23(9):438–44.

[18] Ruggeri L, Capanni M, Casucci M, et al. Role of natural killer cell alloreactivity in HLA-mismatched hematopoietic stem cell transplantation. Blood 1999;94(1):333–9.

[19] Torelli GF, Guarini A, Maggio R, et al. Expansion of natural killer cells with lytic activity against autologous blasts from adult and pediatric acute lymphoid leukemia patients in complete hematologic remission. Haematologica 2005;90(6):785–92.

[20] Leung W, Iyengar R, Turner V, et al. Determinants of antileukemia effects of allogeneic NK cells. J Immunol 2004;172(1):644–50.

[21] Mengarelli A, Zarcone D, Caruso R, et al. Adhesion molecule expression, clinical features and therapy outcome in childhood acute lymphoblastic leukemia. Leuk Lymphoma 2001; 40(5–6):625–30.

[22] Miller JS, Soignier Y, Panoskaltsis-Mortari A, et al. Successful adoptive transfer and in vivo expansion of human haploidentical NK cells in patients with cancer. Blood 2005;105(8): 3051–7.

[23] Koehl U, Esser R, Zimmermann S, et al. Ex vivo expansion of highly purified NK cells for immunotherapy after haploidentical stem cell transplantation in children. Klin Padiatr 2005; 217(6):345–50.

[24] Koehl U, Sorensen J, Esser R, et al. IL-2 activated NK cell immunotherapy of three children after haploidentical stem cell transplantation. Blood Cells Mol Dis 2004;33(3):261–6.

[25] Havran WL, Boismenu R. Activation and function of gamma delta T cells. Curr Opin Immunol 1994;6(3):442–6.

[26] Boismenu R, Havran WL. An innate view of gamma delta T cells. Curr Opin Immunol 1997; 9(1):57–63.

[27] Duval M, Yotnda P, Bensussan A, et al. Potential antileukemic effect of gamma delta T cells in acute lymphoblastic leukemia. Leukemia 1995;9(5):863–8.

[28] Dolstra H, Fredrix H, van der Meer A, et al. TCR gamma delta cytotoxic T lymphocytes expressing the killer cell-inhibitory receptor p58.2 (CD158b) selectively lyse acute myeloid leukemia cells. Bone Marrow Transplant 2001;27(10):1087–93.

[29] Lamb LS Jr, Henslee-Downey PJ, Parrish RS, et al. Increased frequency of TCR gamma delta + T cells in disease-free survivors following T cell-depleted, partially mismatched, related donor bone marrow transplantation for leukemia. J Hematother 1996;5(5):503–9.

[30] Schilbach KE, Geiselhart A, Wessels JT, et al. Human gammadelta T lymphocytes exert natural and IL-2-induced cytotoxicity to neuroblastoma cells. J Immunother 2000;23(5):536–48.

[31] Otto M, Barfield RC, Iyengar R, et al. Human gammadelta T cells from G-CSF-mobilized donors retain strong tumoricidal activity and produce immunomodulatory cytokines after clinical-scale isolation. J Immunother 2005;28(1):73–8.

[32] Otto M, Barfield RC, Martin WJ, et al. Combination immunotherapy with clinical-scale enriched human {gamma}{delta} T cells, hu14.18 antibody, and the immunocytokine Fc-IL7 in disseminated neuroblastoma. Clin Cancer Res 2005;11(23):8486–91.

[33] Prigione I, Corrias MV, Airoldi I, et al. Immunogenicity of human neuroblastoma. Ann N Y Acad Sci 2004;1028:69–80.

[34] Goulmy E. Human minor histocompatibility antigens: new concepts for marrow transplantation and adoptive immunotherapy. Immunol Rev 1997;157:125–40.

[35] Marijt WAE, Heemskerk MHM, Kloosterboer FM, et al. Hematopoiesis-restricted minor histocompatibility antigens HA-1- or HA-2-specific T cells can induce complete remissions of relapsed leukemia. Proc Natl Acad Sci U S A 2003;100(5):2742–7.

[36] Mutis T, Verdijk R, Schrama E, et al. Feasibility of immunotherapy of relapsed leukemia with ex vivo-generated cytotoxic T lymphocytes specific for hematopoietic system-restricted minor histocompatibility antigens. Blood 1999;93(7):2336–41.

[37] Walter EA, Greenberg PD, Gilbert MJ, et al. Reconstitution of cellular immunity against cytomegalovirus in recipients of allogeneic bone marrow by transfer of T-cell clones from the donor. N Engl J Med 1995;333(16):1038–44.

[38] Peggs KS, Verfuerth S, Pizzey A, et al. Adoptive cellular therapy for early cytomegalovirus infection after allogeneic stem-cell transplantation with virus-specific T-cell lines. Lancet 2003;362(9393):1375–7.

[39] Rauser G, Einsele H, Sinzger C, et al. Rapid generation of combined CMV-specific CD4 + and CD8 + T-cell lines for adoptive transfer into recipients of allogeneic stem cell transplants. Blood 2004;103(9):3565–72.

[40] Cobbold M, Khan N, Pourgheysari B, et al. Adoptive transfer of cytomegalovirus-specific CTL to stem cell transplant patients after selection by HLA-peptide tetramers. J Exp Med 2005;202(3):379–86.

[41] Feuchtinger T, Lang P, Hamprecht K, et al. Isolation and expansion of human adenovirus-specific CD4 + and CD8 + T cells according to IFN-[gamma] secretion for adjuvant immunotherapy. Exp Hematol 2004;32(3):282–9.

[42] Papadopoulos EB, Ladanyi M, Emanuel D, et al. Infusions of donor leukocytes to treat Epstein-Barr virus-associated lymphoproliferative disorders after allogeneic bone marrow transplantation. N Engl J Med 1994;330(17):1185–91.

[43] Rooney CM, Smith CA, Ng CYC, et al. Infusion of cytotoxic T cells for the prevention and treatment of Epstein-Barr virus-induced lymphoma in allogeneic transplant recipients. Blood 1998;92(5):1549–55.

[44] Gottschalk S, Rooney CM, Heslop HE. Post-transplant lymphoproliferative disorders. Annu Rev Med 2005;56:29–44.

[45] Weinstock DM, Ambrossi GG, Brennan C, et al. Preemptive diagnosis and treatment of Epstein-Barr virus-associated post transplant lymphoproliferative disorder after hematopoietic stem cell transplant: an approach in development. Bone Marrow Transplant 2006;37(6): 539–46.

[46] van Esser JWJ, van der Holt B, Meijer E, et al. Epstein-Barr virus (EBV) reactivation is a frequent event after allogeneic stem cell transplantation (SCT) and quantitatively predicts EBV-lymphoproliferative disease following T-cell-depleted SCT. Blood 2001;98(4):972–8.

[47] Rooney CM, Loftin SK, Holladay MS, et al. Early identification of Epstein-Barr virus-associated post-transplantation lymphoproliferative disease. Br J Haematol 1995;89(1): 98–103.

[48] van Esser JWJ, Niesters HGM, van der Holt B, et al. Prevention of Epstein-Barr virus-lymphoproliferative disease by molecular monitoring and preemptive rituximab in high-risk patients after allogeneic stem cell transplantation. Blood 2002;99(12):4364–9.

PEDIATRIC CLINICS
OF NORTH AMERICA

ELSEVIER
SAUNDERS

Pediatr Clin N Am 53 (2006) 699–713

Therapies and Vaccines for Emerging Bacterial Infections: Learning from Methicillin-resistant *Staphylococcus aureus*

Chandy C. John, MD, MS[a,b,*],
John R. Schreiber, MD[a,b]

[a]*Department of Pediatrics, University of Minnesota Medical School, 420 Delaware Street SE, Minneapolis, MN 55455, USA*
[b]*University of Minnesota Children's Hospital, 420 Delaware Street SE, Minneapolis, MN 55455, USA*

Few emerging bacterial infections have had a more dramatic impact in recent years than methicillin-resistant *Staphylococcus aureus* (MRSA). *S aureus* infections have been a serious health problem for humans for millennia. The discovery of penicillin was initially a major breakthrough in combating these infections, but resistance to penicillin developed rapidly through *S aureus* beta-lactamase production. Methicillin, a beta-lactamase stable penicillin, was subsequently developed and used successfully against *S aureus*. Methicillin resistance emerged in 1961 [1], but MRSA remained for many years an almost exclusively nosocomial infection.

• Outbreaks of community-acquired MRSA (CA-MRSA) were reported as early as the 1980s [2], but CA-MRSA remained a relatively unusual phenomenon until the late 1990s, when reports of CA-MRSA outbreaks [3,4] and distinct clinical syndromes associated with CA-MRSA (furunculosis and severe necrotizing pneumonia) began to appear [5,6]. CA-MRSA is now a pathogen of major significance in many areas of the world. •

The publication of the complete genomes of different nosocomial MRSA [7,8], CA-MRSA [9], and community-acquired methicillin-susceptible *S aureus* (CA-MSSA) [7] isolates has greatly increased the understanding of differences and similarities between CA-MRSA, nosocomial MRSA, and

_____

* Corresponding author. Department of Pediatrics, University of Minnesota, 420 Delaware Street SE, 850 Mayo, MMC-296, Minneapolis, MN 55455.
E-mail address: ccj@umn.edu (C.C. John).

doi:10.1016/j.pcl.2006.05.004   *pediatric.theclinics.com*

MSSA and the potential roles of different virulence factors. Molecular biology has played a critical role in distinguishing CA-MRSA infections from nosocomial MRSA infections and has provided insight into potential pathogenic mechanisms that might explain the clinical syndromes associated with CA-MRSA. This understanding in turn has guided both treatment and prevention strategies against MRSA. This article outlines the molecular biology of MRSA, how molecular biology has contributed to the understanding of MRSA infections, current therapy and prevention of MRSA, and the prospects for a vaccine against *S aureus*.

The molecular biology of methicillin-resistant *Staphylococcus aureus*

Mechanism of Staphylococcus aureus *beta-lactam resistance*

S aureus resistance to penicillin is mediated by production of beta-lactamases. Methicillin resistance is mediated by alterations in penicillin-binding proteins, specifically penicillin-binding protein-2a (PBP-2a). PBP-2a alterations are encoded by the *mecA* gene, which is carried on the staphylococcal cassette chromosome (SCC) *mec* [10]. Five types of SCC*mec* have been described to date. Types I and IV have the *mec*A gene as the only determinant of resistance, whereas types II and III contain several determinants for resistance to non–beta-lactam antibiotics. In nosocomial strains of MRSA, SCC*mec* types are almost always type II and III. Development of these strains generally has occurred in response to antibiotic pressure. Most CA-MRSA infections have been type IV and consequently have had less antibiotic resistance than nosocomial MRSA. SCC*mec* type IV is much smaller than SCC*mec* types II and III and hence is more easily transmissible to other staphylococci [10]. The SCC*mec* type IV element was seen frequently seen in strains of *Staphylococcus epidermidis* long before it became common in *S aureus* [11], and transfer across staphylococcal species may have led to the form of MRSA seen in CA-MRSA. As discussed later, in MRSA outbreaks, determination of SCC type has helped to determine whether MRSA was community acquired or nosocomial in origin.

Virulence factors in methicillin-resistant Staphylococcus aureus

Molecular biology has allowed identification of numerous virulence factors in *S aureus*, some of which are seen more frequently in MRSA. The best-described virulence factors, which probably are responsible for some of the distinctive clinical characteristics of CA-MRSA infection, are the Panton-Valentine leukocidin (*PVL*) genes. The *PVL* genes encode a leukotoxin with two separate secreted proteins of the S and F class, LukS-PVL and LukF-PVL. The *PVL* genes and the hemolysins (α- and γ-hemolysin) are the pore-forming toxins of staphylococci. *PVL* cause pore formation and cell lysis of neutrophils, monocytes, and macrophages [12] and also are responsible for cell activation through membrane calcium channels

[13]. These actions lead to local inflammation, chemotaxis, neutrophil infiltration, and secretion of degenerative enzymes and generation of superoxide ions, which causes tissue necrosis [10]. The LukS-PVL/LukF-PVL combination encoded by *PVL* has been shown to be a potent inducer of inflammatory mediators from human granulocytes in vitro [14] and caused dermonecrotic lesions in a rabbits injected intradermally with *PVL* [15,16]. α-Hemolysin, another pore-forming toxin, also is produced more frequently by CA-MRSA strains, acts on many cell types and has produced dermonecrosis in rabbits [17]. The role of γ-hemolysin in clinical disease is unclear.

A number of other virulence factors are released by *S aureus*. These factors and their putative effects have been summarized nicely in a recent review by Zetola and colleagues [10]. Among the best-known *S aureus* virulence factors is toxic shock syndrome toxin 1, but the *tst* gene that encodes this toxin is not present in most CA-MRSA. Other toxins that can produce a toxic shock–like syndrome, the staphylococcal enterotoxins, have been identified in cases of severe CA-MRSA infections, however. Staphylococcal enterotoxins B and C were identified in case series of CA-MRSA in children in Minnesota and North Dakota [18], and the genes that encode staphylococcal enterotoxins A and H were found in isolates from a series of four children who had severe pneumonia or sepsis caused by MRSA or MSSA [19]. The sepsislike presentation of many of the patients from whom these isolates were obtained suggests that enterotoxins may play a role in the pathogenesis of some forms of severe CA-MRSA disease. Other virulence factors of potential importance include the bacteriocins, which kill bacteria closely related to the producing strain, and collagen-adhesin protein, which may facilitate adherence to respiratory epithelium in necrotizing pneumonia. Although the *PVL* gene has been present in very high frequencies in almost all CA-MRSA studies, including those of severe disease, the frequencies of staphylococcal enterotoxin genes and the *cna* gene in CA-MRSA infections have been highly variable. For example, in one study of adolescents who had *S aureus* sepsis (12 CA-MRSA, 2 CA-MSSA), all 12 of the MRSA isolates had *lukS-PVL* and *lukF-PVL* genes, but none had *cna* or *tst* genes, and only one had genes encoding staphylococcal enterotoxins [20].

Molecular typing of methicillin-resistant Staphylococcus aureus

Identification of specific MRSA isolates by a variety of typing methods has significantly advanced study of the epidemiology of MRSA infections. A number of methods are now available to type MRSA isolates. For many years pulsed field gel electrophoresis has been the standard method of MRSA typing [21,22], but other methods that have been used include assessment of single nucleotide polymorphisms [23], multilocus sequence typing [24], polymerase chain reaction restriction fragment length polymorphisms [25], and DNA oligonucleotide arrays [26]. Use of these typing methodologies, in combination with assessment of SCCmec type and presence of virulence factor genes, has allowed evaluation of the clonality of infections during outbreaks [22] and comparison of relatedness and presence of virulence factors in isolates from different eras of antibiotic susceptibility [27]. Robinson and colleagues [27] demonstrated that *PVL* was present in almost all of the 80/81 strain penicillin-resistant isolates from the 1950s and 1960s that caused outbreaks of skin lesions, sepsis, and severe pneumonia, and that the 80/81 strain is highly related to one of six major genotypes of *PVL*-positive CA-MRSA. For this MRSA genotype, genotyping has allowed tracing of its history and likely origin.

The contribution of molecular biology to understanding
methicillin-resistant Staphylococcus aureus *infection*

Defining methicillin-resistant Staphylococcus aureus*:*
community-acquired versus nosocomial methicillin-resistant
Staphylococcus aureus

CA-MRSA and nosocomial or health care–associated (HCA) MRSA are now distinguished more by molecular and clinical epidemiologic characteristics than strictly by history. Epidemiologic studies of MRSA have clearly shown that some health-care exposures are not identified in standard exclusion criteria for CA-MRSA [28], so that individuals may be misclassified as having CA-MRSA when their MRSA was health-care associated. In addition, it is difficult to come up with precise questions or time points that exclude HCA exposures. Some authors have suggested that infections be termed "community-onset" rather than "community-acquired" if they occurred while the patient was in the community [10]. Finally, hospital outbreaks of MRSA with a CA-MRSA phenotype (susceptible to multiple antibiotics, SCC*mec* type IV, *PVL* positive) have also been reported, further muddying the waters [29]. For these reasons, CA-MRSA is best identified by presence of SCC*mec* type IV, with *PVL* and antibiotic susceptibility patterns as further confirmatory evidence. If CA-MRSA makes further inroads into nosocomial infection, new terminology may be required to distinguish CA-MRSA from HCA-MRSA.

Clinical presentations of community-acquired methicillin-resistant
Staphylococcus aureus *infection in children*

The two clinical syndromes that have been widely identified with CA-MRSA are skin and soft tissue infections (SSTIs), often with abscess or furuncle formation, and severe necrotizing pneumonia, usually following influenza. MRSA-associated SSTIs account for the majority of infections and occur more frequently in young children [30,31], although other groups, including athletes [32], Native Americans [33], men who have sex with men [34], and intravenous drug users [35], are also at higher risk (Table 1), and

Table 1
Clinical characteristics of community-acquired and health-care associated methicillin-resistant
S aureus

Characteristic	Community-acquired MRSA	Health care associated MRSA
Exposure	Community	Health-care associated
Vulnerable populations	Children, athletes, older adults, Native Americans, intravenous drug users	Persons with extensive health care facility exposure, hemodialysis patients, immunocompromised patients, patients with indwelling intravascular catheters, patients in intensive care units
Clinical presentation	Furunculosis, necrotizing pneumonia	Intravascular catheter infection, surgical wound infection, ventilator-associated pneumonia
Antibiotic susceptibility	Usually susceptible to multiple non-beta lactam antibiotics, including clindamycin	Usually resistant to multiple non beta lactam antibiotics, including clindamycin

Abbreviation: MRSA, methicillin-resistant *S aureus*.

many cases of CA-MRSA SSTI occur in adults. As noted in the section on virulence factors in MRSA, the majority cases of CA-MRSA with SSTI are positive for *PVL* genes [36], and the leukocidal effects of *PVL* are thought to be responsible for the characteristic furuncles seen in this condition, with their areas of skin necrosis. The skin necrosis has been mistaken for spider bites, and the spider-bite appearance may actually be a clue that the patient has MRSA. In a Los Angeles county prison in late 2002, an outbreak of suspected spider bites was in fact an outbreak of dermonecrotic MRSA infections spread from one prisoner to others [34]. Earlier that year, an astute clinician in Cleveland, Ohio, noticed that a number of children were coming in with what their parents termed "spider bites," but there was no documentation of a spider bite, and culture of abscesses from the area of necrotic skin grew MRSA (C. Hoyen, personal communication, 2002). Finally, a case series of MRSA infections thought to be secondary to spider bites was reported from the Houston, Texas, Veteran's Affairs Medical Center [37]. A letter in response to this case series pointed out that the "spider bites" probably represented dermonecrotic MRSA infection [38]. *PVL*-negative MRSA causing these infections has been reported [39], but almost all MRSA causing cellulitis and abscess or furuncles has been *PVL*-positive, and clinical and in vitro studies lend support to *PVL* as a causative factor in these clinical manifestations. Two studies of musculoskeletal infections have demonstrated that complications occur more often in individuals who have *PVL*-positive CA-MRSA than in individuals who have *PVL*-negative CA-MRSA [39,40]. In addition, *PVL* has been shown to cause in vitro pore formation and cell lysis of neutrophils [12,13] and may also cause apoptosis through the mitochondrial pathway [41]. Together, these findings suggest that *PVL* is involved in the pathogenesis of CA-MRSA SSTI and musculoskeletal infections and is not simply a marker of CA-MRSA infection.

Necrotizing pneumonia, generally occurring after influenza, is the other well-described clinical manifestation of CA-MRSA infection and can affect otherwise healthy adults [6,42,43] and children [44,45] as well as premature neonates [46]. Necrotizing pneumonia caused by CA-MRSA is character-ized by hemoptysis, leukopenia, concomitant furunculosis or SSTI, and a fulminant course. This presentation is much less common than SSTI but is far more deadly, with mortality rates as high as 37% [44]. Severe non-nec-rotizing pneumonias caused by CA-MRSA also have been reported in chil-dren [45]. Other clinical syndromes, including musculoskeletal infections, endocarditis, bacteremia, brain abscess, and sinusitis, also have been re-ported with CA-MRSA but less frequently than SSTI or necrotizing pneumonia.

Current therapy and prevention of methicillin-resistant Staphylococcus aureus infection

Antibiotics

Antibiotic therapy for MRSA depends on the severity of illness and the health-care–associated exposures of the patient (Fig. 1). CA-MRSA and HCA-MRSA typically have distinct antibiotic profiles. CA-MRSA usually is susceptible to multiple non–beta-lactam antibiotics, including clindamy-cin, trimethoprim-sulfamethoxazole, and doxycycline, whereas HCA-MRSA often is resistant to clindamycin and, depending on the area, may also be resistant to trimethoprim-sulfamethoxazole and doxycycline [47]. Both CA-MRSA and HCA-MRSA are almost always susceptible to vanco-mycin, linezolid, and daptomycin, although vancomycin resistance has been rarely reported, most often in patients who have been receiving chronic van-comycin therapy [48,49].

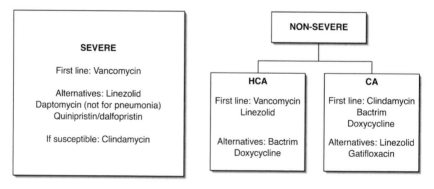

Fig. 1. Antibiotic treatment of methicillin-resistant Staphylococcus aureus. CA, community-acquired; HCA, health care–associated.

For severely ill patients who have MRSA infection, vancomycin, a glycopeptide antibiotic, is currently the initial antibiotic of choice, regardless of health care exposure history [50]. As clinical trials continue with newer antibiotics, this preference may change. Vancomycin requires high peak levels and does not penetrate well into soft tissues, and it is inferior to beta-lactam therapy for treatment of MSSA bacteremia [51–53]. In a pooled analysis comparing vancomycin with the newer oxazolidinone antibiotic linezolid, however, vancomycin demonstrated similar outcomes in patients who had staphylococcal bacteremia [54].

In contrast, for nosocomial MRSA and possibly CA-MRSA pneumonia, there is evidence that vancomycin, which has poor lung tissue penetration, may be inferior to linezolid. Outcomes were better for linezolid than vancomycin in two retrospective, double-blind adult studies of nosocomial MRSA pneumonia [55], and linezolid may become the drug of choice for this condition. Current American Thoracic Society guidelines for adults who have ventilator-associated MRSA pneumonia include linezolid as an alternative to vancomycin therapy [56]. For CA-MRSA necrotizing pneumonia, data on linezolid use are more limited [57]. In one case series of four patients who had necrotizing MRSA pneumonia and were doing poorly on vancomycin therapy, clinical status improved when treated with clindamycin or linezolid [58]. The authors of the latter study speculated that the clinical improvement with clindamycin resulted from its inhibition of exotoxin production and that linezolid, which also acts to inhibit bacterial protein synthesis and which has been shown in vitro to reduce S aureus virulence factor production [59], may have similar effects in vivo. Linezolid is generally well tolerated, although neutropenia and thrombocytopenia may be seen with prolonged therapy. Linezolid also can be given orally, providing an oral agent with which a patient can complete therapy as an outpatient. Linezolid is currently extremely expensive, however.

If a patient has true CA-MRSA (ie, no risk factors for HCA-MRSA, as discussed later), clindamycin may be a reasonable alternative for severe infection, although clindamycin resistance varies by region. Most experts would require susceptibility information before they administered clindamycin as the sole treatment for severe MRSA infection, and S aureus isolates that are erythromycin resistant must always be tested for inducible clindamycin resistance, usually by the "D" test. Other options to consider in severe infection include daptomycin (except for pneumonia) and quinipristin/dalfopristin. Both have excellent gram-positive coverage, including coverage of almost all MRSA, but both are expensive, and quinipristin/dalfopristin has numerous side effects that limit its use. Concerns about overuse of daptomycin have led to a general consensus that it should be used for severe MRSA infections only if there are contraindications to vancomycin use or vancomycin has failed to eradicate MRSA [50]. In addition, daptomycin is inactivated by surfactant and so should not be used for pneumonia.

For individuals who have nonsevere infections, initial therapy is guided by the presence or absence of HCA exposures. HCA exposures include hospitalization within the past 2 years, outpatient visit within the past year, nursing home admission within the past year, antibiotic use within the past year, hemodialysis, chronic illness, intravenous drug use, and close contact with persons with risk factors [10]. Individuals with any of these risk factors should be considered to have HCA exposure. First-line therapy for these individuals who have nonsevere infection could include vancomycin, linezolid, trimethoprim-sulfamethoxazole, or doxycycline. The choice of agent will depend on the nature of the infection, the history of antibiotic use, and the antimicrobial susceptibility pattern of HCA-MRSA in the area. For true non-severe CA-MRSA infection, clindamycin and trimethoprim-sulfamethoxazole are good options for treatment, again depending on the local susceptibility patterns for CA-MRSA. Doxycycline is another option for children older than 8 years of age. Linezolid has an excellent track record for treatment of SSTI [60,61], but its expense and the availability of equally efficacious, less expensive alternatives for most patients make it a second-line choice for nonsevere MRSA infections. Gatifloxacin and moxifloxacin had good in vitro activity against MRSA in some studies [62] and can be considered if other options are not feasible and CA-MRSA in the community is usually susceptible to these antibiotics.

Novel antibiotics that show promise for treatment of MRSA infection include the lipoglycopeptide dalbavancin [63] and the glycylcycline tigecycline [64]. Dalbavancin's long half-life allows a dosing schedule of a single dose 1000 mg on day 1 and 500 mg on day 8; in this dosing schedule dalbavancin was as efficacious as linezolid for the treatment of SSTI [63]. Tigecycline has both gram-positive and gram-negative activity and may become an option for hospitalized individuals who have complex infections. A concise review of drug therapy for MRSA was recently published by Ellis and Lewis [65].

Abscess drainage for skin and soft tissue infections

A critical part of treatment of CA-MRSA SSTIs is drainage of any abscesses that form. One study in children showed that even with ineffective antibiotic treatment against CA-MRSA, drainage effectively took care of abscesses smaller than 5 cm in diameter [66]. The authors suggest that for abscesses smaller than 5 cm, drainage alone, without adjunctive antibiotic therapy, may be adequate treatment.

Adjunctive treatment for staphylococcal sepsis

At present, the only adjunctive therapy frequently used in cases of staphylococcal toxic syndrome or sepsis is intravenous immunoglobulin (IVIG). Studies have suggested its benefit in streptococcal toxic shock syndrome [67,68], and a review of IVIG treatment in bacterial sepsis also suggested a reduction in mortality with its use [69]. In vitro studies suggest that a higher dose of IVIG may be required to neutralize staphylococcal toxins than is required to neutralize streptococcal toxins [70], but clinical trials in humans have used IVIG dosing similar to that given in streptococcal toxic shock syndrome (generally a total dose of 2 g/kg, given over 2 or 3 days) [67].

Eradication of methicillin-resistant Staphylococcus aureus *colonization*

In cases of recurrent or severe MRSA infection, eradication of MRSA colonization may be desirable. Unfortunately, neither of the topical therapies currently recommended for elimination of colonization (nasal mupirocin or chlorhexidine baths) is highly effective [71–73]. Combinations of mupirocin with antibiotic treatment (novobiocin and rifampin [74] or minocycline and rifampin [75]) may be more effective than mupirocin alone in eradication of MRSA colonization. In ICUs and other areas where risk of MRSA infection and spread is high, adherence to strict handwashing procedures and appropriate isolation precautions for MRSA is critical.

Future prospects: vaccines against *Staphylococcus aureus*

Given the potential increasing resistance of MRSA to antimicrobials, the emergence of vancomycin tolerance, and the difficulty in treating serious MRSA infections even with appropriate antibiotics, there have been increased research efforts to find effective passive and active immunization strategies against MRSA and other staphylococcal infections.

Several epitopes of *S aureus* have been chosen as potential targets for active and passive immunization. The recent characterization of the capsular polysaccharides of *S aureus* has been of particular interest in vaccine development. Because antibodies against capsular polysaccharides of other human pathogens such as pneumococcus have been found to be protective, the capsular polysaccharides *S aureus* have been used in pilot vaccines to induce anticapsular antibodies [76]. Serotypes 5 and 8 were chosen because of epidemiologic data suggesting that the majority of isolates from infected hospitalized patients were of this phenotype [77]. Because polysaccharides are T-independent antigens that do not elicit T-cell help, do not elicit booster responses with repeated doses, and are poor immunogens in children under the age of 24 months, these capsular polysaccharides were conjugated to the protein from *Pseudomonas aeruginosa* exotoxin A to convert the polysaccharides to more of the characteristics of T-dependent antigens to elicit T-cell help. These conjugate vaccines were found to elicit high titers of anticapsular antibodies in animals with booster responses after multiple immunizations, and these antibodies were opsonic for killing of homologous serotypes of staphylococcus [78]. This combination vaccine was used as a single dose in a randomized, double-blind, phase III clinical trial in adult patients who had end-stage renal disease and were receiving hemodialysis, because this patient group has an unusually high incidence of serious infections with S aureus [76]. Partial immunity was achieved for approximately 40 weeks postimmunization, with a significant reduction in S aureus bacteremia. By 54 weeks postimmunization, however, there were no differences in bacteremia rates between the vaccinated and unvaccinated patient groups [76]. Because conjugate vaccines owe their advantage to their ability to induce booster responses to subsequent doses (unlike pure polysaccharide vaccines), a follow-up study gave another dose of conjugate vaccine 2 to 3 years after the first dose. Although the titers achieved did not match those obtained after the first dose, antibodies elicited were opsonic against the pathogen and stayed in the serum much longer than after the initial immunization [79]. Future studies may use several doses of vaccine much as multiple doses of conjugate vaccines are used in infants to achieve high, sustained protective antibody levels against pneumococcus and *Haemophilus influenzae* type b. Finally, serotype 336, not included in the original vaccine, seems to be an increasing cause of serious S aureus infections. Thus, second-generation vaccines will need to include this and perhaps other serotypes [77].

Another alternative to including multiple serotypes of capsular polysaccharides in conjugate vaccines is to use other antigens that are commonly found across all serotypes that may also induce protective antibodies. Both S aureus and S epidermidis synthesize the surface polysaccharide Poly-N-Acetyl-β-(1-6)-Glucosamine. Recent studies have shown that this antigen induces antibodies that opsonize a wide variety of staphylococcal strains for killing by phagocytes and protected animals from fatal staphylococcal infections [80]. Other potential targets include cell wall–associated proteins that are crucial for bacterial attachment to the host, such as clumping factor. Clumping factor, as well as other adhesion molecules, is present on a wide variety of S aureus and S epidermidis strains, and antibodies against clumping factor are protective in animal models of methicillin-resistant staphylococcal infections [81].

Despite the encouraging results of the staphylococcal polysaccharide protein conjugate vaccines, active immunization against S aureus may be of limited utility in the patient groups at highest risk of infection, because these patients often are functionally immunocompromised. Thus, passive immunization with high-titer immune globulin or monoclonal antibodies offers another alternative to active immunization. A blinded, randomized multicenter study of intravenous S aureus–immune globulin containing high titers of anticapsular antibodies to types 5 and 8 recently completed a phase II trial in 206 very low birth weight neonates [82]. Infusion of the hyperimmune globulin resulted in high serum levels of anticapsular antibodies, with no difference in side effects compared with saline placebo. Efficacy, however, still remains to be proven. Finally, two passive immunoprophylaxis preparations are in clinical trials to prevent coagulase-negative staphylococcal infections, which also are caused by strains that are commonly resistant to methicillin. The first, a mouse/human chimeric monoclonal antibody against lipoteichoic acid, and the second, a human polyclonal hyperimmune globulin against bacterial proteins that recognize host adhesion molecules, are in clinical trials to determine safety and efficacy [83,84].

Increasing antimicrobial resistance and spread of MRSA into the community has mandated new interest in the prevention of staphylococcal infections through immunization. Promising vaccines using a variety of targets on the bacteria, particularly capsular polysaccharides linked chemically to protein carrier molecules, soon may be useful as aids in the prevention of MRSA infections. Further studies in human trials, however, will determine whether the current generation of vaccines has adequate protective efficacy in target populations at highest risk of staphylococcal infections.

References

[1] Jevons MP. "Celbenin"-resistant staphylococci. BMJ 1961;1:124–5.

[2] Saravolatz LD, Markowitz N, Arking L, et al. Methicillin-resistant Staphylococcus aureus. Epidemiologic observations during a community-acquired outbreak. Ann Intern Med 1982; 96(1):11–6.

[3] Lindenmayer JM, Schoenfeld S, O'Grady R, et al. Methicillin-resistant Staphylococcus aureus in a high school wrestling team and the surrounding community. Arch Intern Med 1998; 158(8):895–9.

[4] Maguire GP, Arthur AD, Boustead PJ, et al. Emerging epidemic of community-acquired methicillin-resistant Staphylococcus aureus infection in the Northern Territory. Med J Aust 1996;164(12):721–3.

[5] Baggett HC, Hennessy TW, Rudolph K, et al. Community-onset methicillin-resistant Staphylococcus aureus associated with antibiotic use and the cytotoxin Panton-Valentine leukocidin during a furunculosis outbreak in rural Alaska. J Infect Dis 2004;189(9):1565–73.

[6] Francis JS, Doherty MC, Lopatin U, et al. Severe community-onset pneumonia in healthy adults caused by methicillin-resistant Staphylococcus aureus carrying the Panton-Valentine leukocidin genes. Clin Infect Dis 2005;40(1):100–7.

[7] Holden MT, Feil EJ, Lindsay JA, et al. Complete genomes of two clinical Staphylococcus aureus strains: evidence for the rapid evolution of virulence and drug resistance. Proc Natl Acad Sci U S A 2004;101(26):9786–91.

[8] Kuroda M, Ohta T, Uchiyama I, et al. Whole genome sequencing of meticillin-resistant Staphylococcus aureus. Lancet 2001;357(9264):1225–40.

[9] Baba T, Takeuchi F, Kuroda M, et al. Genome and virulence determinants of high virulence community-acquired MRSA. Lancet 2002;359(9320):1819–27.

[10] Zetola N, Francis JS, Nuermberger EL, et al. Community-acquired meticillin-resistant Staphylococcus aureus: an emerging threat. Lancet Infect Dis 2005;5(5):275–86.

[11] Wisplinghoff H, Rosato AE, Enright MC, et al. Related clones containing SCCmec type IV predominate among clinically significant Staphylococcus epidermidis isolates. Antimicrob Agents Chemother 2003;47(11):3574–9.

[12] Meunier O, Falkenrodt A, Monteil H, et al. Application of flow cytometry in toxinology: pathophysiology of human polymorphonuclear leukocytes damaged by a pore-forming toxin from Staphylococcus aureus. Cytometry 1995;21(3):241–7.

[13] Finck-Barbancon V, Duportail G, Meunier O, et al. Pore formation by a two-component leukocidin from Staphylococcus aureus within the membrane of human polymorphonuclear leukocytes. Biochim Biophys Acta 1993;1182(3):275–82.

[14] Konig B, Prevost G, Konig W. Composition of staphylococcal bi-component toxins determines pathophysiological reactions. J Med Microbiol 1997;46(6):479–85.

[15] Cribier B, Prevost G, Couppie P, et al. Staphylococcus aureus leukocidin: a new virulence factor in cutaneous infections? An epidemiological and experimental study. Dermatology 1992;185(3):175–80.

[16] Ward PD, Turner WH. Identification of staphylococcal Panton-Valentine leukocidin as a potent dermonecrotic toxin. Infect Immun 1980;28(2):393–7.

[17] van der Vijver JC, van Es-Boon MM, Michel MF. A study of virulence factors with induced mutants of Staphylococcus aureus. J Med Microbiol 1975;8(2):279–87.

[18] Centers for Disease Control and Prevention. Four pediatric deaths from community-acquired methicillin-resistant Staphylococcus aureus–Minnesota and North Dakota, 1997–1999. MMWR Morb Mortal Wkly Rep 1999;48(12):707–10.

[19] Mongkolrattanothai K, Boyle S, Kahana MD, et al. Severe Staphylococcus aureus infections caused by clonally related community-acquired methicillin-susceptible and methicillin-resistant isolates. Clin Infect Dis 2003;37(8):1050–8.

[20] Gonzalez BE, Martinez-Aguilar G, Hulten KG, et al. Severe Staphylococcal sepsis in adolescents in the era of community-acquired methicillin-resistant Staphylococcus aureus. Pediatrics 2005;115(3):642–8.

[21] Chavez-Bueno S, Bozdogan B, Katz K, et al. Inducible clindamycin resistance and molecular epidemiologic trends of pediatric community-acquired methicillin-resistant Staphylococcus aureus in Dallas, Texas. Antimicrob Agents Chemother 2005;49(6):2283–8.

[22] Naimi TS, LeDell KH, Boxrud DJ, et al. Epidemiology and clonality of community-acquired methicillin-resistant Staphylococcus aureus in Minnesota, 1996–1998. Clin Infect Dis 2001;33(7):990–6.

[23] Stephens AJ, Huygens F, Inman-Bamber J, et al. Methicillin-resistant Staphylococcus aureus genotyping using a small set of polymorphisms. J Med Microbiol 2006;55(Pt 1):43–51.

[24] Berglund C, Molling P, Sjoberg L, et al. Multilocus sequence typing of methicillin-resistant Staphylococcus aureus from an area of low endemicity by real-time PCR. J Clin Microbiol 2005;43(9):4448–54.

[25] Mitani N, Koizumi A, Sano R, et al. Molecular typing of methicillin-resistant Staphylococcus aureus by PCR-RFLP and its usefulness in an epidemiological study of an outbreak. Jpn J Infect Dis 2005;58(4):250–2.

[26] Monecke S, Ehricht R. Rapid genotyping of methicillin-resistant Staphylococcus aureus (MRSA) isolates using miniaturised oligonucleotide arrays. Clin Microbiol Infect 2005; 11(10):825–33.

[27] Robinson DA, Kearns AM, Holmes A, et al. Re-emergence of early pandemic Staphylococcus aureus as a community-acquired meticillin-resistant clone. Lancet 2005;365(9466):1256–8.

[28] Buck JM, Como-Sabetti K, Harriman KH, et al. Community-associated methicillin-resistant Staphylococcus aureus, Minnesota, 2000–2003. Emerg Infect Dis 2005;11(10):1532–8.

[29] Bratu S, Eramo A, Kopec R, et al. Community-associated methicillin-resistant Staphylococcus aureus in hospital nursery and maternity units. Emerg Infect Dis 2005;11(6):808–13.

[30] Dietrich DW, Auld DB, Mermel LA. Community-acquired methicillin-resistant Staphylococcus aureus in southern New England children. Pediatrics 2004;113(4):e347–52.

[31] Fridkin SK, Hageman JC, Morrison M, et al. Methicillin-resistant Staphylococcus aureus disease in three communities. N Engl J Med 2005;352(14):1436–44.

[32] Begier EM, Frenette K, Barrett NL, et al. A high-morbidity outbreak of methicillin-resistant Staphylococcus aureus among players on a college football team, facilitated by cosmetic body shaving and turf burns. Clin Infect Dis 2004;39(10):1446–53.

[33] Groom AV, Wolsey DH, Naimi TS, et al. Community-acquired methicillin-resistant Staphylococcus aureus in a rural American Indian community. JAMA 2001;286(10):1201–5.

[34] Centers for Disease Control. Outbreaks of community-associated methicillin-resistant Staphylococcus aureus skin infections–Los Angeles County, California, 2002–2003. MMWR Morb Mortal Wkly Rep 2003;52(5):88.

[35] Qi W, Ender M, O'Brien F, et al. Molecular epidemiology of methicillin-resistant Staphylococcus aureus in Zurich, Switzerland (2003): prevalence of type IV SCCmec and a new

SCCmec element associated with isolates from intravenous drug users. J Clin Microbiol 2005;43(10):5164–70.

[36] Yamasaki O, Kaneko J, Morizane S, et al. The association between Staphylococcus aureus strains carrying Panton-Valentine leukocidin genes and the development of deep-seated follicular infection. Clin Infect Dis 2005;40(3):381–5.

[37] Fagan SP, Berger DH, Rahwan K, et al. Spider bites presenting with methicillin-resistant Staphylococcus aureus soft tissue infection require early aggressive treatment. Surg Infect (Larchmt) 2003;4(4):311–5.

[38] Miller LG, Perdreau-Remington F, Rieg G, et al. Necrotizing fasciitis caused by community-associated methicillin-resistant Staphylococcus aureus in Los Angeles. N Engl J Med 2005; 352(14):1445–53.

[39] Martinez-Aguilar G, Avalos-Mishaan A, Hulten K. Community-acquired, methicillin-resistant and methicillin-susceptible Staphylococcus aureus musculoskeletal infections in children. Pediatr Infect Dis J 2004;23(8):701–6.

[40] Bocchini CE, Hulten KG, Mason EO Jr, et al. Panton-Valentine leukocidin genes are associated with enhanced inflammatory response and local disease in acute hematogenous Staphylococcus aureus osteomyelitis in children. Pediatrics 2006;117(2):433–40.

[41] Genestier AL, Michallet MC, Prevost G, et al. Staphylococcus aureus Panton-Valentine leukocidin directly targets mitochondria and induces Bax-independent apoptosis of human neutrophils. J Clin Invest 2005;115(11):3117–27.

[42] Boussaud V, Parrot A, Mayaud C, et al. Life-threatening hemoptysis in adults with community-acquired pneumonia due to Panton-Valentine leukocidin-secreting Staphylococcus aureus. Intensive Care Med 2003;29(10):1840–3.

[43] Frazee BW, Salz TO, Lambert L, et al. Fatal community-associated methicillin-resistant Staphylococcus aureus pneumonia in an immunocompetent young adult. Ann Emerg Med 2005;46(5):401–4.

[44] Gillet Y, Issartel B, Vanhems P, et al. Association between Staphylococcus aureus strains carrying gene for Panton-Valentine leukocidin and highly lethal necrotising pneumonia in young immunocompetent patients. Lancet 2002;359(9308):753–9.

[45] Gonzalez BE, Hulten KG, Dishop MK, et al. Pulmonary manifestations in children with invasive community-acquired Staphylococcus aureus infection. Clin Infect Dis 2005;41(5): 583–90.

[46] McAdams RM, Mazuchowski E, Ellis MW, et al. Necrotizing staphylococcal pneumonia in a neonate. J Perinatol 2005;25(10):677–9.

[47] Naimi TS, LeDell KH, Como-Sabetti K, et al. Comparison of community- and health care-associated methicillin-resistant Staphylococcus aureus infection. JAMA 2003;290(22): 2976–84.

[48] Smith TL, Pearson ML, Wilcox KR, et al. Emergence of vancomycin resistance in Staphylococcus aureus. Glycopeptide-Intermediate Staphylococcus aureus Working Group. N Engl J Med 1999;340(7):493–501.

[49] Tenover FC, Weigel LM, Appelbaum PC, et al. Vancomycin-resistant Staphylococcus aureus isolate from a patient in Pennsylvania. Antimicrob Agents Chemother 2004;48(1): 275–80.

[50] Kowalski TJ, Berbari EF, Osmon DR. Epidemiology, treatment, and prevention of community-acquired methicillin-resistant Staphylococcus aureus infections. Mayo Clin Proc 2005; 80(9):1201–7.

[51] Chang FY, Peacock JE Jr, Musher DM, et al. Staphylococcus aureus bacteremia: recurrence and the impact of antibiotic treatment in a prospective multicenter study. Medicine (Baltimore) 2003;82(5):333–9.

[52] Khatib R, Johnson LB, Fakih MG, et al. Persistence in Staphylococcus aureus bacteremia: incidence, characteristics of patients and outcome. Scand J Infect Dis 2006;38(1):7–14.

[53] Siegman-Igra Y, Reich P, Orni-Wasserlauf R, et al. The role of vancomycin in the persistence or recurrence of Staphylococcus aureus bacteraemia. Scand J Infect Dis 2005;37(8):572–8.

[54] Shorr AF, Kunkel MJ, Kollef M. Linezolid versus vancomycin for Staphylococcus aureus bacteraemia: pooled analysis of randomized studies. J Antimicrob Chemother 2005;56(5): 923–9.

[55] Wunderink RG, Rello J, Cammarata SK, et al. Linezolid vs vancomycin: analysis of two double-blind studies of patients with methicillin-resistant Staphylococcus aureus nosocomial pneumonia. Chest 2003;124(5):1789–97.

[56] Guidelines for the management of adults with hospital-acquired, ventilator-associated, and healthcare-associated pneumonia. Am J Respir Crit Care Med 2005;171(4):388–416.

[57] Kaplan SL, Afghani B, Lopez P, et al. Linezolid for the treatment of methicillin-resistant Staphylococcus aureus infections in children. Pediatr Infect Dis J 2003;22(9 Suppl):S178–85.

[58] Micek ST, Dunne M, Kollef MH. Pleuropulmonary complications of Panton-Valentine leukocidin-positive community-acquired methicillin-resistant Staphylococcus aureus: importance of treatment with antimicrobials inhibiting exotoxin production. Chest 2005;128(4): 2732–8.

[59] Bernardo K, Pakulat N, Fleer S, et al. Subinhibitory concentrations of linezolid reduce Staphylococcus aureus virulence factor expression. Antimicrob Agents Chemother 2004; 48(2):546–55.

[60] Weigelt J, Itani K, Stevens D, et al. Linezolid versus vancomycin in treatment of complicated skin and soft tissue infections. Antimicrob Agents Chemother 2005;49(6):2260–6.

[61] Itani KM, Weigelt J, Li JZ, et al. Linezolid reduces length of stay and duration of intravenous treatment compared with vancomycin for complicated skin and soft tissue infections due to suspected or proven methicillin-resistant Staphylococcus aureus (MRSA). Int J Antimicrob Agents 2005;26(6):442–8.

[62] Metzler K, Hansen GM, Hedlin P, et al. Comparison of minimal inhibitory and mutant prevention drug concentrations of 4 fluoroquinolones against clinical isolates of methicillin-susceptible and -resistant Staphylococcus aureus. Int J Antimicrob Agents 2004;24(2):161–7.

[63] Jauregui LE, Babazadeh S, Seltzer E, et al. Randomized, double-blind comparison of once-weekly dalbavancin versus twice-daily linezolid therapy for the treatment of complicated skin and skin structure infections. Clin Infect Dis 2005;41(10):1407–15.

[64] Ellis-Grosse EJ, Babinchak T, Dartois N, et al. The efficacy and safety of tigecycline in the treatment of skin and skin-structure infections: results of 2 double-blind phase 3 comparison studies with vancomycin-aztreonam. Clin Infect Dis 2005;41(Suppl 5):S341–53.

[65] Ellis MW, Lewis JS II. Treatment approaches for community-acquired methicillin-resistant Staphylococcus aureus infections. Curr Opin Infect Dis 2005;18(6):496–501.

[66] Lee MC, Rios AM, Aten MF, et al. Management and outcome of children with skin and soft tissue abscesses caused by community-acquired methicillin-resistant Staphylococcus aureus. Pediatr Infect Dis J 2004;23(2):123–7.

[67] Darenberg J, Ihendyane N, Sjolin J, et al. Intravenous immunoglobulin G therapy in streptococcal toxic shock syndrome: a European randomized, double-blind, placebo-controlled trial. Clin Infect Dis 2003;37(3):333–40.

[68] Kaul R, McGeer A, Norrby-Teglund A, et al. Intravenous immunoglobulin therapy for streptococcal toxic shock syndrome–a comparative observational study. The Canadian Streptococcal Study Group. Clin Infect Dis 1999;28(4):800–7.

[69] Alejandria MM, Lansang MA, Dans LF, et al. Intravenous immunoglobulin for treating sepsis and septic shock. Cochrane Database Syst Rev 2002;1:CD001090.

[70] Darenberg J, Soderquist B, Normark BH, et al. Differences in potency of intravenous polyspecific immunoglobulin G against streptococcal and staphylococcal superantigens: implications for therapy of toxic shock syndrome. Clin Infect Dis 2004;38(6):836–42.

[71] Harbarth S, Dharan S, Liassine N, et al. Randomized, placebo-controlled, double-blind trial to evaluate the efficacy of mupirocin for eradicating carriage of methicillin-resistant Staphylococcus aureus. Antimicrob Agents Chemother 1999;43(6):1412–6.

[72] Kampf G, Jarosch R, Ruden H. Limited effectiveness of chlorhexidine based hand disinfectants against methicillin-resistant Staphylococcus aureus (MRSA). J Hosp Infect 1998;38(4): 297–303.

[73] Loeb M, Main C, Walker-Dilks C, et al. Antimicrobial drugs for treating methicillin-resistant Staphylococcus aureus colonization. Cochrane Database Syst Rev 2003;4:CD003340.

[74] Walsh TJ, Standiford HC, Reboli AC, et al. Randomized double-blinded trial of rifampin with either novobiocin or trimethoprim-sulfamethoxazole against methicillin-resistant Staphylococcus aureus colonization: prevention of antimicrobial resistance and effect of host factors on outcome. Antimicrob Agents Chemother 1993;37(6):1334–42.

[75] Darouiche R, Wright C, Hamill R, et al. Eradication of colonization by methicillin-resistant Staphylococcus aureus by using oral minocycline-rifampin and topical mupirocin. Antimicrob Agents Chemother 1991;35(8):1612–5.

[76] Shinefield H, Black S, Fattom A, et al. Use of a Staphylococcus aureus conjugate vaccine in patients receiving hemodialysis. N Engl J Med 2002;346(7):491–6.

[77] Roghmann M, Taylor KL, Gupte A, et al. Epidemiology of capsular and surface polysaccharide in Staphylococcus aureus infections complicated by bacteraemia. J Hosp Infect 2005; 59(1):27–32.

[78] Fattom A, Schneerson R, Szu SC, et al. Synthesis and immunologic properties in mice of vaccines composed of Staphylococcus aureus type 5 and type 8 capsular polysaccharides conjugated to Pseudomonas aeruginosa exotoxin A. Infect Immun 1990;58(7):2367–74.

[79] Fattom A, Fuller S, Propst M, et al. Safety and immunogenicity of a booster dose of Staphylococcus aureus types 5 and 8 capsular polysaccharide conjugate vaccine (StaphVAX) in hemodialysis patients. Vaccine 2004;23(5):656–63.

[80] Maira-Litran T, Kropec A, Goldmann DA, et al. Comparative opsonic and protective activities of Staphylococcus aureus conjugate vaccines containing native or deacetylated Staphylococcal Poly-N-acetyl-beta-(1–6)-glucosamine. Infect Immun 2005;73(10):6752–62.

[81] Hall AE, Domanski PJ, Patel PR, et al. Characterization of a protective monoclonal antibody recognizing Staphylococcus aureus MSCRAMM protein clumping factor A. Infect Immun 2003;71(12):6864–70.

[82] Benjamin DK, Schelonka R, White R, et al. A blinded, randomized, multicenter study of an intravenous Staphylococcus aureus immune globulin. J Perinatol 2006;26:290–5.

[83] Bloom B, Schelonka R, Kueser T, et al. Multicenter phase II study to assess safety and preliminary efficacy of Veronate, a donor selected anti-staphylococcal immune globulin in very low birth weight infants [abstract]. Pediatr Res 2004;55:392.

[84] Weisman LE, Fisher GW, Mandy GT, et al. Safety and pharmacokinetics of an anti-lipoteichoic acid humanized mouse chimeric antibody in healthy adults [abstract]. Pediatr Res 2002;51:270A.

ELSEVIER
SAUNDERS

PEDIATRIC CLINICS
OF NORTH AMERICA

Pediatr Clin N Am 53 (2006) 715–725

Genetic Aspects of the Etiology and Treatment of Asthma

John R. Meurer, MD, MBA[a,b,c,*],
James V. Lustig, MD[a,b,d], Howard J. Jacob, PhD[a,b]

[a]Medical College of Wisconsin and Children's Research Institute,
8701 Watertown Plank Road, Milwaukee, WI 53226, USA
[b]Downtown Health Center, 1020 North 12th Street,
Milwaukee, WI 53233, USA
[c]Fight Asthma Milwaukee Allies, Children's Hospital and Health System,
9000 West Wisconsin Avenue, MS 790, Milwaukee, WI 53201, USA
[d]Children's Hospital of Wisconsin, 9000 West Wisconsin Avenue, Milwaukee, WI 53201, USA

The primary objective of this article is to provide a review of the genetic aspects of the etiology and treatment of asthma for pediatric practitioners who are experienced in asthma diagnosis and management but lack expertise in genetics and immunology. This work is substantiated by reports in the literature and by our research and clinical experience in the fields of asthma, general and community pediatrics, allergy, immunology, and human and molecular genetics.

Context

The genetics of asthma is important in pediatric practice. Asthma is the most common chronic disorder in children and adolescents, the leading cause of hospitalizations in children under 15 years of age, and the leading cause of school absences [1]. Current clinical knowledge of the genetic aspects of asthma is needed to understand the epidemiology, pathogenesis, natural history, diagnosis, and management of children with asthma.

Dr. Meurer has received unrestricted grant support from GlaxoSmithKline, AstraZeneca, Merck, Schering Plough, Sepracor, and Novartis as director of continuing medical education programs in asthma diagnosis and management. Dr. Jacob serves on the board of directors of Physiogenix, Inc., where he is a founder and major shareholder. Physiogenix does not conduct any asthma research and is focused on developing new rat models of human diseases.

* Corresponding author. Downtown Health Center, 1020 North 12th Street, Milwaukee, WI 53233.
E-mail address: jmeurer@mcw.edu (J.R. Meurer).

Identifying the genes associated with asthma offers a means to better define its pathogenesis, with the promise of improving preventive strategies, diagnostic tools, and therapies [2].

Evidence acquisition

The data sources used for this review focused on computerized databases. We searched Ovid MEDLINE 1996 to February 2006 and Evidence Based Medicine Reviews, including the Cochrane Database of Systematic Reviews, Database of Abstracts of Reviews of Effects, and Cochrane Central Register of Controlled Trials, all through the first quarter of 2006, and the American College of Physicians Journal Club from 1991 to February 2006. We also used a pertinent chapter on genetics of asthma in a popular textbook of pediatric allergy [3].

Our search strategy focused on the keywords asthma and genetics. We limited articles to humans and English language in the years 2001 to 2006. We extracted pertinent review articles and original articles focused on the etiology or therapy, prevention, and control of asthma. We included the highest-quality evidence available in peer-reviewed medical journals, and the most recent systematic reviews. We focused on information relevant to pediatric clinical practice rather than technical data in genetic studies.

Evidence synthesis

MEDLINE listed 1007 articles on asthma genetics from 1996 through February 2006. The following section synthesizes the major findings of our review of the genetic aspects of the etiology and treatment of asthma for pediatric practitioners.

Genetics studies of asthma provide a greater understanding of disease pathogenesis. The identification of novel genes and associated pathways delineates new pharmacologic targets for developing therapeutics. Asthma genetic research may improve diagnostics that could identify susceptible individuals allowing early life screening and targeting of preventive therapies to at-risk individuals. Asthma pharmacogenetics can subclassify disease on the basis of drug-metabolizing polymorphisms and genetic modifiers, permitting targeting of specific therapies. Such data also may determine the likelihood of an individual's responding to a particular therapy and permit the development of comprehensive individualized treatment plans [3].

Human genetics and the etiology of asthma

Asthma is a phenotypically heterogeneous inflammatory airway disease associated with intermittent respiratory symptoms, bronchial hyperresponsiveness, and reversible airflow obstruction [4]. Genetic factors, predominantly atopy and parental history of asthma, are key components in the development of asthma [5]. Asthma and atopy are related conditions most likely involving multiple genes that interact with each other and the environment [6]. Genetic predisposition varies with race and ethnicity (ie, genes associated with asthma in one population may not be associated or may be less frequently associated with asthma in another population) [7]. The frequency of high-risk variants in candidate genes can differ between African Americans, Puerto Ricans, and Mexican Americans, and this might contribute to the differences in disease prevalence. Maintenance of certain allelic variants in the population over time might reflect selective pressures in previous generations [8].

The contribution of genetics to asthma has been examined in a wide variety of studies, ranging from epidemiologic association and twin studies to molecular analysis through high throughput cloning and microarray gene expression experiments [9]. Twin studies have indicated a considerable genetic component of asthma. This component most likely consists of genes of additive effect. Twin studies also have shown that individual specific environmental factors are important [10]. Epidemiologic studies provide evidence that the interaction of multiple genetic and environmental factors contributes to the causation of asthma. Patients who have asthma vary in age of onset, course, sensitivity to specific environmental precipitants, and response to therapy. Consequently, the relative contribution of genetic factors also may vary considerably among patients.

The prevalence of asthma has risen dramatically in the past two decades, suggesting that environmental risk factors have a key role. The high incidence of asthma in urban populations compared with a significantly lower incidence in rural populations strengthens this premise. Asthma, but not other manifestations of allergy, is less commonly reported among farm-reared children [11]. Control of environmental risk factors and improved treatment are the primary public health strategies for the prevention of asthma [12].

Several risk factors have been identified in the pathophysiology of asthma, including sensitization and exposure to cockroaches, house dust mites, and the mold *Alternaria tenuis*, among other aeroallergens. Viral respiratory infections, primarily those caused by respiratory syncytial virus, are a significant risk factor for the development of childhood wheezing in the first decade of life [5].

Symptoms of wheeze and persistent cough in the first year of life are associated with indoor allergens, such as cockroaches and persistent mold; air contaminants, such as exposure to tobacco smoke and to gas and wood-burning stoves; and maternal history of asthma [13].

A cohort study with assessment of exposure before the onset of asthma strengthened the evidence regarding the independent effects of parental atopy and exposure to molds on the development of asthma. A population-based, 6-year prospective cohort study of 1984 children 1 to 7 years of age found that 7.2% of children developed asthma during the study period, resulting in an incidence rate of 125 cases per 10,000 person-years. Parental atopy and the presence of mold odor in the home reported at baseline were independent determinants of asthma incidence, but no apparent interaction was observed [14].

Maternal history of asthma influences the relation between day care–related exposures and childhood asthma. In children without a maternal history of asthma, day care attendance in early life was associated with a decreased risk for asthma and recurrent wheezing at the age of 6 years, and with a decreased risk for any wheezing after the age of 4 years. This finding could imply that the impact of environmental components within the home or the benefit of exposure to different environments is important. Among children with a maternal history of asthma, day care in early life had no protective effect on asthma or recurrent wheezing at the age of 6 years. Instead it was associated with an increased risk for wheezing in the first 6 years of life, suggesting a greater contribution of genetics [15].

Asthma and chronic obstructive pulmonary disease

Asthma and chronic obstructive pulmonary disease (COPD) are common respiratory diseases that are caused by the interaction of genetic susceptibility with environmental factors. Environmental influences are important in both diseases, and although there are differences in genetic susceptibilities, there are also similarities [16]. The Dutch hypothesis, formulated in the 1960s, holds that the various forms of airway obstruction are different expressions of a single disease entity. It suggests that genetic factors (such as airway hyperresponsiveness and atopy), endogenous factors (such as age and sex), and exogenous factors (such as allergens, infections, and smoking) all play a role in the pathogenesis of chronic nonspecific lung disease [17]. Family studies pointed toward susceptibility loci for both asthma- and COPD-related phenotypes in the same chromosomal region. There is evidence for a gene–environment interaction with passive smoking for asthma patients compared with individual smoking for COPD patients. One candidate gene, interleukin-13, has shown similar results for both asthma and COPD [16].

To prove the Dutch hypothesis of genetic and environmental interactions in the development of asthma and COPD definitively, longitudinal genetic studies must be performed. Such studies must also include subjects with a range of airway obstruction phenotypes that do not necessarily meet the current strict definitions of asthma or COPD (ie, the extremes of these conditions that are used in clinical studies) [16].

Molecular genetics and the etiology of asthma

Sophisticated paradigms depict asthma as a disorder of complex genetic and environmental interactions that affect the developing immune system and ultimately result in the episodic release of pro-contractile mediators, including leukotrienes and prostaglandins, causing susceptible individuals to wheeze [18]. Initiation and regulation of allergic inflammation is influenced by many factors, including cell type, membrane receptors, and mediators generated. The altered response of targeted airway smooth muscle is an important factor in the subsequent expression of asthma. The genetic regulation and association of genetic polymorphisms has enhanced our understanding of host susceptibility [19].

The asthmatic response is characterized by elevated production of IgE, cytokines, and chemokines; mucus hypersecretion; airway obstruction; eosinophilia; and enhanced airway hyperreactivity to spasmogens. Clinical and experimental investigations have demonstrated a strong correlation between the presence of $CD4^+$ T helper 2 (Th2) cells, eosinophils, and disease severity, suggesting an integral role for these cells in the pathophysiology of asthma [20].

Physiological studies have led to the characterization of genetic variants associated with asthma or atopic airway inflammation in several biologic pathways potentially related to asthma. Genetic variants are present, for example, in the beta-adrenergic receptor, cytokines associated with the secretion of IgE and airway inflammation, and transferase presumed to be involved in the detoxification of inhaled irritants. One study reported gene–environment interaction in which the effect of smoking on the risk for asthma was increased by a specific beta-adrenergic receptor genotype [12].

Airway inflammation is a key factor in the mechanisms of asthma. Investigative bronchoscopy with segmental antigen challenge and induced sputum analyses to evaluate features of airway inflammation related to asthma severity have added insights into our understanding of these mechanisms [9].

Asthma genetics uses genetic mapping techniques to localize gene loci linked to asthma and physiologic studies followed by positioning cloning to identify genes that affect the disease process. Various mapping techniques have identified several genes and chromosome regions associated with asthma [4,21]. Different populations of patients might have different asthma profiles, and the association of specific genetic markers might be limited to specific traits and groups of patients [19]. For example, gene mapping and positional cloning have yielded information about a metalloproteinase, ADAM-33, that may have a role in inflammatory responses or smooth muscle hypertrophy or hyperreactivity [22]. ADAM-33 is an asthma susceptibility gene with lung-specific factors that regulate the susceptibility of lung epithelium and fibroblasts to remodeling in response to allergic inflammation [3].

Several chromosomal regions influencing asthma and atopy have been genetically mapped, and a role for several candidate genes has been established [2]. The number of candidate genes and implicated chromosomal regions remains large [4]. Position cloning is used to identify complex trait susceptibility genes. The approach involves the collection of well-pheno-typed cohorts (either through family-based or case-control designs), the generation of high-density, single nucleotide polymorphism linkage dis-equilibrium maps, and the application of powerful statistical methods to localize narrow regions of genetic association with disease. PHF11 and DPP10 genes relating to asthma were identified using this approach [23]. Atopic children may have a cytokine imbalance or dysregulation in which the transition from Th2-type to Th1-type immunity is delayed [5]. Chemo-kines, including thymus and activation-regulated cytokine, are important in the regulation of inflammation and IgE synthesis and have a role in asthma [9].

Surprisingly few of the genes associated with asthma involve known asthma mediators. The best-established asthma genes include disintegrin and ADAM 33, dipeptidyl peptidase 10, PHD finger protein 11, and the prostanoid DP1 receptor. Identification of these unsuspected genes has led to models of asthma pathogenesis that expand previous concepts of asthma as solely a disease of smooth muscle abnormalities, inflammatory cell pres-ence, and airway structural changes [18].

Th2 cells may induce asthma through the secretion of an array of cyto-kines (IL-4, -5, -9, -1) that activate inflammatory and residential effector pathways. In particular, IL-4 and IL-13 are produced at elevated levels in the asthmatic lung and may regulate hallmarks of the disease. The potency of IL-13 in promoting airway hyperreactivity and mucus hypersecretion and the ability of IL-13 blockade to abrogate critical aspects of experimental asthma suggest that is may be a critical cytokine in disease pathogenesis [20].

Extensive studies also have shown a central role for chemokines in or-chestrating aspects of the asthmatic response. Chemokines are potent leuko-cyte chemoattractants, cellular activating factors, and histamine-releasing factors, which makes them particularly important in the pathogenesis of al-lergic inflammation. In particular, the eotaxin subfamily of chemokines and their receptor (CC chemokine receptor 3) have emerged as central regulators of the asthmatic response [20].

Goblet cell hyperplasia has been established as a pathologic characteristic of asthma. Abnormalities in goblet cell number are accompanied by changes in stored and secreted mucin. The functional consequences of these changes in mucin stores and secretion can contribute to multiple clinical abnormal-ities in patients with asthma, including sputum production, airway narrow-ing, inflammation, exacerbations, and accelerated loss in lung function. $CD4^+$ T cells and their Th2 cytokine products are important mediators of goblet cell hyperplasia, and MUC5AC is the dominant mucin gene that is expressed in goblet cells [24].

Genetic factors almost certainly play a role in determining susceptibility to air pollutants, such as those involved with antioxidant defenses. The best studied of these in the context of air pollution risks are glutathione-S-trans-ferase polymorphisms [25].

Genetics and the treatment of asthma

Pharmacogenomics is the study of the relationship between patterns of genetic variability, or polymorphisms, in sets of genes and individual variability in the response to pharmacotherapy. An estimated 70% to 80% of variability in individual responses to therapy may have a genetic basis. Mechanisms that may have heritable variations that can alter therapeutic and toxic responses to drugs include absorption, distribution, metabolism, excretion, interaction with biologic pathways, and unintended targets [26].

Although genes coding for some key treatment targets contain little polymorphic variation, like the muscarinic M2 and M3 receptors, other genes whose products are important targets of asthma treatment contain extensive genetic variation. The best examples of the latter are the beta(2)-adrenoceptor and 5-lipooxygenase (ALOX5) genes [27]. Genetic variability in both of these genes may account in part for interindividual variability in treatment response [28].

Polymorphisms of the beta(2)-adrenergic receptor may influence airway responses to regular inhaled beta-agonist treatment [29]. Albuterol (R)- and (S)-enantiomers may have distinct effects on airway relaxation and regulation of inflammation, suggesting that mono-isomeric therapy may have therapeutic advantages [9]. In one study, levalbuterol decreased the need for asthma hospitalization; however, the length of stay was similar in racemic albuterol and levalbuterol groups [30].

Treatment with anti-leukotriene drugs results in clinical improvement in many, though not all, patients with asthma. Polymorphisms of two genes in the leukotriene pathway, the gene and the synthase gene, have been demonstrated to have pharmacogenetic associations with asthma. Polymorphisms of the ALOX5 promoter gene and the leukotriene C_4 synthase gene have been associated with changes in the function of these genes, leading to association studies of the polymorphisms' effects on responses to leukotriene modifier therapy [26]. A genotype that limits expression of ALOX5 is associated with reduced leukotriene C_4 production by eosinophils and is predictive of moderate to severe asthma in children. Children with asthma having a genetic variant that impairs their ability to express ALOX5 have more severe disease than those bearing genotypes that have more efficient baseline expression of ALOX5 [31]. For example, no difference in clinical response to montelukast treatment was observed between aspirin-intolerant asthmatics and aspirin-tolerant asthmatics [32].

It is hoped that linkage and association studies will define new therapeutic targets for asthma, but until then, studies have focused on improving response to beta(2)-adrenoceptor agonist and leukotriene modifier therapy. Genetic polymorphism may account for interindividual differences in toxicity and efficacy of asthma medications. An initial approach will be the use of panels of polymorphisms to calculate the relative risk–benefit ratio of a particular therapeutic course for an individual patient [26]. To date, analysis of single nucleotide alterations, polymorphisms, and limited sets of closely linked genetic polymorphisms or haplotypes are inconclusive in delineating how genotype predictors can be used to optimize current asthma therapies based on each patient's genetic profile [33]. Positional cloning and chromosomal walking to detect subtle regional variations may lead to individualized therapies.

Asthma treatment with inhaled steroids demonstrates significant person-to-person variability. Genetic variation could contribute to this response to inhaled glucocorticosteroids. The approach of a test and validation strategy to assess steroid pathway candidate genes can identify replicated treatment responses. Researchers at the Channing Laboratory of Harvard University genotyped 131 single nucleotide polymorphisms in 14 candidate genes in the steroid pathway in an 8-week clinical trial of 470 adults with moderate to severe asthma. They then validated findings in a second population of individuals with childhood asthma in a 4-year clinical trial of inhaled steroids and a third population of adults with asthma. One gene, corticotrophin-releasing hormone receptor 1, demonstrated multiple single nucleotide polymorphisms associations within each of the three populations [34]. Individuals homozygous for the variants of interest manifested a doubling to quadrupling of the lung function response to corticosteroids compared with lack of the variants [35]. Further research in the children demonstrated that TBX21, which encodes for the transcription factor expressed in T cells, may be an important determinant of pharmacogenetic response to the therapy of asthma with inhaled corticosteroids [36].

The future of asthma genetics research

An expert working group of the National Heart, Lung, and Blood Institute identified the genetics, gene–environment interactions, and pharmacogenetics as one of six of the top priority areas for research in asthma [37]. Asthma genetics research is still in the early stages and faces some technical problems. Such studies will require the identification of standardized definitions of asthma phenotypes, intermediate biologic measures associated with the risk for asthma, well-defined populations in unbiased studies with sufficient power to detect small effects, and the methods to concurrently measure both environmental and genetic risk factors. Any reported association between a genetic variant and asthma risk cannot be considered established until the results of the study have been replicated [12].

Determining associations between genes and asthma is just the first step in the translation of genomic research into clinical insights. This effort will require increasing attention to the study of the functions of proteins, or proteomics, including the characterization of the proteins identified as a result of genomic research [12].

Ongoing research is focused on identifying which children who have wheezing early will progress to childhood asthma. Several prospective epidemiologic studies are investigating the relations among cytokine dysregulation, respiratory tract infections, and allergen exposure and sensitization in the development of asthma. Identifying the pathogenic mechanisms could enable clinicians to identify children at high risk and thereby to treat childhood asthma more effectively [5].

Corticosteroids are the most potent anti-inflammatory agents used to treat chronic inflammatory diseases, such as asthma. About 5% of asthmatic patients do not respond well, or at all, to corticosteroid therapy, however. Although this phenomenon is uncommon, it poses a difficult therapeutic problem because few alternative therapies are available and these patients account for one half of the health care costs of asthma. If the mechanisms for corticosteroid insensitivity are understood they may in turn provide insight into the key mechanisms of corticosteroid action and allow a rational way to treat these individuals whose disease is severe [38].

Pharmacogenomic assays will be readily available in clinical laboratories by 2010. Considering the rapid fall in the cost of genotyping at multiple loci simultaneously, it is unlikely that the technology will limit the introduction of this methodology; rather, the design and execution of clinical trials in multiple populations will be the rate-limiting step. We advocate obtaining genetic material in all clinical asthma trials and consideration of prospective genotype-stratified clinical trials. Such association studies and biologically informative pharmacogenomic trials over the next decade should allow us to minimize drug side effects but also to maximize drug efficacy [26].

Although the claims for immediate impact of genomics have sometimes been overstated, the ultimate consequences of the integration of genomics into medical research and practice are likely to be revolutionary. By providing insights into the networks and pathways of biology, genomics has already begun to alter the fundamental understanding of health and diseases such as asthma. By providing more sophisticated knowledge of biology at the individual level and of disease typology, genomics has already begun to personalize health care. By widening the number of potential drug targets and better identifying those children a specific drug is likely to benefit and those it is likely to harm, genomics already has begun to expand the pharmacotherapeutic regimen. By changing societal discussion of race, ethnicity, and disparities, genomics already has begun to influence society [39].

Summary

This article provides a clinical review of the genetic aspects of the etiology and treatment of asthma for pediatric practitioners. Asthma and chronic obstructive pulmonary disease are common respiratory diseases that are caused by the interaction of genetic susceptibility with environmental factors. The asthmatic response is characterized by elevated production of IgE, cytokines, and chemokines; mucus hypersecretion; airway obstruction; eosinophilia; and enhanced airway hyperreactivity to spasmogens.

The contribution of genetics to asthma has been examined in epidemiologic association and twin studies and genetic mapping techniques and positioning cloning. The best-established asthma genes include disintegrin and ADAM 33, dipeptidyl peptidase 10, PHD finger protein 11, and the prostanoid DP1 receptor. Polymorphisms of the beta(2)-adrenergic receptor may influence airway responses to inhaled beta-agonists. Polymorphisms of the 5-lipooxegenase promoter gene and the leukotriene C_4 synthase gene may have effects on responses to leukotriene modifier therapy. TBX21, which encodes for the transcription factor expressed in T cells, may affect response to inhaled corticosteroids.

By providing insights into the networks and pathways of biology, genetics already has begun to alter the fundamental understanding of health and diseases such as asthma. Within a few years, practitioners may apply sophisticated knowledge of biology at the individual level and of disease typology to expand the pharmacotherapeutic regimen and to personalize diagnosis and management.

References

[1] American Academy of Allergy, Asthma, and Immunology. Pediatric asthma: promoting best practice, guide for managing asthma in children. Milwaukee, WI: AAAAI; 1999.

[2] Cookson WO. Asthma genetics. Chest 2002;121(3 Suppl):7S–13S.

[3] Holloway JW, Cakebread JA, Holgate ST. The genetics of allergic disease and asthma. In: Leung DYM, Sampson HA, Geha RS, et al, editors. Pediatric allergy: principles and practice. St. Louis, MO: Mosby; 2003. p. 23–38.

[4] Collaborative Study on the Genetics of Asthma. A genome-wide search for asthma susceptibility loci in ethnically diverse populations. Nat Genet 1997;15(4):389–92.

[5] Lemanske RJ Jr. Issues in understanding pediatric asthma: epidemiology and genetics. JACI 2002;109(Suppl 6):S521–4.

[6] Blumenthal JB, Blumenthal MN. Genetics of asthma. Med Clinics N Am 2002;86(5): 937–50.

[7] Ghosh B, Sharma S, Nagarkatti R. Genetics of asthma: current research paving the way for development of personalized drugs. Indian J Med Res 2003;117:185–97.

[8] Barnes KC. Genetic epidemiology of health disparities in allergy and clinical immunology. J Allergy Clin Immunol 2006;117:243–54.

[9] Busse WW, Rosenwasser LJ. Mechanisms of asthma. JACI 2003;111(3 Suppl):S799–804.

[10] Koppelman GH, Los H, Postma DS. Genetic and environment in asthma: the answer of twin studies. Eur Respir J 1999;13(1):8–14.

[11] Adler A, Tager I, Quintero DR. Decreased prevalence of asthma among farm-reared children compared with those who are rural but not farm-reared. JACI 2005;115(1):67–73.

[12] Burke W. Genomics as a probe for disease biology. N Engl J Med 2003;349(10):969–74.

[13] Belanger K, Beckett W, Triche E, et al. Symptoms of wheeze and persistent cough in the first year of life: associations with indoor allergens, air contaminants, and maternal history of asthma. Am J Epid 2003;158(3):195–202.

[14] Jaakkola JJ, Hwang BF, Jaakkola N. Home dampness and molds, parental atopy, and asthma in childhood: a 6-year population-based cohort study. Environ Health Perspect 2005;113(3):357–61.

[15] Celedon JC, Wright RJ, Litonjua AA, et al. Day care attendance in early life, maternal history of asthma, and asthma at age of 6 years. AJRCCM 2003;167(9):1239–43.

[16] Meyers DA, Larj MJ, Lange L. Genetics of asthma and COPD: similar results for different phenotypes. Chest 2004;126(2 Suppl):105S–10S.

[17] Postma DS, Boezen HM. Rationale for the Dutch hypothesis: allergy and airway hyper-responsiveness as genetic factors and their interaction with environment in the development of asthma and COPD. Chest 2004;126(Suppl 2):96S–104S.

[18] Lilly CM, Palmer LJ. Genetic studies seek to advance our knowledge by identifying the differences in our genetic make-up that cause us to be susceptible. Am J Respir Cell Mol Biol 2005;33(3):224–6.

[19] Bochner BS, Busse WW. Allergy and asthma. JACI 2005;15(5):953–9.

[20] Zimmermann N, Hershey GK, Foster PS, et al. Chemokines in asthma: cooperative interaction between chemokines and IL-13. JACI 2003;111(2):227–42.

[21] Daniels SE, Bhattacharrya S, James A, et al. A genome-wide search for quantitative trait loci underlying asthma. Nature 1996;383(6597):247–50.

[22] Shapiro SD, Owen CA. ADAM-33 surfaces as an asthma gene. N Engl J Med 2002;347(12): 936–8.

[23] Weiss ST, Raby BA. Asthma genetics 2003. Hum Mol Genet 2004;13(Spec 1):R83–9.

[24] Fahy JV. Goblet cell and mucin gene abnormalities in asthma. Chest 2002;122(Suppl 6): 320S–6S.

[25] Peden DB. Epidemiology and genetics of asthma risk associated with air pollution. JACI 2005;115(2):213–9.

[26] Wechsler ME, Israel E. How pharmacogenetics will play a role in the management of asthma. AJRCCM 2005;172:12–8.

[27] Hines RN, McCarver DG. Pharmacogenetics and the future of drug therapy. Pediatr Clin North Am 2006;53(4):591–619.

[28] Fenech A, Hall IP. Pharmacogenetics of asthma. Br J Clin Pharm 2002;53(1):3–15.

[29] Israel E, Drazen JM, Liggett SB, et al. Effect of polymorphism of the beta(2)-adrenergic receptor on response to regular use of albuterol in asthma. Int Arch All Immunol 2001; 124(1–3):183–6.

[30] Carl JC, Myers TR, Kirchner HL, et al. Comparison of racemic albuterol and levalbuterol for treatment of acute asthma. J Pediatr 2003;143:731–6.

[31] Kalayci O, Birben E, Sackesen C, et al. ALOX5 promotor genotype, asthma severity and LTC4 production by eosinophils. Allergy 2006;61:97–103.

[32] Mastalerz L, Nizankowska E, Sanak M, et al. Clinical and genetic features underlying the response of patients with bronchial asthma to of the treatment with a leukotriene receptor antagonist. Eur J Clin Invest 2002;32(12):949–55.

[33] Wallace AM, Sandford AJ. Therapeutic response to asthma medications: genotype predictors. Treat Respir Med 2004;3(3):161–71.

[34] Weiss ST, Lake SL, Silverman ES, et al. Asthma steroid pharmacogenetics: a study strategy to identify replicated treatment responses. Proc Am Thor Soc 2004;1(4):364–7.

[35] Tantisira KG, Lake S, Silverman ES, et al. Corticosteroid pharmacogenetics: association of sequence variants in CRHR1 with improved lung function in asthmatics treated with inhaled corticosteroids. Hum Mol Genet 2004;13(13):1353–9.

[36] Tantisira KG, Hwang ES, Raby BA, et al. TBX21: a functional variant predicts improvement in asthma with the use of inhaled corticosteroids. Proc Natl Acad Sci USA 2004; 101(52):18099–104.

[37] Busse WW, Banks-Schlegel S, Noel P, et al. Future research directions in asthma: an NHLBI working group report. ARJCCM 2004;170(6):683–90.

[38] Adcock IM, Lane SJ. Corticosteroid-insensitive asthma: molecular mechanisms. J Endocrinol 2003;178(3):347–55.

[39] Guttmacher AE, Collins FS. Realizing the promise of genomics in biomedical research. JAMA 2005;294(11):1399–402.

ELSEVIER
SAUNDERS

PEDIATRIC CLINICS
OF NORTH AMERICA

Pediatr Clin N Am 53 (2006) 727–749

Inflammatory Bowel Disease—Environmental Modification and Genetic Determinants

Subra Kugathasan, MD[a],*,
Devendra Amre, MBBS, PhD[b]

[a]Department of Pediatrics, Medical College of Wisconsin,
8701 Watertown Plank Road, Milwaukee, WI 53226, USA
[b]Department of Pediatrics, University of Montreal, Research Center,
Saint-Justine Hospital, 3175, Cote-Ste-Catherine, Montreal, PQ H3T 1C5, Canada

Crohn's disease (CD) and ulcerative colitis (UC), collectively known as inflammatory bowel disease (IBD), are increasing in incidence among children and negatively impact their growth, education, and social well-being. The currently proposed genetic model for IBD phenotypes emphasizes complex interactions between environmental factors and promoting and modifying genetic determinants, resulting in the clinical expression of the disease in the gastrointestinal (GI) tract of genetically predisposed individuals. Complex disease such as IBD is controlled by multiple risk factors that interact and evolve together. A major breakthrough in understanding the pathogenesis of CD occurred with the identification of the first IBD susceptibility gene, *CARD15*. More recently, many more single nucleotide polymorphisms (SNPs) in at least eight susceptibility loci from several chromosomes have been associated with IBD. The most consistent environmental factors believed to be associated in the etiology of CD are smoking, perinatal events, childhood infections, microbial agents, diet, and domestic hygiene. Complex diseases such as IBD cannot be understood in terms of a simple disease model; instead, they inherently and intrinsically are characterized by complex networks of interacting genetic and environmental causal agents that are embedded in pathways connecting the genome with disease-related phenotypes. Clarification of these genes and environmental interactions will require well-designed clinical studies in carefully phenotyped

---

* Corresponding author.
   E-mail address: skuga@mcw.edu (S. Kugathasan).

0031-3955/06/$ - see front matter © 2006 Elsevier Inc. All rights reserved.
doi:10.1016/j.pcl.2006.05.009   *pediatric.theclinics.com*

population-based cohorts to identify the lifetime gene–gene and gene–environmental interactions that determine the susceptibility and eventual outcome of IBD (Fig. 1). Studies such as International HapMap Project and the promise of whole genome association scans likely will lead to major advances during the next decade.

Introduction: interaction of environmental and genetics in pediatric inflammatory bowel disease

Is there an environmental cause for pediatric IBD when there is a strong link between genetics and IBD? This is perhaps the key question that has been dominating research in the pathogenesis of IBD for the past 20 years. Numerous reviews on the topic emphasize the importance of this research and highlight the complexity of defining the specific risk factors [1–3]. Various lines of evidence suggest that the environment could play an important role. The most convincing evidence is based on observations from twin studies. Monozygotic twins (MZ) show concordance rates ranging from 36% to 58% for CD and 8% to 16% for UC. Dizygotic twins (DZ) show average concordance rates of 4% for CD and UC [4]. Although the higher concordance observed among MZ twins compared with DZ twins suggests contributions from genetic risk factors, the high concordance is confounded by shared environmental risk factors and shared genetic risk factors. In addition, the approximately 50% lack of concordance for CD and nearly 80% lack of concordance for UC among monozygotic twins strongly suggests that a large proportion of CD and UC cases are linked to environmental exposures. In general, about 30% to 40% of adults who have IBD have a family history of IBD, whereas about 20% to 30% of children who have IBD have a family member affected with IBD [4]. These proportions

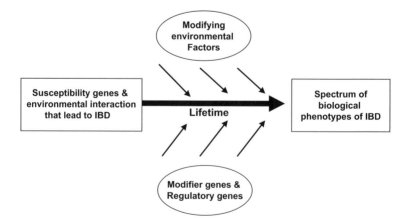

Fig. 1. Lifetime interactions between genetic and environmental interactions continue to play roles in IBD susceptibility and different phenotypes.

suggest that IBD is more or less a sporadic disease, wherein most of the affected individuals do not have a positive family history. Even among those who do have a family history of disease, the associations may be a result of shared environmental or genetic risk factors. Unfortunately, the scientific community has tended to dissect the evidence to support schools of thought and added fuel to a largely redundant debate on whether nature or nurture is more important for predisposition to IBD. The following paragraphs will examine the role of environment and genes as risk factors for IBD, and argue that the pathogenesis of IBD almost certainly is mediated by a network of effects, meaning that neither genetic nor environmental agents are separate causes of the disease state, but instead, it is their interactions that determine the risk.

Epidemiological descriptive studies

Descriptive studies performed during the latter half of the 20th century revealed that the incidence of CD varies in different geographical populations. The highest rates are observed in European and North American populations, with the lowest rates seen among Japanese and New Zealanders [5]. These discrepancies probably reflect differences in exposure to either environmental or genetic factors. A study of the time trends in disease incidence has shown that the incidence of CD has increased substantially in most developed countries such as Scotland, Denmark, the United Kingdom, the United States, and Japan [5,6]. Such increases over time could be a result of exposures to infections, changing dietary habits (this may change the microflora of the gut), changing hygiene practices, use of medications, vaccinations, or other factors. Studies evaluating birth cohort patterns and clustering of UC based on time and geography support an infectious etiology for IBD [7–9]. Studies on migrant populations have provided further support for the influence of environmental factors in CD etiology. For example, Jayanthi and colleagues [10] compared the incidence of CD during two time periods (1970s and 1980s) between indigenous Caucasians and South Asians who migrated to the United Kingdom at an early age [10]. They reported that the incidence among Caucasians was slightly higher during the 1970s but that during the 1980s, incidence among South Asians increased to that of Caucasians, suggesting environmental triggers. Although it is difficult to disentangle the role of specific environmental or genetic risk factors based on this evidence, some studies do suggest a role for environmental triggers. The rapid increase in disease rates within a short period after World War II could be attributed to the exposure to infectious agents [6]. Perhaps more indicative of the role for infectious agents are the observations on the temporal and geographical clustering of CD cases and the seasonal variation in the incidence of disease [7,11]. The observation of the development of IBD in married couples adds further support for the presence of infectious agents or dietary exposures [12]. A role for gene–environmental interactions recently was suggested through observations made by Mont-gomery and colleagues [13]. When studying the incidence of IBD in a cohort of individuals born within a week of each other, the authors reported that the incidence of IBD was significantly higher among South Asians compared with the indigenous European population even after controlling for potentially confounding variables [13]. Based on the idea that infant mortality is a good indicator of early life events and is strongly inversely correlated with IBD (infant mortality is very high among the South Asian populations), the authors postulated that South Asians probably have greater genetic predisposition that is unmasked only in the presence of environmental exposures. It could be speculated that these exposures prob-ably relate to perinatal and early childhood infections. There is evidence from Japan that the incidence of CD is increasing with changes in dietary habits [14].

Specific risk factors

More direct evidence on the role of specific environmental risk factors can be obtained from analytic observational studies such as cohort, cross-sectional, and case-control studies. Although some IBD studies have specif-ically targeted the pediatric population, much of the evidence is for adult populations. The following paragraphs briefly review the three environmen-tal risk factors most commonly investigated for their role in IBD pathogen-esis: diet, infections (including hygiene and appendectomy), and smoking.

Diet

Examining dietary elements for their potential association with IBD is natural considering that the GI tract is exposed to a plethora of antigens, most of which are acquired from diet. Thus, it is not surprising that numer-ous investigators have explored whether dietary consumption of fats, vege-tables, fruits, and carbohydrates in particular are related to IBD. The evidence across these different studies is extremely inconsistent. The evi-dence is far more consistent for dietary carbohydrate consumption, where most studies show elevated risks for IBD with higher consumption of refined carbohydrates [15]. It is possible that this consistency is a reflection of diet after disease onset (reverse causality) rather than pre-illness diet. The Gilat and colleagues [16] study was based entirely on children and adolescents. An international study on children younger than 20 years used a dietary assess-ment that was part of a large inquiry that included variables measuring in-fections and hygiene. Cases were mostly prevalent (less than 5 years since diagnosis). No details were available on the dietary questionnaire used. Findings revealed a higher consumption of whole wheat bread and lower consumption of oatmeal cereals among CD cases. Vegetable/fruit consump-tion was not associated with CD.

Infections/hygiene

The environmental exposures that have generated the most interest and controversy have been the associations between infections and hygiene and IBD. To date, most of the studies performed are prevalent case-control studies with retrospective information on exposures ascertained through interviews. Different markers of infection and hygiene exposures have been used. Several case-control studies specifically have studied patients younger than 20 years of age [16–20]. In one of the first studies among children, Gilat and colleagues [16] reported elevated risks for UC but not CD from recurrent respiratory tract infections within the first 10 years after birth and lower risks from varicella for UC (70% versus 79% in controls, $P < .01$) but not for CD. For both UC and CD, no associations with other viral/bacterial infections or with hygiene-related variables (eg, number of siblings, bedroom sharing, and home environment) were observed. Koletzko and colleagues [17,18] reported that diarrhea during infancy was associated with CD and UC. Rigas and colleagues [19] found a nonsignificant trend for decreasing risks with breast feeding, birth order, and sibship size for both UC and CD. In a population-based case-control study, Baron and colleagues [20] reported increased risk for UC with bedroom sharing, diseases during pregnancy, and smallpox vaccination (no estimate provided). Risks were elevated for CD from breast feeding and BCG vaccination, whereas drinking tap water was protective. No relationship was seen with other hygiene-related exposures (crude analysis). In the authors' own recent case-control study [21], they observed that children who were diagnosed with infection by a physician, who owned a pet, and who stayed in crowded homes had elevated risks for CD.

By and large, evidence from the six studies performed among children suggests that infections and related hygiene exposures in early childhood may increase risk for UC or CD. These findings are consistent with observations made for adult-onset IBD except for two studies. In one case-control study, based on subjects between 16 and 87 years of age, Gent and colleagues [22] reported that the availability of hot water (odds ratio [OR] = 5.0, 95% confidence interval [CI] = 1.4 to 17.3), use of a separate bathroom (OR = 3.3, 95% CI = 1.3 to 8.3), and a sewage system (OR = 2.6, 95% CI = 0.9 to 7.3) were associated with increased risks for CD [22]. No associations with UC were obvious, however. In another study, Duggan and colleagues [23] reported that the nonavailability of hot water before age 11 was associated with significant protection (OR = 0.56, 95% CI = 0.3 to 0.9) from CD [23]. Other studies evaluating markers of hygiene suggest lower prevalence of *Helicobacter pylori* in IBD [24–26], while others suggest no associations [27,28]. The only study evaluating serology for hepatitis A virus found no associations with UC or CD [29].

Appendectomy as a risk factor for UC has been a subject of detailed study. Strong inverse associations with UC (OR: 0.31, 95% CI: 0.26 to

0.37) were shown in a meta-analysis [30]. Appendectomy for possible appendicitis (rather than incidental) confers protection [31]. The evidence for CD is less clear, although a recent study has shown that appendectomy enhances the risk for acquiring CD [32]. In the only study among children, Gilat and colleagues [16] reported lower prevalence of appendectomy among patients who had UC and a higher prevalence among patients who had CD compared with controls [16]. Information on antibiotic use and risk for IBD in children is also unclear. Gilat and colleagues [16] reported no associations with CD or UC. Many studies also have explored other surrogate markers of infection such as breast feeding [16,18–21]. By and large, breast feeding has been found to be protective, although Baron and colleagues [20] have reported elevated risks. The risks from day care attendance, birth order, sibship size, and owning a pet are also inconsistent.

Smoking

Smoking is perhaps the only environmental exposure that consistently has been associated with risks for IBD. Nonetheless, it has been shown to be positively associated with CD and negatively associated with UC. The mechanisms underlying these diametrically opposite effects, however, are unclear. Calkins and colleagues [33] used meta-analysis to show that life-long nonsmokers had an approximately threefold elevated risk for UC compared with smokers [33]. The lower risk also was shown to be associated with the number of cigarettes smoked, and that former smokers tend to lose their protection on cessation. Although the association between smoking and IBD is confirmed for adult-onset IBD, evidence for pediatric onset IBD is limited. Three of the five studies among children evaluated this exposure. Rigas and colleagues [19] did not find any association between maternal smoking and both CD and UC. Baron and colleagues [20] reported an association between passive smoking (either by parents or care givers) for UC or CD, whereas Amre and colleagues [21] did not find any association between maternal smoking and CD. They reported that children who smoked had a tendency for an elevated risk for CD, but these findings were based on small numbers.

Environmental risk factors for pediatric inflammatory bowel disease: what is new, and where do we stand?

The evidence for specific environmental factors contributing to pediatric onset is limited and inconsistent. The observed differences between studies could have resulted largely from differences in study designs used and the varying tools implemented to measure the relevant exposures. Given the comparatively low incidence of pediatric IBD, most of the studies were case-control studies with exposure ascertained using questionnaires. Misclassification of exposure is a serious possibility, especially for dietary and infection-related exposures, and differences in their rates across studies would lead to varying degrees of associations. Given the differing IBD phenotypes in children as compared with adults, it is paramount that comprehensive dietary evaluations be performed using validated questionnaires and newly diagnosed patients. In the absence of the latter, any investigation will be prone to misclassification, recall bias, and reverse causality. On the other hand, varying results across geographically diverse populations could indicate that the observed heterogeneity is a true heterogeneity resulting from differential susceptibility to similar environmental insults mediated by potential genetic variants, a reflection of the presence of gene–environment interactions.

Genetic determinants in inflammatory bowel disease—available evidence

A major breakthrough in understanding the pathogenesis of CD occurred with the identification of the first IBD susceptibility gene, *CARD15,* also known as *NOD2* [34]. *CARD15* is a cytoplasmic molecule involved in sensing unique microbial cell wall components. Three SNPs within the *CARD15/NOD2* mutations (R702W, G908R, and 1007fsinsC) are established independent risk factors for CD in Caucasians [35,36]. Interestingly, *CARD15/NOD2* mutations are absent or very rare in Asians (Japanese, Chinese, and Korean), Arabs, Africans, and African Americans [34]. Even among Caucasian patients who have CD, a great amount of genetic heterogeneity exists. The *CARD15/NOD2*-dependent population-attributable risk is mild to modest among Northern European populations (Irish, Norwegians, Scots, Fins), as compared with populations residing in the lower latitudes (Germans and Italians). Individuals with one of the three major disease-associated alleles have a two- to fourfold increased risk for developing CD, whereas homozygous or compound heterozygous carriers have an up to 40-fold increase in genotype-relative risk [37]. Despite their strong association with CD, genetic alterations of the *CARD15/NOD2* gene are neither sufficient nor necessary for the development of CD. This is based on the observation that 1% to 5% of the general Caucasian population is homozygous, and 10% to 20% is heterozygous for CD-associated mutations. Additionally, up to 70% of patients who have CD do not have *CARD15/NOD2* alleles mutated [37]. Furthermore, CARD15/NOD2-deficient mice do not develop intestinal inflammation spontaneously [38]. Based on haplotype analysis, emerging data suggest that *CARD15/NOD2* mutations might have arisen recently [34].

Besides the *CARD15/NOD2* gene, particular interest has been focused on other replicated IBD loci such as the IBD5 region on chromosome 5. The locus first was identified in a genome-wide linkage scan, and the association of the IBD5-risk haplotype with CD subsequently was confirmed by three other independent groups [39–41]. By using fine mapping, linkage disequilibrium methods, and haplotype analysis, the IBD5 region subsequently was replicated and narrowed to an 11-SNP haplotype of 250 kb. Two novel polymorphisms in the solute carrier family *22A4/22A5* (*SLC22A4/A5*) genes within this region were identified in the Canadian population and proposed as two CD-associated alleles carried by the same haplotype, *SLC22A-TC*. *SLC22A4* and *SLC22A5* encode the organic cation transporters 1 and 2, respectively. Interestingly, the IBD5 locus was associated most strongly with the early onset of CD (maximum LOD score of 3.9 in CD children under 16 years at disease onset), but only a modest effect was seen when adult-onset CD was included (maximum LOD score 2.4) from the initial studies, thereby raising the hope that IBD5 may represent an early-onset CD gene [42]. Recent studies from pediatric-onset CD cohorts, however, showed that the effect of IBD5 risk is only modest and lower compared with adult-onset CD. Consistent with previously reported epistatic interactions between the *IBD5* and *IBD1* loci (encompassing the *CARD15/NOD2* gene), the disease risk was enhanced in the presence of both CD-associated *SLC22A4-A5* and *CARD15/NOD2* mutations [43].

By using a positional cloning approach, Stoll and colleagues [44] identified disease-associated variants responsible for the previously described linkage of CD with chromosome 10q23. The investigators described three IBD-associated genetic variations in the disk large homolog 5 (*DLG5*) gene, a gene encoding a scaffolding protein involved in maintaining epithelial integrity death/proliferation. The authors also examined the gene–gene interaction between *DLG5* and *CARD15,* and showed an association between the 113A variant and the presence of *CARD15* variants. A recent article by Daly and colleagues [45] further supports that *DLG5* does confer IBD susceptibility. Recently, Friedrichs and colleagues [46] published a report using multi-variate logistic regression analysis to examine several large IBD cohorts from Germany, Italy, and Quebec, Canada. The authors found that the *DLG5* variant is a modest susceptibility risk factor for CD (OR 1.5). More interesting though, was the finding that a dramatic increase in risk was seen for men (OR 2.49) but not for women (OR 1.0).

Despite the critical protective role of certain toll-like receptors (TLRs) at the intestinal mucosal interface, only minor genetic variations affecting the TLR signaling pathway have been identified in IBD [47]. Furthermore, a complex intronic polymorphism of the *CARD4/NOD1* gene recently was linked to CD development [48]. *CARD4/NOD1* confers cellular responsiveness to the unique PGN motif, suggesting a more general involvement of bacterial component sensing in this inflammatory disease.

Many other IBD loci (IBD3, IBD4, and IBD6–9) and alleles have been proposed throughout the human genome. Many susceptibility variants can be expected to confer low relative risks, and independent replication of their association will require a population-based analysis. Modifying loci on 4q23–25 and on 7q have been unraveled, with a suggested role of the *NF-κB1* gene expression and of the multi-drug resistance 1 gene (*MDR1*), respectively [34]. *mdr1* −/− mice have been shown to develop spontaneous colitis [49]. Recently, Brant and colleagues [50] reported a significant association within the common *Ala893* polymorphism in a multi-center North American cohort. Given the pharmacogenetic significance of *MDR1*, combined with its importance in mediating intestinal epithelial homeostasis, unveiling the role of these transporter genes will provide important insights into the pathogenesis and treatment of IBD.

In addition to genetic approaches, structural and functional studies of the candidate genes are required. Evaluation of genes that are coexpressed under same condition also is required to gain insight into the pathways involved. It is necessary to carry out additional expression studies of the candidate genes in healthy and diseased tissue to determine whether they are involved in the pathogenesis of IBD, since these genes may alter protein function and expression. For the genes of interest, animal models, such as knock-out or transgenic mice, could be used to further assess the function and the roles of these genes.

New strategies for mapping genes in inflammatory bowel disease—whole genome association approach and HapMap project

Up until now, the search for IBD genes up primarily has been based on linkage mapping and has not harnessed the full power of linkage disequilibrium (LD) (association) mapping on a genome-wide scale. When susceptibility loci are identified, they span larger chromosomal segments and contain a large number of candidate genes. Consequently, there is a need to develop further mapping strategies to overcome these limitations. On the flip side, LD mapping is not guaranteed to identify susceptibility variants if multiple rare susceptibility alleles exist within a given disease locus, or if there is extensive LD around the disease locus. The latter has been the case for the IBD5 locus in CD, where it is difficult, if not impossible, to distinguish one SNP as the etiological variant over others in strong LD with it. Using a high-density set of markers in an association study is likely to have greater power to localize genes with small-to-moderate effects. Following the seminal work by Risch and Merikangas [51], genome-wide association analyses are likely to be a powerful approach for disease mapping. The recent success of the whole-genome LD mapping approach in age-related macular degeneration, another complex disease, is of great interest [52]. Here alleles of relatively large effect were found in the presence of marginal evidence of linkage. Completion of phase 2 of the International HapMap Project, which will allow intelligent selection of a subset of SNPs that will capture most of the information about human genetic variation provided by all common SNPs, combined with high-throughput genotyping technologies such as the Illumina (Santa Clara, California) or Affymetrix (San Diego, California) platforms, should facilitate the discovery of pediatric-onset IBD genes. The greatest challenges that must be overcome for a whole-genome LD (association) mapping approach is the substantial cost and dealing with the problem of multiple comparisons when interpreting the significance of results [53].

Genetic discoveries and their clinical significance in inflammatory bowel disease

Complex diseases such as IBD are controlled by multiple risk factors that evolve and interact with each other. From environmental exposure to the clinical and biological expression of IBD-related phenotypes, there are multiple processing steps controlled by the host and the environment. The currently proposed genetic model for IBD phenotypes emphasizes complex interactions between environmental factors and promoting/modifying genetic determinants, resulting in the clinical expression of the disease at the GI tract of genetically predisposed individuals. Specific mutations that occur in disease-promoting genes influence the development of distinct clinical phenotypes, whereas mutations in the modifying genes influence specific features of the disease phenotype such as disease penetrance, progression, complications, or response to treatment. *CARD15/NOD2* mutations have been studied extensively in genotype–phenotype correlation studies. Consistently, *CARD15/ NOD2* variants are associated with a younger age at onset, the presence of ileal involvement, and a tendency to develop strictures or fistulas [35,36]. Furthermore, a significant gene dosage effect has been observed for CD site and complications [36]. For instance, at least 95% of the patients homozygous for *CARD15/NOD2* mutations present with ileal lesions [34]. Existing data remain conflicting as to whether *CARD15/NOD2* carriage is associated with a more severe disease course, suggesting that this feature depends on modifying genes or environmental risk factors. The authors have shown that stricturing complications leading to early surgery were found more frequently in patients with the 1007fs mutation within the *CARD15* gene compared with those children without mutations [54]. Children with this mutation had a 6.6-fold increased risk for developing a stricturing phenotype requiring surgery. Genotyping at presentation might identify a subgroup of CD children who are at risk for more rapid development of complications, hence enabling these patients to benefit from the early use of more aggressive therapies.

The results from genotype–phenotype analysis using other IBD susceptibility genes are ongoing. In the Newman and colleagues study, the *SLC22A4-TC* diplotype did not influence the age of disease diagnosis [43]. Given the epistatic effect (ie, the interaction of two or more genes controlling the expression of a phenotype) between *CARD15/NOD2* and *SLC22A4-TC* with ileal involvement in CD, genetic effects of this *SLC22A4-A5* and *CARD15/NOD2* mutation may result from a common physiopathologic mechanism in the ileum. The presence of the *SLC22A-TC* diplotype was not associated with UC in the presence or absence of *CARD15/NOD2* risk alleles. Newman and colleagues [43] indicate that the *SLC22A-TC* diplotype constitutes a CD-specific variant that acts together with *CARD15/ NOD2* risk alleles to induce a predisposition to CD and ileal involvement among patients who have CD. The studies conducted to date have indicated no correlation between *DLG5* and any particular phenotypes.

Data on *CARD15/NOD2* in people have shown a gene dosage effect consistent with a recessive model and a predisposition to the development of lesions in the terminal ileum where Paneth's cells are abundant. Mice lacking CARD15/NOD2 showed a defect in defense against per os infection by *Listeria monocytogenes*, which was paralleled by a decreased expression of particular Paneth's cell-derived cryptdins [38]. Consistent with these data, CD patients homozygous for *CARD15/NOD2* mutations showed decreased expression of Paneth's cell α-defensins HD-5 and HD-6 [34]. Further work should clarify to what extent such immunodeficiencies might affect the microbial flora and promote intestinal infection and inflammation. Ongoing studies using clinically relevant enteropathogens and humanized flora might help to identify the essential priming or triggering environmental risk factor(s) in the development of CD-related phenotypes in *CARD15/NOD2* knock-out animals.

The innate immune system has an important role in preventing bacterial-induced intestinal inflammation and repelling pathogenic infection. Given the nature of the CD-susceptibility gene identified to date, it seems reasonable to postulate that impaired bacterial PGN sensing is a major primary event leading to local inflammation or hyper-responsiveness of the innate immune system or abnormal activation of T and B cells. The physiological function of the other susceptibility genes in Paneth's cells' function, intestinal immunity, or death remains speculative.

Gene–environment interactions in a complex disease model

The term complex disease is attributed to diseases or outcomes that have a genetically inherited component but an expression of the phenotype dependent on interactions with multiple genes or multiple environmental factors (examples include diabetes, most cardiovascular diseases, most neuron-psychological traits such as depression or schizophrenia, and most cancers). The terminology has been developed to contrast complex diseases from diseases that are predominantly caused by inheritance of dysfunctional single genes (monogenic diseases). Even the most common monogenic disorders, however, such as the thalassemias, are likely multifactorial, with the expression of a particular phenotype depending on interactions with other genetic and nongenetic factors [55]. In spite of the ambiguity in terminology, it is believed widely that most complex diseases are the result of interactions between genes and the environment. There has been an ongoing debate, however, on the definition, measurement, interpretation, and public health importance of gene–environment interactions.

Studying gene–environment interactions

Statistical interactions between two factors (gene and an environmental factor here) is said to exist when the effects of genotype on disease risk depend on the level of exposure to an environmental risk factor, or vice versa. The definition, however, depends on the measures used to assess risk. When risk ratios are used (ie, the ratio of disease incidence among exposed to the disease incidence among unexposed), the interaction corresponds with a multiplicative model for the joint effects of two or more risk factors in which the risk ratio between subjects exposed and unexposed to a risk factor (environmental for example) does not vary according to strata defined by exposure to another risk factor (for example genotypes). Statistical interaction is said to be present when there is a lack of fit to the multiplicative model. If the effect measure used were the rate difference, interaction would be defined as a lack of fit to an additive model for the joint effects of the two risk factors. Table 1 showcases an example for assessing interaction on the two scales. It also showcases an example where interactions assessed by the two different models would give different results, thereby adding to the complexity in interpreting findings. It has been suggested that dependence on the specific model would be limited when at least one of the two study factors does not have an effect on disease in the absence of the other study factor, because the presence of interaction according to one model would imply presence of interaction on another model.

Interpretation and utility

In addition to the difficulties in defining and measuring interactions, another important issue is the difference between biological and statistical interaction. Although, this is a well-understood caveat, it is not so obvious in practice. If interactions at the biological level were known, there would be no point in studying them statistically. Hence, on most occasions in the absence of a priori knowledge, once statistical interactions are determined, attempts are made to provide biological explanations to the relationships observed. Many statistical interactions, however, could arise because of chance and may not have any biological significance, thereby limiting their value. Nonetheless, if significant gene–environment interactions are detected, these individuals should be advised to reduce exposure to known environmental factors associated with disease. Studying gene–environment

Table 1
Assessing gene–environment interactions

A	Environmental exposure		B	Environmental exposure	
Gene	Absent	Present	Gene	Absent	Present
Absent	1.0 $(R00)$	2.0 $(R01)$	Absent	1.0	4.0
Present	3.0 $(R10)$	6.0 $(R11)$	Present	4.0	16.0

Interaction on the multiplicative scale is present when R_{01} R_{10} # R_{11}, whereas interaction on the additive scale is said to exist when R_{11}# R_{01} + R_{10}. In example A, there is no interaction on the multiplicative scale or additive scale between the environmental exposure and the gene. In example B, interaction is absent on the multiplicative scale but present on the additive scale. The entries in the table are risks for disease per 100,000 person-years (example is hypothetical).

interactions could thus influence public health as advocated by Khoury and colleagues [56].

Gene–environment interactions in inflammatory bowel disease pathogenesis

One of the general descriptions with regards to the etiopathogenesis of IBD commonly used is that IBD is the result of interactions between multiple genetic, environmental, and immunological mediators. Much of this perhaps stems from studies performed among animals. Currently, there seems to be limited or no epidemiological evidence of such interactions among humans. The difficulties are understandable given that there it is not clear which interactions to target and which interactions are biologically possible. Furthermore, given the multitude of the potential scenarios, it is not clear which scenario fits with the pathogenesis of IBD. Some efforts have been made to evaluate whether interactions between smoking and loci linked to IBD are associated with IBD. For example, Pierik and colleagues [57] studied potential interactions between smoking and the IBD4 locus (chromosome 14q11) using a family-based design from families recruited through an international collaboration that included 13 centers across the world [57]. The mean age of diagnosis of affected sibling pairs was 21.7 years. A significant distortion in mean allele sharing (MAS) was observed among CD-affected sibling pairs for four markers within the IBD4 locus. The MAS was significantly higher among those families where all or at least one sibling smoked compared with nonsmoking CD families. Based on these findings, they proposed that gene–environmental interactions are associated with CD. One of the proposed mechanisms underlying these interactions was the possibility that the IBD4 locus harbors susceptibility genes for both CD and smoking or two different susceptibility genes (each for CD and smoking) in linkage disequilibrium. These findings need to be replicated to confirm the associations.

Despite the fact that direct epidemiological evidence for the presence of potential gene–environment interactions in IBD etiology is limited, other lines of evidence point to the presence of such interactions. For example, the heterogeneity in risks from environmental exposures (diet, hygiene) across different populations may be related to the presence of gene–environment interactions. Table 2 provides an explanation on how the heterogeneity could be the result of gene–environment. The authors recently [58] postulated a plausible gene–environment interaction model related to dietary consumption, variants in the xenobiotic metabolizing enzyme genes, and risk for IBD (Fig. 2). In this model, the authors proposed that the potential dietary contributions to IBD etiology are likely related to the individual's capacity to metabolize dietary components. Even if individuals in the population were to have diets above or below established norms, only those individuals whose normal physiological processes are overwhelmed because of inherent genetic susceptibilities are likely to be prone to IBD. Xenobiotic metabolizing enzyme genes are a family of genes involved in the metabolism

Table 2
Illustration of how differences in results in different geographical areas can indicate presence of G × E

	Risk from environmental factor (E) (odds ratios)
Example of interaction on the multiplicative scale[a]	
Absence of DNA variant (G−)	1.0
Presence of DNA variant (G+)	3.0
Varying associations between environmental factors and inflammatory bowel disease across populations indicative of presence of gene-environment interactions[b]	
Absence of genetic variant (G−) (populations showing no risks)	1.0
Presence of genetic (G+) (population showing elevated risks)	2.0

[a] Among those who have the genetic variant, the odds ratio between environmental exposure and disease is 3.0. By comparison, in the absence of the genetic variant, the environmental exposure does not confer any risk for disease. The differences in the odds ratios according to strata defined by the gene suggest the presence of interaction on the multiplicative scale.

[b] In this hypothetical example, populations in which no associations with the environmental exposure may have a very low prevalence of potential genes associated with disease. At the same time, populations showing positive associations with the environmental risk factor and disease may have a large proportion of individuals with the at-risk genetic variant.

of a range of endogenous and exogenous substrates. They are classified broadly as phase 1 enzymes such as the cytochrome P-450 (CYP) enzymes, metabolism by which leads to production of intermediary metabolites that get detoxified further by phase 2 enzymes such as glutathione S-transferases that make the intermediary product water-soluble by means of a conjugation process enabling the successful elimination. Essentially, the function of these enzymes is to detoxify potential toxins. Nonetheless, on many occasions, the detoxification process leads to production of intermediates that bear inflammatory and tissue-damaging potential (by release of reactive oxygen species). Individuals show extensive variability in the activities and levels of these enzymes that are determined genetically. In addition, many of the enzymes are expressed in the GIT, and the genes coding them are present in locations of the genome that have shown linkage with IBD. The authors have postulated that individuals possessing variant forms of particular XME enzymes, and whose diets are high in fat and low in vegetables and fruits, are more likely to be at risk for IBD. Currently, studies are underway to investigate this hypothesis.

Mendelian randomization and complex diseases

Although the exact contributions of gene–environment to IBD pathogenesis and to other complex diseases remain unexplored, one important contribution of studying genetic associations could be the ability to overcome

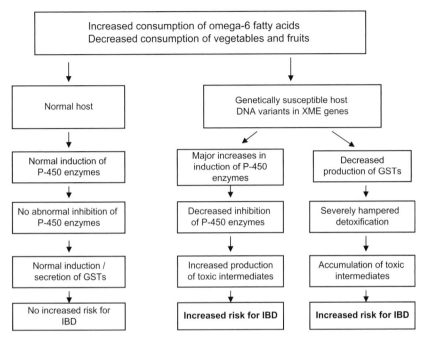

Fig. 2. Interactions between dietary elements, xenobiotic metabolizing enzymes, and risk for IBD.

limitations of classic epidemiology (investigation of associations of non-genetic risk factors with disease risk) by exploiting the concept of Mendelian randomization. This concept, first put forward by Katan [59] and later conceptualized further by Davey-Smith and Ebrahim [60], is based on the observations that the distributions of genotypes at birth occur according to Mendelian laws, and thus, groups formed are akin to random allocation [59]. Such groups (with differing genotypes) are unlikely to differ systematically with the exception of linkage disequilibrium. Hence, any associations studied between genotypes and disease, especially using the case-parent design, is equivalent to a randomized clinical trial. The latter also will be true for well-designed case-control studies (where confounding caused by population stratification has been controlled for). This concept of Mendelian randomization can be applied to studying whether environmental risk factors are causally related to disease. When measuring potential associations between environmental factors and disease, major concerns are related to misclassification of exposure and reverse causality (wherein any association between the factor and disease may have occurred because of changes in the risk factor brought about by disease). If genetic polymorphisms produce phenotypic differences (eg, blood levels of cholesterol, homocysteine, fibrinogen, or organophosphates) that mirror the biological effects of modifiable environmental exposures (eg, low folate diet enhancing blood levels of homocysteine), which in turn alter disease risk, the different polymorphisms should be related to disease risk to the extent predicted by their influence on the phenotype. Common polymorphisms that have well-characterized biological function therefore can be used to study the effect of a suspected exposure on disease risk. The advantages would be that any associations studied would not be susceptible to confounding caused by socioeconomic or behavioral characteristics, as the SNPs would not be expected to be associated with these potential confounding variables.

Another important method where this concept can be used and that is relevant to IBD pathogenesis is studying the causal association between dietary exposures and certain disease endpoints. Because dietary exposures are difficult to measure, and any associations with disease are prone to misclassification and confounding/reverse causality, studying associations between functional polymorphisms in genes that alter the metabolism or bioavailability of dietary components and disease could provide insights into the causal relationship between dietary exposures and disease. For example, the methylene tetrahydrofolate gene (*MTHFR*) determines the levels of homocysteine (a product of dietary folate metabolism), an intermediary product thought to be associated with neural tube defects (NTDs) in various observational epidemiological studies [61]. As the levels of homocysteine can be influenced by potential confounding variables such as smoking, however, it was unclear whether homocysteine was causally related to NTD. By reporting associations between the *MTHFR* genotypes that enhance production of homocysteine and risk for NTD, researchers have provided strong evidence that maternal dietary folate consumption (or lack thereof, in this case) is causally related to NTD risk [62]. Other examples of the application of Mendelian randomization have shown a link between dietary folate, homocysteine, and coronary heart disease by studying associations between the *MTHFR* gene and risk for coronary heart disease [63].

Mendelian randomization and potential mechanisms in inflammatory bowel disease pathogenesis

The concept of Mendelian randomization may play a crucial role in delineating potentially causal environmental risk factors for IBD. Dietary factors long have been studied and implicated, but much of the available evidence is susceptible to misclassification of consumption patterns and reverse causality. Thus, traditional observations studies would be limited with respect to establishing a causal relationship between dietary components and IBD. From dietary factors, the role of polyunsaturated fatty acids has received the greatest attention. In vivo and in vitro experiments consistently have shown that a balance between ω-3 and ω-6 fatty acids may be crucial for maintaining physiological inflammation, and perturbations of this balance between these fatty acids may underlie the chronic inflammation characteristic of IBD [64]. Similarly, clinical trials have provided some evidence on the beneficial effects of ω-3 fatty acids in IBD [65]. Diets of North American populations are heavily loaded in favor of ω-6 fatty acids. Metabolism of ω-6 fatty acids leads to the production of arachidonic acid, which in turn leads to the production of leucotriene β4, which a potent mediator of inflammation. On the other hand, metabolism of ω-3 fatty acids leads to the production of fatty acids such as eicosapentaenoic acid (EPA) and docosahexaenoic acid (DHA) [66], which lead to the production of leucotriene β_5, which has a much reduced capacity to mediate inflammation (10% of $LT\beta_4$). These findings suggest that a balance between specific fatty acids may be important in IBD pathogenesis. Nonetheless, epidemiological evidence for the latter is limited because of the inherent difficulty of measuring consumption of different fatty acids. Hence, establishing a casual link between fatty acids and IBD is difficult. Despite this, if polymorphisms in certain genes that code key enzymes that metabolize intermediate substrates in the fatty acid metabolism pathway could be targeted and studied for associations with IBD, this would provide important evidence for the role of fatty acids in the pathway to the inflammation characteristic of IBD. The concept of Mendelian randomization could be used for clarifying the associations between fatty acids and IBD. Genes involved in the catabolism and conversion of $LT\beta_4$ to $LT\beta_5$, and whose variants confer interindividual variability in the ability to convert $LT\beta_4$ to $LT\beta_5$, could be targeted. As mentioned previously, $LT\beta_5$ has a reduced potential for inflammatory activity. Certain genes belonging to the XME family of genes specifically catalyze the conversion of $LT\beta_4$ to $LT\beta_5$. Association between these genotypes (or haplotypes) and IBD will provide evidence that fatty acids (or their metabolites) are linked to IBD pathogenesis. The authors are in the process of evaluating these associations (Fig. 3).

The implementation of the concept of Mendelian randomization, however, comes with certain caveats. Two of these are of primary importance. First, the assumption is that the genetic variants are not associated with the disease (ie, the genotypes do not influence disease by means of alternative pathways). Second, and perhaps more importantly, with regards to genes that alter the function, activity, and concentration of enzymes involved in metabolic pathways, the alteration should be specific, meaning that the same gene should not be involved in altering the metabolic pathways of a range of substrates (pleiotropy). The latter caveat is applicable to dietary substrates and the enzymes that are involved in their metabolism. Many XMEs have a range of substrates, and hence studying genetic polymorphisms associated with them may not specifically delineate the causal pathway related to one particular substrate. It may be necessary to study a combination of genes (that affect the same substrate) for associations with IBD. Thus, Mendelian randomization, and its application as far as IBD is concerned, will be limited to specific exposures and less applicable for nonspecific exposures. One may consider clarifying the role of infections with IBD using this concept. Genetic polymorphisms in cytokine genes may

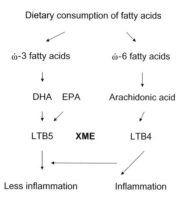

Fig. 3. Mendelian randomization and IBD pathogenesis. Diets higher in ω-6 fatty acids lead to production of arachidonic acid, which leads to the production of LTB-4, a potent mediator of inflammation. Metabolism of ω-3 fatty acids leads to the production of EPA and DHA, which produce LTB5, which has 10% of the inflammatory potential of LTB4. Xenobiotic enzymes (XME) that convert LTB4 to LTB5 will reduce the capacity for inflammation and may protect from IBD. Studying the association between the XME gene and IBD may provide evidence for a link between fatty acids and IBD.

appear to be prime targets for assessing the role of infections in the causal pathway of IBD. The relationship, however, between infections and cytokines is nonspecific, and any genetic associations studied are unlikely to provide further clarifications on the link between infections and IBD. Another exposure–disease relationship that could be targeted would be the link between smoking and IBD. As observational studies have shown opposite effects of smoking in CD and UC, targeting genes that are involved in the metabolism of nicotine (the constituent in smoke that potentially could mediate the link between smoking and inflammation) may provide insights on the causal nature of the association between smoking and IBD. Similarly, the exact role of oral contraceptives in IBD also could be amenable to evaluation using Mendelian randomization.

Challenges in the way forward; genotype by environmental interactions

There is little argument that a complex disease like IBD is the result of life-long interactions between genetic and environmental susceptibilities. There is paucity of research, however, incorporating genotype-by-interaction into human genetic studies. Despite the importance of gene–environmental interactions, most studies make an early and prominent assumption that no genotype-by-environment interactions exist. In fact, one explanation for the research falling short of earlier expectations in IBD is the inability to incorporate gene–environmental interactions in study designs and statistical analysis. There are many underlying reasons for the shortage of gene–environmental interaction studies. The greatest difficulty is the ability to measure an individual's exposure to his or her environment. Although there have been revolutionary advances in measuring genetic variation over the last decade, measurement of environmental factors still are based largely on questionnaires and indirect measurements. The second reason is the fear of further exponential explosions in the number of variables with which one must contend. There is a lack of appreciation for good study design for estimating gene–environmental interactions. Arguably, the best study designs are those based on environmental modifications, such as diet or cigarette smoking. Such studies, however, are expensive and difficult to execute in larger cohorts. Lastly, the inability to directly incorporate environmental factors into genetic studies is cultural. Most investigators who have the capability to perform state-of-the art genotyping technologies and use HapMap data effectively are likely to consider the results of diet habits and recall questionnaires to be soft and uninformative, and therefore not worthy of further serious considerations.

Pediatric versus adult inflammatory bowel disease—why are children with inflammatory bowel disease an ideal population to study gene—environmental interactions?

Studying gene–gene and gene–environmental interactions to understand the pathogenesis in a genetically complex trait such as IBD presents challenges with substantial resource allocation. Therefore, selecting the right population to study gene–environmental interactions for IBD susceptibility and outcome is critically important. Although the pathogenesis of CD is likely to be same in pediatric and adult populations, compared with adults with IBD, pediatric-onset IBD is not compounded by numerous and prolonged environmental exposures, thereby providing an ideal opportunity to narrow down the exposure in measurable terms. For example, the prevalence of smoking or passive smoking—a major confounding variable in studies of IBD—is substantially lower in the pediatric population. If incident cases of IBD are studied, the environmental factors are relatively easy to track compared with adult IBD, where long-standing disease with multiple environmental exposures is present. In addition, family members of pediatric index cases, particularly parents and siblings, are often times more readily available for enrollment into studies than family members of adult subjects. These family-based studies, in particular transmission disequlibrium testing (TDT), a gold standard test for genetic associations, can be performed easily when DNA from family trios and siblings is available. This type of analysis eliminates the problems of traditional case-control studies such as spurious associations and genetic heterogeneity [67]. Lastly, pediatric patients are usually followed prospectively from the time of diagnosis, thus the environmental exposures and evolving phenotypes can be monitored and recorded accurately.

Summary

Complex disease such as IBD is controlled by multiple risk factors that evolve and interact with each other In a genetically susceptible host, there are multiple processing steps controlled by the host and the environment, from environmental exposure to the clinical and biological expression of IBD-related phenotypes. It should be obvious to most people that if new genetic discoveries are to attain their potential promise in IBD, the barriers to relax the assumptions of genotype-by-environment interactions need immediate attention. The first design issue in studying a complex disorder such as IBD is to identify and characterize the right population. Investigators should recognize this problem rather than simply work with convenient samples. For various reasons, children with newly diagnosed IBD (incident cases) are suited ideally to carry out such investigations. Technical advances of the HapMap project and the promise of whole-genome association scans have been impressive, driving down the cost of SNP genotyping while driving up the quality and completeness of the data to a degree far exceeding initial expectations. There is no single optimal design that will identify genetic and environmental factors that contribute to IBD risk most efficiently. Disease-oriented investigators who think that just by genotyping their cohorts they will produce a clean genomic solution to identifying genetic risks have been misled. The pathogenesis of IBD almost certainly is mediated by a network of effects, meaning that neither genetic nor environmental agents are separate causes of the disease state, but instead their interactions determine the risk. Investigators aimed at clarifying these interactions ultimately will lead to a clearer understanding of the underlying mechanisms of IBD, which will provide insight for improved prevention and treatment.

References

[1] Ekbom A. The epidemiology of IBD: a lot of data but little knowledge. How shall we proceed? Inflamm Bowel Dis 2004;10(Suppl 1):S32–4.

[2] Loftus EV Jr, Sandborn WJ. Epidemiology of inflammatory bowel disease. Gastroenterol Clin North Am 2002;31(1):1–20.

[3] Tamboli CP, Cortot A, Colombel JF. What are the major arguments in favour of the genetic susceptibility for inflammatory bowel disease? Eur J Gastroenterol Hepatol 2003;15(6):587–92.

[4] Russell RK, Satsangi J. IBD: a family affair. Best Pract Res Clin Gastroenterol 2004;18(3): 525–39.

[5] Farrokhyar F, Swarbrick ET, Irvine EJ. A critical review of epidemiological studies in inflammatory bowel disease. Scand J Gastroenterol 2001;36(1):2–15.

[6] Russel MG, Stockbrugger RW. Epidemiology of inflammatory bowel disease: an update. Scand J Gastroenterol 1996;31(5):417–27.

[7] Ekbom A, Helmick C, Zack M, Adami HO. The epidemiology of inflammatory bowel disease: a large, population-based study in Sweden. Gastroenterology 1991;100(2):350–8.

[8] Delco F, Sonnenberg A. Exposure to risk factors for ulcerative colitis occurs during an early period of life. Am J Gastroenterol 1999;94(3):679–84.

[9] Chowers Y, Odes S, Bujanover Y, et al. The month of birth is linked to the risk of Crohn's disease in the Israeli population. Am J Gastroenterol 2004;99(10):1974–6.

[10] Jayanthi V, Probert CS, Pinder D, et al. Epidemiology of Crohn's disease in Indian migrants and the indigenous population in Leicestershire. Q J Med 1992;82(298):125–38.

[11] Miller DS, Keighley A, Smith PG, et al. Crohn's disease in Nottingham: a search for time-space clustering. Gut 1975;16(6):454–7.

[12] Comes MC, Gower-Rousseau C, Colombel JF, et al. Inflammatory bowel disease in married couples: 10 cases in Nord Pas de Calais region of France and Liege county of Belgium. Gut 1994;35(9):1316–8.

[13] Montgomery SM, Morris DL, Pounder RE, et al. Paramyxovirus infections in childhood and subsequent inflammatory bowel disease. Gastroenterology 1999;116(4):796–803.

[14] Shoda R, Matsueda K, Yamato S, et al. Epidemiologic analysis of Crohn's disease in Japan: increased dietary intake of n-6 polyunsaturated fatty acids and animal protein relates to the increased incidence of Crohn's disease in Japan. Am J Clin Nutr 1996;63(5):741–5.

[15] Cashman KD, Shanahan F. Is nutrition an aetiological factor for inflammatory bowel disease? Eur J Gastroenterol Hepatol 2003;15(6):607–13.

[16] Gilat T, Hacohen D, Lilos P, et al. Childhood factors in ulcerative colitis and Crohn's disease. An international cooperative study. Scand J Gastroenterol 1987;22(8):1009–24.

[17] Koletzko S, Sherman P, Corey M, et al. Role of infant feeding practices in development of Crohn's disease in childhood. BMJ 1989;298(6688):1617–8.

[18] Koletzko S, Griffiths A, Corey M, et al. Infant feeding practices and ulcerative colitis in childhood. BMJ 1991;302(6792):1580–1.

[19] Rigas A, Rigas B, Glassman M, et al. Breast feeding and maternal smoking in the etiology of Crohn's disease and ulcerative colitis in childhood. Ann Epidemiol 1993;3(4):387–92.

[20] Baron S, Turck D, Leplat C, et al. Environmental risk factors in paediatric inflammatory bowel diseases: a population-based case control study. Gut 2005;54(3):357–63.

[21] Amre DK, Lambrette P, Law L, et al. Investigating the hygiene hypothesis as a risk factor in pediatric onset Crohn's disease; case control study. Am J Gastroenterol 2006;101:1–7.

[22] Gent AE, Hellier MD, Grace RH, et al. Inflammatory bowel disease and domestic hygiene in infancy. Lancet 1994;343(8900):766–7.

[23] Duggan AE. Usmani I, Neal KR, et al. Appendectomy, childhood hygiene, *Helicobacter pylori* status, and risk of inflammatory bowel disease: a case control study. Gut 1998;43(4):494–8.

[24] el-Omar E, Penman I, Cruikshank G, et al. Low prevalence of *Helicobacter pylori* in inflammatory bowel disease: association with sulphasalazine. Gut 1994;35(10):1385–8.

[25] Halme L, Rautelin H, Leidenius M, et al. Inverse correlation between *Helicobacter pylori* infection and inflammatory bowel disease. J Clin Pathol 1996;49(1):65–7.

[26] Vare PO, Heikius B, Silvennoinen JA, et al. Seroprevalence of *Helicobacter pylori* infection in inflammatory bowel disease: is *Helicobacter pylori* infection a protective factor? Scand J Gastroenterol 2001;36(12):1295–300.

[27] Parente F, Molteni P, Bollani S, et al. Prevalence of *Helicobacter pylori* infection and related upper gastrointestinal lesions in patients with inflammatory bowel diseases. A cross-sectional study with matching. Scand J Gastroenterol 1997;32(11):1140–6.

[28] Basset C, Holton J, Bazeos A, et al. Are *Helicobacter* species and enterotoxigenic *Bacteroides fragilis* involved in inflammatory bowel disease? Dig Dis Sci 2004;49(9):1425–32.

[29] Feeney MA, Murphy F, Clegg AJ, et al. A case-control study of childhood environmental risk factors for the development of inflammatory bowel disease. Eur J Gastroenterol Hepatol 2002;14(5):529–34.

[30] Koutroubakis IE, Vlachonikolis IG, Kouroumalis EA. Role of appendicitis and appendectomy in the pathogenesis of ulcerative colitis: a critical review. Inflamm Bowel Dis 2002;8(4):277–86.

[31] Smithson JE, Radford-Smith G, Jewell GP. Appendectomy and tonsillectomy in patients with inflammatory bowel disease. J Clin Gastroenterol 1995;21(4):283–6.

[32] Andersson RE, Olaison G, Tysk C, et al. Appendectomy is followed by increased risk of Crohn's disease. Gastroenterology 2003;124(1):40–6.

[33] Calkins BM. A meta-analysis of the role of smoking in inflammatory bowel disease. Dig Dis Sci 1989;34(12):1841–54.

[34] Chamaillard M, Iacob R, Desreumaux P, et al. Advances and perspectives in the genetics of inflammatory bowel diseases. Clin Gastroenterol Hepatol 2006;4(2):143–51.

[35] Ahmad T, Armuzzi A, Bunce M, et al. The molecular classification of the clinical manifestations of Crohn's disease. Gastroenterology 2002;122(4):854–66.

[36] Abreu MT, Taylor KD, Lin YC, et al. Mutations in NOD2 are associated with fibrostenosing disease in patients with Crohn's disease. Gastroenterology 2002;123(3):679–88.

[37] Hugot JP, Chamaillard M, Zouali H, et al. Association of NOD2 leucine-rich repeat variants with susceptibility to Crohn's disease. Nature 2001;411(6837):599–603.

[38] Kobayashi KS, Chamaillard M, Ogura Y, et al. Nod2-dependent regulation of innate and adaptive immunity in the intestinal tract. Science 2005;307(5710):731–4.

[39] Giallourakis C, Stoll M, Miller K, et al. IBD5 is a general risk factor for inflammatory bowel disease: replication of association with Crohn's disease and identification of a novel association with ulcerative colitis. Am J Hum Genet 2003;73(1):205–11.

[40] Negoro K, McGovern DP, Kinouchi Y, et al. Analysis of the IBD5 locus and potential gene–gene interactions in Crohn's disease. Gut 2003;52(4):541–6.

[41] Mirza MM, Fisher SA, King K, et al. Genetic evidence for interaction of the 5q31 cytokine locus and the CARD15 gene in Crohn's disease. Am J Hum Genet 2003;72(4):1018–22.

[42] Rioux JD, Silverberg MS, Daly MJ, et al. Genomewide search in Canadian families with inflammatory bowel disease reveals two novel susceptibility loci. Am J Hum Genet 2000;66(6):1863–70.

[43] Newman B, Gu X, Wintle R, et al. A risk haplotype in the Solute Carrier Family 22A4/22A5 gene cluster influences phenotypic expression of Crohn's disease. Gastroenterology 2005;128(2):260–9.

[44] Stoll M, Corneliussen B, Costello CM, et al. Genetic variation in DLG5 is associated with inflammatory bowel disease. Nat Genet 2004;36(5):476–80.

[45] Daly MJ, Pearce AV, Farwell L, et al. Association of DLG5 R30Q variant with inflammatory bowel disease. Eur J Hum Genet 2005;13(7):835–9.

[46] Friedrichs F, Brescianini S, Annese V, et al. Evidence of transmission ratio distortion of DLG5 R30Q variant in general and implication of an association with Crohn's disease in men. Hum Genet 2006;119(3):305–11.

[47] Torok HP, Glas J, Tonenchi L, et al. Polymorphisms of the lipopolysaccharide-signaling complex in inflammatory bowel disease: association of a mutation in the toll-like receptor 4 gene with ulcerative colitis. Clin Immunol 2004;112(1):85–91.

[48] McGovern DP, Hysi P, Ahmad T, et al. Association between a complex insertion/deletion polymorphism in NOD1 (CARD4) and susceptibility to inflammatory bowel disease. Hum Mol Genet 2005;14(10):1245–50.

[49] Panwala CM, Jones JC, Viney JL. A novel model of inflammatory bowel disease: mice deficient for the multiple drug resistance gene, mdr1a, spontaneously develop colitis. J Immunol 1998;161(10):5733–44.

[50] Brant SR, Panhuysen CI, Nicolae D, et al. MDR1 Ala893 polymorphism is associated with inflammatory bowel disease. Am J Hum Genet 2003;73(6):1282–92.

[51] Risch N, Merikangas K. The future of genetic studies of complex human diseases. Science 1996;273(5281):1516–7.

[52] Klein RJ, Zeiss C, Chew EY, et al. Complement factor H polymorphism in age-related macular degeneration. Science 2005;308(5720):385–9.

[53] Clark AG, Boerwinkle E, Hixson J, et al. Determinants of the success of whole-genome association testing. Genome Res 2005;15(11):1463–7.

[54] Kugathasan S, Collins N, Maresso K, et al. CARD15 gene mutations and risk for early surgery in pediatric-onset Crohn's disease. Clin Gastroenterol Hepatol 2004;2(11):1003–9.

[55] Weatherall DJ. Single-gene disorders or complex traits: lessons from the thalassaemias and other monogenic diseases. BMJ 2000;321(7269):1117–20.

[56] Khoury MJ, Wagener DK. Epidemiological evaluation of the use of genetics to improve the predictive value of disease risk factors. Am J Hum Genet 1995;56(4):835–44.

[57] Pierik M, Yang H, Barmada MM, et al. The IBD international genetics consortium provides further evidence for linkage to IBD4 and shows gene–environment interaction. Inflamm Bowel Dis 2005;11(1):1–7.

[58] Amre DK, Seidman EG. DNA variants in cytokine and NOD2 genes, exposures to infections and risk for Crohn's disease. Paediatr Perinat Epidemiol 2003;17(3):302–12.

[59] Katan MB. Apolipoprotein E isoforms, serum cholesterol, and cancer. Lancet 1986;1(8479):507–8.

[60] Davey Smith G, Ebrahim S. Mendelian randomization: can genetic epidemiology contribute to understanding environmental determinants of disease? Int J Epidemiol 2003;32(1):1–22.

[61] Botto LD, Yang Q. 5,10-Methylenetetrahydrofolate reductase gene variants and congenital anomalies: a HuGE review. Am J Epidemiol 2000;151(9):862–77.

[62] Scholl TO, Johnson WG. Folic acid: influence on the outcome of pregnancy. Am J Clin Nutr 2000;71(Suppl 5):1295S–303S.

[63] Klerk M, Verhoef P, Clarke R, et al. MTHFR 677C → T polymorphism and risk of coronary heart disease: a meta-analysis. JAMA 2002;288(16):2023–31.

[64] Belluzzi A, Boschi S, Brignola C, et al. Polyunsaturated fatty acids and inflammatory bowel disease. Am J Clin Nutr 2000;71(Suppl 1):339S–42S.

[65] MacLean CH, Mojica WA, Newberry SJ, et al. Systematic review of the effects of n-3 fatty acids in inflammatory bowel disease. Am J Clin Nutr 2005;82(3):611–9.

[66] Calder PC, Grimble RF. Polyunsaturated fatty acids, inflammation and immunity. Eur J Clin Nutr 2002;56(Suppl 3):S14–9.

[67] Spielman RS, Ewens WJ. The TDT and other family-based tests for linkage disequilibrium and association. Am J Hum Genet 1996;59(5):983–9.

ELSEVIER
SAUNDERS

PEDIATRIC CLINICS
OF NORTH AMERICA

Pediatr Clin N Am 53 (2006) 751–765

Application of Genetic Approaches to Ocular Disease

Mark S. Ruttum, MD[a],*, Linda M. Reis, MS[b],
Elena V. Semina, PhD[c]

[a]*Medical College of Wisconsin, 925 North 87th Street, Milwaukee, WI 53226, USA*
[b]*Children's Hospital of Wisconsin, P.O. Box 1997, MS 716, Milwaukee, WI 53201, USA*
[c]*Medical College of Wisconsin, 8701 Watertown Plank Road, Milwaukee, WI 53226, USA*

During the last decade, there has been an exponential increase in genetic studies of ocular disorders. These studies have identified numerous genes responsible for monogenic ocular conditions, and, in some cases, resulted in identification of multiple genes contributing to the disease. Further analysis of these genes in animal and cell culture models is now underway and will lead to a better understanding of the mechanisms of ocular development at the genetic and cellular level. Gene cloning and animal model approaches continue to play an essential role in genetic studies and are beginning to be enhanced by recently developed genomic and proteomic tools. These technologies are likely to provide valuable clues about the pathogenesis of human ocular diseases and facilitate the development of therapeutic agents [1–4] (Fig. 1). An overview of genetic approaches with examples of their application to the study of eye disease is provided.

Identification and studies of genetic factors

Linkage studies and gene identification

The first step in human genetic studies typically involves recruitment of families with multiple individuals affected with the same condition. The presence of multiple affected individuals suggests a genetic cause of the disease, and genetic linkage approaches can be employed to identify the DNA fragment that contains the disease-causing gene. To perform this analysis, DNA samples from affected and unaffected family members are used to screen multiple genetic markers with known locations within human genome

* Corresponding author.
  E-mail address: mruttum@mcw.edu (M.S. Ruttum).

0031-3955/06/$ - see front matter © 2006 Elsevier Inc. All rights reserved.
doi:10.1016/j.pcl.2006.05.010

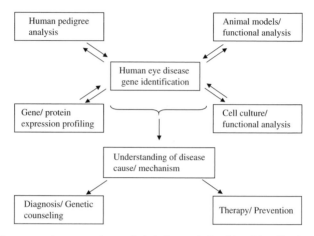

Fig. 1. Different genetic approaches and their inter-relationships. Identification and under-standing of genetic interactions that play role in human eye disease will improve genetic coun-seling and eventually lead to a better treatment and prevention of these conditions.

for co-inheritance with the disease phenotype in the family. Another way to narrow the genomic region containing a disease gene is through analysis of cytogenetic abnormalities such as chromosome rearrangements and dele-tions in affected individuals. This approach was instrumental in the identi-fication of genes for several ocular disorders, including the *SOX2* gene, which is associated with human anophthalmia [5], and the *PITX2* and *FOXC1* genes, which are involved in Axenfeld-Rieger syndrome [6,7]. As soon as the genomic region that contains the gene of interest is identified, expression and mutation studies in candidate genes located in the region can be undertaken to determine the disease-causing gene.

For single-gene (monogenic or Mendelian) disorders, a large pedigree with a distinct and reliable phenotype is likely to provide researchers with a successful identification of the disease-containing region. For conditions that are caused by a complex interaction of several genes (polygenic inher-itance) or by a combination of genetic and environmental factors (multifac-torial inheritance), linkage/association studies become more complicated and require a large number of carefully selected affected and control samples [8]. The recently developed SNP (simple nucleotide polymorphisms or single DNA bases that differ between individuals) technologies, in combination with multiplexed assays (simultaneous analysis of multiple markers in one experiment), and sample pooling methods (estimating allelic frequencies by analysis of pooled rather than individual DNA samples), provide inves-tigators with tools allowing a previously unprecedented level of analysis for linkage studies [9,10].

Identification of the genomic region(s) containing gene(s) for a particular condition through linkage/association studies is the first step in isolating causative gene(s). Positional gene cloning is a method used to identify disease genes by their chromosomal position. In this technique, no prediction about a potential disease gene is put forward before the search, and the causative gene is identified based on its position within the region of interest. The initial genetic markers shown to be linked with the disease are used to identify the corresponding genomic segment and to locate additional polymorphic probes within this segment. These new markers can be used in further pedigree analysis to narrow down the region for the disease-causing gene.

An alternative method, candidate gene cloning, has been used in many studies. This approach involves predicting candidate genes based on disease characteristics, a gene's function, expression pattern, or other criteria. Candidate gene cloning is indispensable for conditions where large pedigrees suitable for linkage are rare (ie, anophthalmia) [11,12]. Frequently, genetic studies use a combination of both approaches. The genomic region is defined broadly through linkage or chromosomal analysis, and then function of all known genes within the region of interest is reviewed, and those with a theoretical connection to the disease are selected as candidate genes for mutation analysis in affected pedigrees.

Recent advances in genetic research, including complete sequencing of human and several animal genomes and an abundance of bioinformatics resources that summarize genetic information, have empowered geneticists with invaluable tools for human disease gene cloning. An example of such resources includes the Genome Browser at the University of California, Santa Cruz (http://genome.ucsc.edu), which allows investigators to view the human genome sequence, research information about genes, perform comparative interspecies analysis, link to multiple other databases, and much more. Another example is the International HapMap Consortium (https://www.hapmap.org) site, which maintains the public database of common variation in the human genome; this information is critical to genetic association studies and finding genes that affect health and disease [13]. The advances in molecular and genetic technology have accelerated greatly elucidation of the genetic contributions to glaucoma [4], congenital and age-related cataracts [14,15], optic neuropathy [16], corneal dystrophy [17], and retinal degeneration [18–20].

Animal and cell culture models

Animal models are used widely in studies of human disease. Genes shown to be involved in an animal phenotype become candidate genes for similar human conditions. Conversely, model organisms can be created with disruption of specific genes known to be associated with the human phenotype, thus providing information about the developmental processes underlying hereditary human disorders. Successful application of these studies is based on the conserved biological functions of multiple molecules in people and animals. At the current stage of human genetic studies, when multiple disease genes have been identified, studies into the mechanisms of their action are becoming increasingly critical. Many factors that are involved in the embryonic development of vertebrate organs are conserved between species [21–23]. Animal models not only provide a valuable tool for gene identification and functional analysis, but also could provide a model for future testing of therapeutic agents [24–27].

For several decades, the laboratory mouse has been a leading research tool for understanding human biology and disease, particularly when technology to create knockout and transgenic animals became available. Further enhancements include completion of sequencing of the mouse genome, generation of elaborate systems for conditional and inducible gene manipulations, and development of sophisticated genomics and proteomics tools. The mouse continues to serve as a unique mammalian system to study genetic and epigenetic factors contributing to development and disease [28–30].

During the last decade, research into the genetics and mechanisms of glaucoma in mouse models has been growing rapidly. Studies of mouse models, spontaneous and derived from human genes associated with different degrees of anterior segment dysgenesis, have had a significant impact on the understanding of developmental and adult glaucoma [31]. Factors that contribute to glaucoma phenotype can be divided into two major risk groups: factors that lead to increased intraocular pressure, and those that affect viability of retinal ganglion cell [4]. Developmental forms of glaucoma that are associated with abnormalities in embryonic development of ocular tissue demonstrate a complexity of phenotype that is similar to the adult form [32,33]. Recently, Dr. Simon John's group at the Jackson Laboratory, University of Maine, identified the tyrosinase gene (Tyr) as a modifier of the drainage structure phenotype in CYP1B1- and FOXC1- deficient mice (genes that are associated with congenital or developmental glaucoma in people), with Tyr deficiency increasing the magnitude of dysgenesis. The severe dysgenesis in eyes lacking CYP1B1 and TYR was alleviated by administering the tyrosinase product dihydroxyphenylalanine (L-dopa). These results suggest that a tyrosinase/L-dopa pathway may modify human glaucoma phenotypes and create new possibilities for therapeutic treatment [34]. Mouse models are likely to be critical to dissecting the complex nature of glaucoma.

Recently, another animal model, a teleost fish zebrafish, is gaining strength as an important addition to the group of model organisms. The zebrafish model provides several advantages compared with mammalian models because of its relatively inexpensive maintenance and powerful genetic screening opportunities supported by the large number of embryos, superior imaging abilities because of transparency, and ex utero embryogenesis and rapid development [35,36]. Genetic screens in zebrafish have identified an impressive collection of photoreceptor cell mutants [37], lens phenotypes [38,39], and other vision mutants [40,41]. Studies into retina and lens development and aberrations have been a traditional strength of the zebrafish model, and recently mechanisms of the anterior segment formation and associated abnormalities also have become a focus of zebrafish genetics. This research has been facilitated by development of tools for intra-ocular pressure measurements in zebrafish and detailed analysis of the embryology of the anterior segment structures in this organism [42,43].

Cell culture models represent an additional opportunity to gain understanding of the pathogenic effects of various genetic alterations [44]. Use of cell culture models allows genetic manipulations to be performed and observed directly in human cells. Cell lines have been created from various human ocular tissues to facilitate these studies.

Global analysis of gene and protein expression

cDNA and protein microarray technology allows a simultaneous assessment of the expression of tens of thousands of gene transcripts or proteins in a given tissue, thus providing a superior level of phenotypic characterization. Gene and protein expression profiling are used largely to identify a particular expression pattern (biomarker) that is characteristic for a specific clinical state—gene discovery and identification of novel genetic pathways and candidate therapeutic targets then can be explored further [45–48]. These techniques have been applied to ocular conditions with good success. A molecular profile for human uveal melanoma has been investigated and provides a basis for development of new therapeutic interventions [49]. Comparison of normal, aged, and cataractous human lenses revealed massive changes in the expression of many genes between the three groups [50]. Other recent studies compared normal and glaucomatous optic nerve/retinal ganglion cells and also identified changes in gene expression. Further investigation of these transcripts and proteins may reveal additional factors related to ocular disease [51,52]. Specialized ocular microarrays developed by Swaroop and colleagues represent a unique resource for characterization of numerous mouse eye mutants [53].

Outcomes of genetics research

Genetic testing/counseling

When a child is born with or develops a debilitating ocular condition, parents often have questions about the etiology, prognosis, and recurrence/inheritance of the condition. A visit to a genetics clinic can help to answer some of these questions. If an accurate genetic diagnosis can be established, more specific genetic counseling can be provided to patients and families. Genetic diagnoses sometimes can be established clinically based on physical features, especially in syndromic causes of ocular disorders such as albinism, Lowe syndrome, and Marfan syndrome. It is often more difficult to establish a precise genetic diagnosis in individuals with isolated ocular abnormalities, such as congenital cataracts or glaucoma. Availability of accurate, reliable genetic tests for isolated ocular conditions will enable families to obtain more specific information about their children's condition and to identify other family members who may be at risk.

The identification of genes involved in ocular disorders is an important first step toward making a genetic diagnosis. Before genetic testing can be offered to affected individuals, sufficient data must be gathered to ensure accurate detection and interpretation of genetic findings [3,54]. It is important that commercial testing is not offered to patients prematurely, before the results can be interpreted accurately. For example, testing for myocillin, a risk factor in primary open angle glaucoma (POAG), recently has become available. One of the variations in the myocillin gene (MYOC.mt1) was shown to increase disease severity in patients with POAG in some studies, whereas other studies failed to find the same association. Therefore, investigators underline the importance of further testing for the role of this variant in the pathogenesis of POAG before the commercially available test may be employed widely [54].

As illustrated previously, interpretation of genetic test results is not always straightforward. A negative test result may not rule out a hereditary cause of an individual's condition, particularly for conditions with multiple genetic and environmental causes, such as congenital cataracts or glaucoma. Furthermore, because genes are shared among family members, genetic testing may reveal information about individuals not involved in the testing process. It is important for families to receive genetic counseling regarding the benefits, risks, and limitations of genetic testing before such testing is undertaken.

Prospects of gene therapy

Gene transfer technology holds great potential for therapeutic applications. As more knowledge is gained about the genes/proteins that play a critical role in ocular cell differentiation, proliferation, migration, and function, introduction of these factors by means of gene transfer techniques may yield new biological treatment options. The application of this technology to ocular disorders is only beginning to be evaluated, and examples of disorders that are being studied include various corneal conditions, retinal disorders, and optic nerve diseases. Several excellent recent articles and reviews discuss the first successes of gene transfer/therapy studies for ocular tissues/diseases, future directions, and potential for medical practice and concerns, including the risks of this treatment versus its potential benefits [55–61].

The cornea has been considered as an excellent candidate for gene therapy because of its accessibility and immune-privileged nature. Several studies reported successful introduction of DNA into corneal cells using various viral vectors and nonviral methods. These studies suggest great potential for this approach, but more research is required to directly evaluate the possibility of gene-based interventions for specific corneal disorders [55,56].

Optic nerve diseases also have been considered a potential target of gene therapy approaches. Success in gene transfer experiments in animal models of glaucoma, optic neuritis, Leber's hereditary optic neuropathy, and optic nerve transection, has been achieved, and the possibility of using similar techniques to treat human disease is being investigated [57–59].

New technology of RNA interference holds a great promise for treatment of all kinds of human disorders, including ocular conditions [62]. The observed significant heterogeneity of mutations demands a mutation-independent therapeutic strategy for many ocular conditions. Cashman and colleagues recently described an application of RNA interference technology to treatment of a highly heterogeneous group of conditions, retinal degenerations, in human embryonic retinoblasts [63].

Genetic studies of ocular disease

The remainder of this article considers how the genetic tools discussed previously have been used to study several monogenic ocular disorders: albinism, congenital cataracts, congenital glaucoma, and retinoblastoma.

Albinism

Oculocutaneous albinism is an autosomal recessive disease that affects melanin metabolism and has significant eye manifestations. It can occur as an isolated finding (OCA) (Fig. 2), or in association with other systemic diseases (eg, Chediak-Higashi syndrome, Hermansky-Pudlak syndrome). There is also an X-linked form of albinism, ocular albinism (OA), which primarily has eye manifestations. This discussion will be concerned only with OCA and OA.

Children with OCA or OA have deficient ocular pigmentation that leads to maldevelopment of the macular region of the retina, misrouting of optic nerve fibers, iris transillumination (Fig. 3), and nystagmus. Strabismus and significant refractive errors are also common. Visual acuity ranges from 20/40 to 20/400.

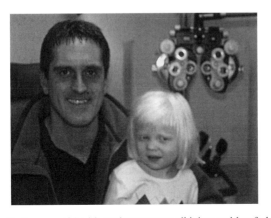

Fig. 2. A young girl with oculocutaneous albinism and her father.

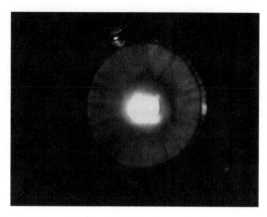

Fig. 3. Iris transillumination defect in a patient with albinism.

Once thought to be a single disease with variable manifestations, linkage analysis from affected families has shown that OCA occurs with mutations in least four different genetic regions; each type of OCA has a different phenotype and visual prognosis [64]. OCA1 is the best studied form of albinism and is caused by a mutation in the tyrosinase gene on chromosome 11q; OCA1 can itself be divided into two forms, OCA1A and OCA1B, which differ in the amount of tyrosinase enzymatic activity. Individuals with OCA1B have residual tyrosinase activity and can develop some ocular and cutaneous pigmentation over time; they also tend to have better visual acuity. OCA2, OCA3, and OCA4 are other forms of oculocutaneous albinism that arise from mutations on chromosomes 15q, 9p, and 5p, respectively [64]. Each of these is associated with a different step in the metabolism of melanin.

Ocular albinism is inherited in an X-linked recessive manner; it has similar ocular findings with OCA but lacks cutaneous involvement. The OA gene, OA1, is located on chromosome Xp and produces a transmembrane protein involved in the biogenesis of melanosomes [65]. Obligate carrier females often show spotty retinal pigmentation and punctuate areas of iris transillumination.

The diagnosis of OCA and OA remains primarily clinical, because the phenotype is so distinctive. The hairbulb assay for tyrosinase activity has been replaced by molecular genetic analysis. Prenatal diagnostic testing seldom is requested.

Congenital cataracts

Isolated hereditary cataracts occur primarily in an autosomal dominant manner, with rare pedigrees showing autosomal recessive or X-linked inheritance (Fig. 4). Congenital cataracts also can be associated with metabolic, renal, musculoskeletal, dermatologic, craniofacial, and infectious etiologies, but those will not be considered in this discussion. One type of inherited

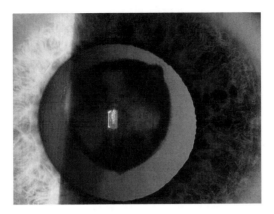

Fig. 4. A hereditary congenital cataract involving the nucleus of the lens.

congenital cataracts was the first autosomal-dominant disease to be genetically mapped in people through its linkage to the Duffy blood group locus on chromosome 1 [66]. To date, 12 loci and 15 specific genes have been identified through linkage analysis as causes of familial congenital cataracts [67].

Until 10 years ago, no specific genes had been identified as causes of inherited cataracts. Because many of the proteins involved in the crystalline lens were known, it made sense to screen the genes responsible for these proteins for mutations that could cause cataracts. If the mutation segregated with the cataract phenotype and was absent in normal individuals, there would be evidence that the gene was responsible for the cataract. This is an example of the candidate gene approach.

Water-soluble crystallins are proteins that are essential in maintaining lens transparency. They comprise 90% of the lens proteins, so the genes coding for them are obvious candidate genes for hereditary cataracts. Crystallins have been subdivided into α, β, and γ forms. Cataract causing mutations have been found on chromosomes 11 and 21 for α-crystallin, chromosomes 17 and 22 for β-crystallin, and chromosome 2 for γ-crystallin [68]. In addition, proteins involved in the crystalline lens cytoskeleton, membrane transport, and protein transcription, have been identified on multiple chromosomes as causes of familial cataracts.

The mouse model has been valuable in the study of inherited cataracts. More than 100 strains have been identified with mostly autosomal-dominant cataracts [68]. All of the mouse crystallin proteins have been implicated in cataract. Other cytoskeletal and transcription factor proteins that cause cataracts also have been discovered, thus marking these as additional candidate genes to be investigated in people.

Congenital glaucoma

Like congenital cataracts, congenital glaucoma exists in a primary form in which it is the only abnormality and also in association with other ocular or systemic manifestations such as Axenfeld-Rieger and Lowe syndromes. The clinical triad of congenital glaucoma consists of epiphora, blepharo-spasm, and photophobia. Infants often present with cloudy and enlarged corneas (Fig. 5). The discussion in this article deals only with the isolated form known as primary congenital glaucoma (PCG), which typically is in-herited in an autosomal-recessive manner.

In PCG, the only observable primary abnormalities are confined to the neural crest-derived anterior chamber angle through which aqueous humor exits the eye to maintain stable intraocular pressure. The cause of anterior chamber angle abnormalities has remained speculative because of inability to track the proposed pathologic mechanisms to any particular molecular defect. Linkage analysis in several large families with the autosomal reces-sive PCG phenotype led to the discovery of a glaucoma gene known as GLC3A on chromosome 2p [69]. A second gene, GLC3B, was found in other families on chromosome 1p [69].

Through the technique of positional cloning of suspected disease genes in this chromosomal region, it was discovered that the GLC3A gene coded for the enzyme cytochrome P4501B1 (CYP1B1) [69]. The gene for this enzyme is expressed in the tissues of the anterior chamber of the eye. Its exact function in eye development is not known; however, it is suspected to be involved in metabolizing molecules used in signaling pathways. Clinical testing for CYP1B1 is not available.

Retinoblastoma

Retinoblastoma, an autosomal dominant disease, is the most common ocular malignancy of childhood, and it is hereditary in about one-third of cases (Fig. 6). Almost all bilateral cases and about 10% of unilateral cases are caused by a germline mutation [70]. The gene for retinoblastoma, RB1, has been localized to chromosome 13q14 through linkage analysis and dele-tion studies [71]. Several different types of mutations have been reported, in-cluding point mutations, deletions, and insertions. About 5% of hereditary

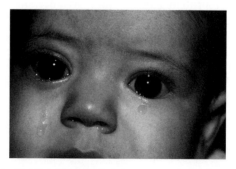

Fig. 5. A young child with bilateral congenital glaucoma. Note the large corneal size and asso-ciated epiphora.

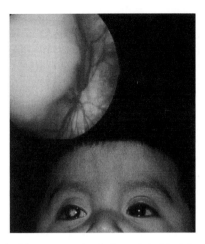

Fig. 6. A child with a retinoblastoma causing leukocoria in his right eye. The tumor abuts the optic nerve.

cases have a karyotypically visible deletion of 13q14 that includes the RB1 gene. This phenotype includes developmental delay, dysmorphic features, and cardiac and renal anomalies, in addition to the retinal tumors [72].

Knudson, observing that patients with bilateral tumors had more tumor foci and presented at an earlier age than those with unilateral tumors, postulated a two-hit model in which those with the germline mutation had one inactive RB1 allele in all the cells in their body and then suffered the loss of the second allele in a retinal cell or cells because of a sporadic mutation, the second hit [73]. In nongerminal (nonhereditary) cases, both RB1 alleles must be inactivated in a single somatic retinal progenitor cell through sporadic mutations.

The RB1 gene codes for a protein that suppresses tumors by regulating certain steps during the cell cycle. Loss of RB1 function allows rapid and uncontrolled cell division. Because all of the body's cells carry the abnormal RB1 allele, children with germline retinoblastoma are subject to other tumors such as sarcomas (especially in radiated tissue) and pineal neuroblastic tumors (so-called trilateral retinoblastoma), which may be an independent primary focus of retinoblastoma [74,75].

Genetic counseling for families with a history of retinoblastoma is important but complex. Empirically derived algorithms are available as an aid to genetic counseling [76]. Both direct (single-strand conformation polymorphism analysis) and indirect (restriction fragment length polymorphisms) methods also can be used to detect small mutations in family members. These tests are costly and may fail to detect any mutation in up to 20% of families with bilateral retinoblastoma [76]. Preimplantation genetic testing has been used to screen embryos for the RB1 mutation. Embryos derived from in vitro fertilization are biopsied at the four- to eight-cell stage; the removed cells then can be tested for the known familial RB1 mutation. Those embryos that are free of disease are transferred; a healthy newborn from a couple in which the father had germline retinoblastoma was reported recently [77].

Summary

This article discussed the impact of genetic approaches in the context of ocular disorders. A similar analysis could be provided for most branches of medicine, as health care increasingly is being shaped by the knowledge gained through genetic studies. These studies provide insight into the developmental and molecular etiology of disease and bring promise of better diagnosis, treatment, and prevention in the future.

Acknowledgments

The authors would like to thank families for their participation in genetic studies and donations of samples and clinical photographs.

References

[1] Graw J. The genetic and molecular basis of congenital eye defects. Nat Rev Genet 2003; 4(11):876–88.
[2] Rosenberg T. Epidemiology of hereditary ocular disorders. Dev Ophthalmol 2003;37:16–33.
[3] MacDonald IM, Tran M, Musarella MA. Ocular genetics: current understanding. Surv Ophthalmol 2004;49(2):159–96.
[4] Libby RT, Gould DB, Anderson MG, et al. Complex genetics of glaucoma susceptibility. Annu Rev Genomics Hum Genet 2005;6:15–44.
[5] Fantes J, Ragge NK, Lynch SA, et al. Mutations in SOX2 cause anophthalmia. Nat Genet 2003;33(4):461–3.
[6] Semina EV, Reiter R, Leysens N, et al. Cloning and characterization of a novel bicoid-related homeobox transcription factor gene, RIEG, involved in Rieger syndrome. Nat Genet 1996;14(4):392–9.
[7] Nishimura DY, Swiderski RE, Alward WL, et al. The forkhead transcription factor gene FKHL7 is responsible for glaucoma phenotypes which map to 6p25. Nat Genet 1998; 19(2):140–7.
[8] Weeks DE, Lathrop GM. Polygenic disease: methods for mapping complex disease traits. Trends Genet 1995;11(12):513–9.
[9] Murray SS, Oliphant A, Shen R, et al. A highly informative SNP linkage panel for human genetic studies. Nature Methods 2004;1(2):113–7.
[10] Kirov G, Nikolov I, Georgieva L, et al. Pooled DNA genotyping on Affymetrix SNP genotyping arrays. BMC Genomics 2006;7(1):27.
[11] Ragge NK, Brown AG, Poloschek CM, et al. Heterozygous mutations of OTX2 cause severe ocular malformations. Am J Hum Genet 2005;76(6):1008–22.
[12] Voronina VA, Kozhemyakina EA, O'Kernick CM, et al. Mutations in the human RAX homeobox gene in a patient with anophthalmia and sclerocornea. Hum Mol Genet 2004; 13(3):315–22.

[13] The International HapMap Consortium. A haplotype map of the human genome. Nature 2005;437:1299–320.

[14] Graw J. Congenital hereditary cataracts. Int J Dev Biol 2004;48(8–9):1031–44.

[15] Hejtmancik JF, Kantorow M. Molecular genetics of age-related cataract. Exp Eye Res 2004; 79(1):3–9.

[16] Votruba M. Molecular genetic basis of primary inherited optic neuropathies. Eye 2004; 18(11):1126–32.

[17] Klintworth GK. The molecular genetics of the corneal dystrophies—current status. Front Biosci 2003;8:d687–713.

[18] Rivolta C, Sharon D, DeAngelis MM, et al. Retinitis pigmentosa and allied diseases: numerous diseases, genes, and inheritance patterns. Hum Mol Genet 2002;11(10):1219–27.

[19] Delyfer MN, Leveillard T, Mohand-Said S, et al. Inherited retinal degenerations: therapeutic prospects. Biol Cell 2004;96(4):261–9.

[20] Klaver CC, Allikmets R. Genetics of macular dystrophies and implications for age-related macular degeneration. Dev Ophthalmol 2003;37:155–69.

[21] Percin EF, Ploder LA, Yu JJ, et al. Human microphthalmia associated with mutations in the retinal homeobox gene CHX10. Nat Genet 2000;25(4):397–401.

[22] Donner AL, Maas RL. Conservation and non-conservation of genetic pathways in eye specification. Int J Dev Biol 2004;48(8–9):743–53.

[23] Kozmik Z. Pax genes in eye development and evolution. Curr Opin Genet Dev 2005;15(4): 430–8.

[24] Young TL. Ophthalmic genetics/inherited eye disease. Curr Opin Ophthalmol 2003;14(5): 296–303.

[25] Bremner R, Chen D, Pacal M, et al. The RB protein family in retinal development and retinoblastoma: new insights from new mouse models. Dev Neurosci 2004;26(5–6):417–34.

[26] Dalke C, Graw J. Mouse mutants as models for congenital retinal disorders. Exp Eye Res 2005;81(5):503–12.

[27] Lindsey JD, Weinreb RN. Elevated intraocular pressure and transgenic applications in the mouse. J Glaucoma 2005;14(4):318–20.

[28] Nishina PM, Naggert JK. Mouse genetic approaches to access pathways important in retinal function. Adv Exp Med Biol 2003;533:29–34.

[29] Mager J, Bartolomei MS. Strategies for dissecting epigenetic mechanisms in the mouse. Nat Genet 2005;37(11):1194–200.

[30] Schweers BA, Dyer MA. Perspective: new genetic tools for studying retinal development and disease. Vis Neurosci 2005;22(5):553–60.

[31] John SW. Mechanistic insights into glaucoma provided by experimental genetics the Cogan lecture. Invest Ophthalmol Vis Sci 2005;46(8):2649–61.

[32] Gould DB, John SW. Anterior segment dysgenesis and the developmental glaucomas are complex traits. Hum Mol Genet 2002;11(10):1185–93.

[33] Gould DB, Smith RS, John SW. Anterior segment development relevant to glaucoma. Int J Dev Biol 2004;48:1015–29.

[34] Libby RT, Smith RS, Savinova OV, et al. Modification of ocular defects in mouse developmental glaucoma models by tyrosinase. Science 2003;299(5612):1578–81.

[35] Goldsmith P, Harris WA. The zebra fish as a tool for understanding the biology of visual disorders. Semin Cell Dev Biol 2003;14(1):11–8.

[36] McMahon C, Semina EV, Link BA. Using zebra fish to study the complex genetics of glaucoma. Comp Biochem Physiol C Toxicol Pharmacol 2004;138(3):343–50.

[37] Tsujikawa M, Malicki J. Genetics of photoreceptor development and function in zebra fish. Int J Dev Biol 2004;48(8–9):925–34.

[38] Vihtelic TS, Hyde DR. Zebra fish mutagenesis yields eye morphological mutants with retinal and lens defects. Vision Res 2002;42(4):535–40.

[39] Vihtelic TS, Yamamoto Y, Springer SS, et al. Lens opacity and photoreceptor degeneration in the zebra fish lens opaque mutant. Dev Dyn 2005;233(1):52–65.

[40] Neuhauss SC. Behavioral genetic approaches to visual system development and function in zebra fish. J Neurobiol 2003;54(1):148–60.

[41] Gross JM, Perkins BD, Amsterdam A, et al. Identification of zebra fish insertional mutants with defects in visual system development and function. Genetics 2005;170(1):245–61.

[42] Link BA, Gray MP, Smith RS, et al. Intraocular pressure in zebra fish: comparison of inbred strains and identification of a reduced melanin mutant with raised IOP. Invest Ophthalmol Vis Sci 2004;45(12):4415–22.

[43] Soules KA, Link BA. Morphogenesis of the anterior segment in the zebra fish eye. BMC Dev Biol 2005;5:12.

[44] Levin LA. Retinal ganglion cells and supporting elements in culture. J Glaucoma 2005;14(4): 305–7.

[45] Wilson AS, Hobbs BG, Speed TP, et al. The microarray: potential applications for ophthalmic research. Mol Vis 2002;8:259–70.

[46] Kittleson MM, Hare JM. Molecular signature analysis: using the myocardial transcriptome as a biomarker in cardiovascular disease. Trends Cardiovasc Med 2005;15(4):130–8.

[47] Mattoon D, Michaud G, Merkel J, et al. Biomarker discovery using protein microarray technology platforms: antibody-antigen complex profiling. Expert Rev Proteomics 2005;2(6): 879–89.

[48] Bertone P, Snyder M. Advances in functional protein microarray technology. FEBS J 2005; 272(21):5400–11.

[49] Seftor EA, Meltzer PS, Kirschmann DA, et al. Molecular determinants of human uveal melanoma invasion and metastasis. Clin Exp Metastasis 2002;19(3):233–46.

[50] Hawse JR, Hejtmancik JF, Horwitz J, et al. Identification and functional clustering of global gene expression differences between age-related cataract and clear human lenses and aged human lenses. Exp Eye Res 2004;79(6):935–40.

[51] Hernandez MR, Agapova OA, Yang P, et al. Differential gene expression in astrocytes from human normal and glaucomatous optic nerve head analyzed by cDNA microarray. Glia 2002;38(1):45–64.

[52] Ivanov D, Dvoriantchikova G, Nathanson L, et al. Microarray analysis of gene expression in adult retinal ganglion cells. FEBS Lett 2006;580(1):331–5.

[53] Farjo R, Yu J, Othman MI, et al. Mouse eye gene microarrays for investigating ocular development and disease. Vision Res 2002;42(4):463–70.

[54] Cohen CS, Allingham RR. The dawn of genetic testing for glaucoma. Curr Opin Ophthalmol 2004;15(2):75–9.

[55] Mohan RR, Sharma A, Netto MV, et al. Gene therapy in the cornea. Prog Retin Eye Res 2005;24(5):537–59.

[56] Rosenblatt MI, Azar DT. Gene therapy of the corneal epithelium. Int Ophthalmol Clin 2004; 44(3):81–90.

[57] Guy J, Qi X, Pallotti F, et al. Rescue of a mitochondrial deficiency causing Leber hereditary optic neuropathy. Ann Neurol 2002;52(5):534–42.

[58] Guy J, Qi X, Hauswirth WW. Adeno-associated viral-mediated catalase expression suppresses optic neuritis in experimental allergic encephalomyelitis. Proc Natl Acad Sci U S A 1998;95(23):13847–52.

[59] Sapieha PS, Peltier M, Rendahl KG, et al. Fibroblast growth factor-2 gene delivery stimulates axon growth by adult retinal ganglion cells after acute optic nerve injury. Mol Cell Neurosci 2003;24(3):656–72.

[60] Martin KR, Quigley HA. Gene therapy for optic nerve disease. Eye 2004;18(11):1049–55.

[61] McFarland TJ, Zhang Y, Appukuttan B, et al. Gene therapy for proliferative ocular diseases. Expert Opin Biol Ther 2004;4(7):1053–8.

[62] Uprichard SL. The therapeutic potential of RNA interference. FEBS Lett 2005;579(26): 5996–6007.

[63] Cashman SM, Binkley EA, Kumar-Singh R. Towards mutation-independent silencing of genes involved in retinal degeneration by RNA interference. Gene Ther 2005;12(15):1223–8.

[64] Oetting WS, Fryer JP, Shriram S, King RA. Oculocutaneous albinism type 1: the last 100 years. Pigment Cell Res 2003;16:307–11.

[65] Oetting WS. New insights into ocular albinism type 1 (OA1): mutations and polymorphisms of the OA1 gene. Hum Mutat 2002;19:85–92.

[66] Donahue RP, Bias WB, Renwick JH, et al. Probable assignment of the Duffy blood group locus to chromosome 1 in man. Proc Natl Acad Sci U S A 1968;61:949–55.

[67] Reddy MA, Francis PJ, Berry V, et al. Molecular genetic basis of inherited cataract and associated phenotypes. Surv Ophthalmol 2004;49:300–15.

[68] Francis PJ, Moore AT. Genetics of childhood cataract. Curr Opin Ophthalmol 2004;15: 10–5.

[69] Sarfarazi M, Stoilov I. Molecular genetics of primary congenital glaucoma. Eye 2000;14: 422–8.

[70] Kivela T, Tuppurainen K, Riikonen P, et al. Retinoblastoma associated with chromosomal 13q14 deletion mosaicism. Ophthalmology 2003;110(10):1983–8.

[71] Sparkes RS, Sparkes MC, Wilson MG, et al. Regional assignment of genes for human esterase D and retinoblastoma to chromosome band 13q14. Science 1980;208:1042–4.

[72] Munier F, Pescia G, Jotterand-Bellomo M, et al. Constitutional karyotype in retinoblastoma. Case report and review of literature. Ophthalmic Paediatr Genet 1989;10:129–50.

[73] Knudson AG Jr. Mutation and cancer: statistical study of retinoblastoma. Proc Natl Acad Sci USA 1971;68:820–3.

[74] Moll AC, Imhof SM, Bouter LM, et al. Second primary tumors in patients with retinoblastoma. A review of the literature. Ophthalmic Genet 1997;18:27–34.

[75] Kivela T. Trilateral retinoblastoma: a meta-analysis of hereditary retinoblastoma associated with primary ectopic intracranial retinoblastoma. J Clin Oncol 1999;17:1829–37.

[76] Abramson DH, Schefler AC. Update on retinoblastoma. Retina 2004;24:828–48.

[77] Xu K, Rosenwaks Z, Beaverson K, et al. Preimplantation genetic diagnosis for retinoblastoma: the first reported liveborn. Am J Ophthalmol 2004;137:18–23.

ELSEVIER
SAUNDERS

PEDIATRIC CLINICS
OF NORTH AMERICA

Pediatr Clin N Am 53 (2006) 767–775

Psychopharmacology: Clinical Implications of Brain Neurochemistry

Russell E. Scheffer, MD

Child and Adolescent Psychiatry and Behavioral Medicine,
Medical College of Wisconsin and Children's Hospital of Wisconsin,
9000 West Wisconsin Avenue, MS 750, Milwaukee, WI 53201, USA

Over the past 50 years much has been learned about the biological basis of psychiatric disorders. Most biological research in psychiatry has been conducted in adults. This has left pediatric psychiatry a relative biological orphan [1,2]. The use of psychopharmacological agents in very young children (eg, preschoolers) is becoming more common. This age range is particularly understudied [3]. The effects of these medications on developmental processes are not well-studied [4]. Many effects of medications may have unintended impacts for patients. There is growing evidence, however, that the consequences of not treating serious psychiatric illnesses outweigh known risks of the medications. Prescription practices should endeavor to limit adverse consequences whenever possible.

This discrepancy between testing of psychopharmacological agents in children and adults is being addressed on many fronts. An important area of improvement is the growth of evidence-based practice related to psychopharmacology. The US Food and Drug Administration (FDA) Modernization Act and Best Pharmaceuticals for Children Act have increased the incentives and funding to study these agents in children.

The brain is by far the most complicated organ in the body. Its malfunction should be of little surprise to anyone. The brain consists of billions of neurons, usually with thousands of interconnections between each. These neurons are organized further into organelles and interconnected into signaling pathways. The possibilities of dysfunction are almost infinite.

Much of the knowledge regarding the mechanisms of action of psychopharmacological agents has been based on the biological interaction of

E-mail address: rscheffer@chw.org

0031-3955/06/$ - see front matter © 2006 Elsevier Inc. All rights reserved.
doi:10.1016/j.pcl.2006.05.012

receptors and ligands at the synapse. These interactions occur very quickly. The onset of action of these agents, however, can take weeks. It is therefore obvious that other factors play a role in the mechanism of action of psychopharmacological agents. These include drug effects on the function of the entire neuron, complex neuronal systems, and numerous brain organelles.

Most currently available psychopharmacological agents work on neuroregulatory neurotransmitters, including dopamine, norepinephrine, serotonin, and others. Neuronal systems that are controlled by these agents are widespread and function in balance with other neurochemicals. These neurochemicals are also responsible for regulating development. This includes serotonin [5], dopamine [6], glutamate, and γ-aminobutyric acid (GABA) [7]. To a great extent, the body attempts to maintain a homeostasis in regards to these chemicals.

These regulatory neurochemicals often are discussed in regards to broad functions. Serotonin has effects throughout the brain and acts to decrease impulsivity and aggression. Norepinephrine commonly acts to stimulate neuronal systems and is involved in alerting responses. Dopamine helps regulate pleasure and assists in reward mechanisms. All of these neurochemicals are distributed widely throughout the brain and have many, sometimes differing, impacts upon behavior and emotion.

The regulatory neurotransmitters are commonly the target of current psychopharmacology. There are a myriad of neuropeptides, hormones, amino acids, and gases (nitric oxide), however, that account for significant amounts of neurotransmission. Although new information is emerging about the roles of these neurotransmitters, few treatments currently target psychiatric illnesses using these mechanisms.

There are various biological processes that regulate an individual's response to psychopharmacological agents (Box 1).

Box 1. Biological processes that may regulate one's response to psychopharmacological agents

Rate and extent of absorption
First pass effects
Metabolism of the agent
Route of excretion
Biological activity of metabolites
Extent that these agents cross the blood-brain barrier
Receptor or site of action affinities
Interactions with other medications and endogenous compounds
Mechanism of receptor interactions
Signal transduction downstream of the receptor
Complex, often conflicting interactions in the brain

Psychopharmacological agents also act in the periphery. These interactions account for many of the adverse events reported by patients. The same neurochemicals that are modified to treat psychiatric conditions also affect the gastrointestinal system, autonomic nervous system, muscle physiology, and many other processes.

Most psychotropic medications are classified as agonists or antagonists. Their actions at receptor sites could be described as partial agonists. This is because there are few psychopharmacological agents that are complete or irreversible agonists or antagonists. Most agents tend to have the net effect of bringing neurochemical activity toward a normal zone.

This point is illustrated in regard to serotonin function in depression and anxiety disorders. Depression is a condition with low serotonin activity. Anxiety disorders typically exhibit high serotonin activity. The selective serotonin reuptake inhibitors (SSRIs) rapidly increase synaptic levels of serotonin. In depression, this results in improved symptoms in 10 to 14 days. The delay is presumably caused by down stream adaptations to this almost instantaneous increase in synaptic serotonin. In anxiety disorders, this rapid increase in synaptic serotonin from an elevated baseline frequently results in temporary increases in anxiety symptoms. Within a few weeks, this resolves, and anxiety symptoms resolve. The SSRI acts as a partial agonist and brings both conditions toward a more normal expression of serotonin function.

The remainder of this article focuses on major diagnostic categories and the neurotransmitter systems affected using current common psychotropic medications.

Major depression

The use of antidepressants in children and adolescents has received much interest in recent years. This has been because of increased concern regarding safety issues following a failure of numerous industry-sponsored registration trials and increased reports of suicidal ideation.

Tricyclic antidepressants (TCAs) have been studied fairly extensively in the past, and, unlike therapy in adults, they were not found to be efficacious. The primary use for these medications remains in the prophylactic treatment of migraines and the use of imipramine in enuresis.

There has been considerable concern about the possibility of overmedicating children and possible harmful adverse effects related to antidepressants. These concerns should not be overlooked; however, since the introduction and wide-spread use of the SSRIs, the trend of suicides has declined. Geographic areas where SSRI prescription is higher have lower youth suicide rates [8].

Psychiatric disorders, including major depression, have suicidality as an inherent risk. That suicidal thoughts or behaviors might arise before, during, or after treatment should not result in a failure to prescribe medications when indicated. One should take steps to monitor patients for adverse effects and the potential for harm to self or others.

The SSRI's primary mechanism of action is believed to be blockade of the serotonin transporter that brings released serotonin back into the neuron. This results in elevated synaptic serotonin levels almost immediately. Industry-sponsored registration trials in children and adolescents have demonstrated little effectiveness because of excessive placebo response. Medication response rates to SSRIs typically have been in the 60% or more range. This is comparable to the rates demonstrated in adult major depression. Placebo response rates frequently have been between 30 and 50%. The upper limits of this range are in excess of those frequently found in adult depression trials. The higher placebo response rate is likely to have many contributing factors. These might include: positive interactions with study personnel, family mobilization for treatment, and children being more sensitive to their environments. Fluoxetine has received FDA approval for major depression in adolescents.

The serotonin/norepinephrine reuptake inhibitors (SNRIs) have not been shown to be particularly useful in clinical trials in children and adolescents. In adults, deficits of norepinephrine neurotransmission have been implicated in the pathophysiology of major depression. This has not been demonstrated conclusively in children.

Anxiety disorders

SSRIs form the mainstay of medication treatment of anxiety disorders. Anxiety disorders frequently are associated with elevated serotonin turnover. The initial blockade of serotonin reuptake results in even higher synaptic levels of serotonin. This information is important, because initial responses to SSRIs in patients who have anxiety disorders can include exacerbations of symptoms. Over time, the moderating effects of the medications result in less anxiety. Fluoxetine, sertraline, and fluvoxamine all have FDA approval in some anxiety disorders. It is important to note that anxiety disorders may be particularly responsive to focused types of psychotherapy (eg, cognitive and behavioral therapy).

Benzodiazepines are used frequently in adults with anxiety disorders. These agents act on chloride channels in similar ways to that of ethanol. Unfortunately, many youth experience a disinhibition on benzodiazepines. Therefore, the use of benzodiazepines in youth is infrequent.

Buspirone acts predominantly upon presynaptic serotonin receptors. This mechanism has been exploited to treat anxiety disorders and to augment the actions of antidepressants. Clinical experience in children has been somewhat better than that in adults. Dosing three times per day is often necessary, and individual doses range from 5 to 20 mg per dose. Buspirone also is used frequently to augment antidepressants and to decrease sexual dysfunction related to SSRIs.

Attention-deficit/hyperactivity disorder

The mainstays of treatment for attention-deficit/hyperactivity disorder (ADHD) are the psychostimulants. These generally can be divided into two classes: those that consist of methylphenidate (MPH) and those with amphetamine (AMPH). These are accompanied by atomoxetine, a nonstimulant FDA-approved for ADHD treatment.

In considering the pharmacological basis of these three interventions, there are some marked differences. These products vary, not only by class, but by delivery system. There are several relatively new stimulant products that result in longer duration of action than those previously available.

The MPH products' primary mechanism of action is to block the reuptake of dopamine (DA). This results in a rapid but short-lived increase in synaptic dopamine. The half life of MPH products is generally 3 to 5 hours.

The amphetamine products have a more complex mechanism of action. AMP blocks the reuptake of norepinephrine (NE) and DA. These actions are similar to combining atomoxetine and MPH (Table 1). In addition, AMPH increases the amount of NE and DA produced, brought into synaptic vesicles, and released at the synapse. These effects result in an increase in the total amount of neurotransmitter available in the synapse.

The differences in mechanism of action seem to imply significant potential differences in response. The more complex mechanism of AMP, which encompasses the mechanisms of both MPH and atomoxetine, might superficially imply better efficacy and more adverse drug reactions. In clinical practice, little difference is noted between MPH and AMP.

Clinical response to psychostimulants (MPH, AMPH) requires a consolidation of brainstem nuclei and their projections to the cortex. This may occur at different times in preschool years. Therefore, when prescribing stimulants to preschoolers who already demonstrate clinical symptoms of ADHD, it is important to keep in mind that their neurodevelopment may not have progressed to the stage that they are able to respond to standard treatments. Often this improves with time and further development. Carrey provided a comprehensive overview of the impact of neurodevelopment on psychiatric illness and the potential implications of treatment [9].

Table 1
Mechanism of action for US Food and Drug Administration-approved attention-deficit/hyperactivity disorder medications

	Methylphenidate	Amphetamines	Atomoxetine
DA reuptake inhibition	X	X	
Increased uptake into and synaptic release of DA/NE		X	
NE reuptake inhibition		X	X

Abbreviations: DA, dopamine; NE, norepinephrine.

Approved delivery systems include: immediate-release, delayed-release, skin patches, and OROS. Delayed-release consists of different beads. The first type of bead is immediate-release. The second releases approximately 4 hours later. This, in effect, results in two doses 4 hours apart with only a single ingestion. OROS provides more consistent release over approximately 8 hours of gut transit. A transdermal patch has been approved recently. Its utility has not yet been demonstrated.

Atomoxetine primarily acts as an NE reuptake inhibitor. This results in a rapid and more long-lasting increase in NE. It demonstrates some dopaminergic activity in the brain also. An advantage to atomoxetine is that its prescription allows for refills. Its demonstrated size is less than that of the stimulants; nonetheless, it is useful in some patients who have ADHD.

There are additional medications that can be used to treat ADHD. These include the a_2 adrenergic agonists clonidine and guanfacine. These agents act at central presynaptic a_2 autoreceptors. They generally are used in one of two situations. The first is for evening activation. It frequently is noted that children who have ADHD have behavior that activates in the early evening. This phenomena occurs even when patients are not on medications, and it can be exacerbated by wear off or rebound effects from stimulants. An evening dosage of an a_2 agonist can take the edge off these phenomena. The second major way in which these agents are used is to treat impulsivity, hyperactivity, and aggression. These can be primary symptoms of ADHD, part of another syndrome, or isolated target symptoms. In the treatment of ADHD, they provide little benefit for the symptoms of inattention.

Bipolar disorder

Mood stabilizers

Lithium salts, carbamazepine, and valproic acid have been mainstays of bipolar disorder treatment for some time. All three agents have FDA approval for the treatment of acute mania in adults. These agents have not been studied definitively in youth who have bipolar disorder. These agents have biological effects that are different than most other psychotropic medications. Their actions are not primarily through receptors at the synapse. The positive action of these agents indirectly impacts upon serotonin, norepinephrine, and dopamine neurotransmission.

Lithium was grandfathered into FDA approval for use in children as young as age 12. There are no published adequate trials of lithium in youth to determine if it is efficacious and safe. Through the Best Pharmaceuticals for Children Act, it will be studied in the 7- to 17-year-old age group in the near future.

Carbamazepine can induce liver enzymes. This can result in lowered levels of psychopharmacological agents and hormonal contraceptives. Its primary indication, along with valproic acid, is in the treatment of seizure disorders.

Valproic acid (VPA) is a branched chain fatty acid. VPA and lithium both have been found to have neuroprotective effects in animals and to induce neurogenesis in adult animals.

Psychotic disorders

Antipsychotics

Antipsychotics are the fastest growing psychopharmacology class in the United States. They are FDA-approved for treating schizophrenia and in most cases for mania in adults. To date, none has received FDA approval in youth.

The older antipsychotics frequently are referred to as typical antipsychotics. The major effect of these agents is in the blockade of dopaminergic neurotransmission. This is primarily at the dopamine 2 receptor.

The atypical antipsychotics block dopamine in different ways. Some agents (eg, risperidone, olanzapine, and ziprasidone) block dopamine receptors tightly, with low dissociation constants. Quetiapine binds loosely for short periods of time. Aripiprazole is considered a partial dopamine agonist. The result of using these atypical antipsychotics is an approximate 30% effective rate of dopamine neurotransmission, while the receptor is otherwise blocked.

Dopamine blockade results in several adverse effects, including: neuromotor adverse effects, akathisia, elevated prolactin, and anhedonia.

Neuromotor adverse effects include dystonic reactions, pseudo-parkinsonism, and tremor. These adverse effects can be very dysphoric for the patient and may result in decreased adherence to the patient's medical regimen.

Akathisia is a sense of motor restlessness, and it often is misinterpreted as increasing agitation, psychosis, and on occasion as symptoms of ADHD. Akathisia is frequently painful and is considered to be one of the most serious and modifiable risk factors for suicide.

Dopamine is also a prolactin inhibitory factor; therefore, the blockade of dopamine results in elevations of prolactin. Elevated prolactin is related to gynecomastia, galactorrhea, sexual dysfunction, osteopenia, amenorrhea, and possibly an increased risk of breast cancer.

Anhedonia results from the blockade of dopamine. Dopamine is required for neurotransmission of many types of pleasurable feelings. Its prolonged blockade, and resulting decrease in pleasurable experiences, is also a risk factor for suicide.

The newer antipsychotics, commonly referred to as atypical antipsychotics, combine dopaminergic blockade with serotonin agonism. This combined activity is thought to decrease the neuromotor adverse effects of the typical antipsychotics. The extent to which they cause neuromotor adverse effects differs by agent.

These agents frequently have actions in the adrenergic, histaminic, and other neurotransmitter systems also. This accounts for some of the adverse events associated with antipsychotics (eg, sedation, orthostatic hypotension).

The relative safety of the atypical antipsychotics has resulted in their prescription for an increasing number of conditions. These conditions include symptoms of severe aggression and impulsivity, mood instability, and stereotyped and self-injurious behavior amongst others. None of the atypical antipsychotics are approved for use in youth. Many studies are underway to determine the efficacy and safety of these agents in youth.

Autism spectrum disorders

No specific treatments exist for the autism spectrum disorders (ASDs, autism, Asperger's disorder, pervasive developmental disorder, not otherwise specified). Various psychopharmacological treatments, however, are used. These interventions are targeted toward symptoms of ADHD, aggression, impulsivity, mood dysregulation, self-injurious behavior, and stereotypic behaviors. Idiosyncratic reactions to psychopharmacologic agents are somewhat more common in ASDs than other conditions. The treatment of ADHD follows that for the typical syndrome. The treatment of aggression includes a_2 adrenergic agonists (clonidine and guanfacine), mood stabilizers, and antipsychotics. Self-injurious and stereotypic behaviors are treated frequently with antipsychotics.

Naltrexone, an opioid antagonist, is used under the theory that self-injurious and stereotypic behaviors result as an unconscious attempt to activate the endogenous opioid systems. By blocking endogenous opioids patients frequently discontinue these behaviors.

Electrocardiograms

Blair and colleagues summarized the evidence for ECG monitoring in pediatric psychopharmacology [10]. This manuscript provides an overview for the approach to evaluating a patient before starting a psychotropic medication. Most concerns revolve around corrected QT interval prolongation with antipsychotics, tricyclic antidepressants, and stimulants when combined with alpha adrenergic agonists. Current practice suggests that personal or family history of cardiac abnormalities or physical findings that are worrisome for cardiac problems would increase the vigilance for ECG monitoring.

Summary

The brain is a complex organ consisting of 100 billion neurons and support cells. Neurons have hundreds to thousands of synaptic connections to other neurons. These interconnections result in local feedback loops and long chains of neurons connected in functional units. The brain is organized further into organelles and ultimately to the peripheral nervous system. Attempts to focally influence specific neurotransmitter systems invariably have impacts upon other neurotransmitter systems. The pharmacological impact upon one neurotransmitter system results in compensatory impact upon other systems.

Children metabolize and use medications differently than adults [11]. In many cases, these differences impact the dosing schedule of medications. This also may help to explain why some agents have not demonstrated effectiveness [12]. There is an exciting future for pharmacogenomic profiling in pediatric neuropharmacology.

Psychopharmacological interventions are being used with increasing frequency in youth. This includes use in very young children, in combinations and other off-label uses. These practices need to be reviewed periodically as the evidence base for there use expands.

References

[1] Riddle MA, Labellarte MJ, Walkup JT. Pediatric psychopharmacology: problems and prospects. J Child Adolesc Psychopharmacol 1998;8(2):87–97.

[2] Walkup JT, Cruz K, Kane S, et al. The future of pediatric psychopharmacology. Pediatr Clin North Am 1998;45(5):1265–78.

[3] DeBar LL, Lynch F, Powell J, et al. Use of psychotropic agents in preschool children: associated symptoms, diagnoses, and health care services in a health maintenance organization. Arch Pediatr Adolesc Med 2003;157(2):150–7.

[4] Greenhill LL, Vitiello B, Abikoff H, et al. Developing methodologies for monitoring long-term safety of psychotropic medications in children: report on the NIMH conference, September 25, 2000. J Am Acad Child Adolesc Psychiatry 2003;42(6):651–5.

[5] Whitaker-Azmitia PM, Druse M, Walker P, et al. Serotonin as a developmental signal. Behav Brain Res 1996;73(1–2):19–29.

[6] Breese GR, Baumeister AA, McCown TJ, et al. Behavioral differences between neonatal and adult 6-hydroxydopamine-treated rats to dopamine agonists: relevance to neurological symptoms in clinical syndromes with reduced brain dopamine. J Pharmacol Exp Ther 1984;231(2):343–54.

[7] Cameron HA, Hazel TG, McKay RD. Regulation of neurogenesis by growth factors and neurotransmitters. J Neurobiol 1998;36(2):287–306.

[8] Olfson M, Shaffer D, Marcus SC, et al. Relationship between antidepressant medication treatment and suicide in adolescents. Arch Gen Psychiatry 2003;60(10):978–82.

[9] Carrey N. Developmental neurobiology: implications for pediatric psychopharmacology. Can J Psychiatry 2001;46(9):810–8.

[10] Blair J, Taggart B, Martin A. Electrocardiographic safety profile and monitoring guidelines in pediatric psychopharmacology. J Neural Transm 2004;111(7):791–815.

[11] Tosyali MC, Greenhill LL. Child and adolescent psychopharmacology. Important developmental issues. Pediatr Clin North Am 1998;45(5):1021–35 [vii.].

[12] Findling RL. Paediatric psychopharmacology: closing the gap between science and practice. Expert Opin Pharmacother 2001;2(4):523–5.

Obesity and Its Therapy: From Genes to Community Action

Joseph A. Skelton, MD[a,b,*], Laure DeMattia, DO[b,c], Lawrence Miller, PsyD[b], Michael Olivier, PhD[d]

[a]Division of Pediatric Gastroenterology and Nutrition, Medical College of Wisconsin,
8701 Watertown Plank Road, PO Box 26509, Milwaukee, WI 53226, USA
[b]The NEW (Nutrition, Exercise, and Weight-management) Kids™ Program,
Children's Hospital of Wisconsin, 9000 West Wisconsin Avenue, Milwaukee, WI 53226, USA
[c]Family and Community Medicine, Medical College of Wisconsin,
8701 Watertown Plank Road, PO Box 26509, Milwaukee, WI 53226, USA
[d]Department of Physiology, Human and Molecular Genetics Center,
Medical College of Wisconsin, 8701 Watertown Plank Road, PO Box 26509,
Milwaukee, WI 53226, USA

The increase in the number of overweight children over the last several decades is obvious to anyone who cares for or works with children. To the general practitioner, this is an especially frustrating problem. Few treatment modalities exist, and despite great knowledge of contributing factors, little can be accomplished in a brief office visit. Additionally, exciting advances in basic science research, beginning with the discovery of leptin in 1994 [1], have not led to novel tools for use in everyday clinical practice. Leptin turned out to be the tip of the iceberg in the scientific investigation of obesity and its comorbidities. To date, more than 600 genes, markers, and regions of chromosomes have been linked to obesity [2]. Does this mean we are closer or further away from finding better ways to treat and prevent obesity?

Traditionally, the biopsychosocial model of obesity as a disease has been considered appropriate, as all elements of the model are relevant (Fig. 1). This model shows disease arising from the overlap of components. In applying this model to obesity research, biologic systems are viewed in isolation, not taking into account their interaction with the environment and behaviors until there is "disease" present. Although strides have been made

* Corresponding author. Division of Pediatric Gastroenterology and Nutrition, Medical College of Wisconsin, 8701 Watertown Plank Road, Milwaukee, WI 53226.

E-mail address: jskelton@mcw.edu (J.A. Skelton).

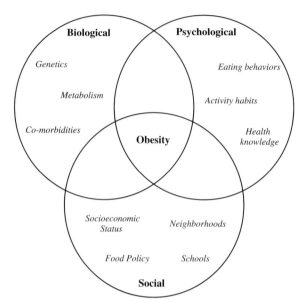

Fig. 1. Biopsychosocial model of obesity.

exploring the pathophysiology of obesity, treatment and prevention have focused on the other two components: psychological and social. The best interventions have been in the fields of dietary management and behavioral
change [3–5]. Drug therapy has been limited, especially in children [6–8]. Genetic testing is applicable to only a small number of those affected by obesity. Exploring the cellular and molecular mechanisms behind obesity while
clinically treating from the other end of the spectrum can result in slow
progress. By integrating basic science with clinical research, treatments
and interventions will be better focused and more quickly translated into
care plans. To facilitate this, a paradigm shift has taken place.

A more comprehensive model of childhood overweight is the Ecological
Systems Theory [9], which helps conceptualize the contributors to obesity
(Fig. 2). Physiologic, behavioral, and environmental components are inter-
twined, and none can be fully considered without understanding the systems
in which they are embedded. Instead of dissecting out the contributors to
weight status, they are viewed holistically. This "clinical" approach can
also be applied to research.

Using an ecological model, known therapies such as cognitive behavioral
modification and modified nutrition can be translated into genetic research.
Investigating the genomics of behavior can allow for targeted interventions
in those predisposed to dysfunctional eating or parenting behaviors. Nutritional genomics could one day identify particular individuals that may require supplementation of essential fatty acids to maintain a healthy
weight. The complex nature of the obesity epidemic is no longer a hindrance

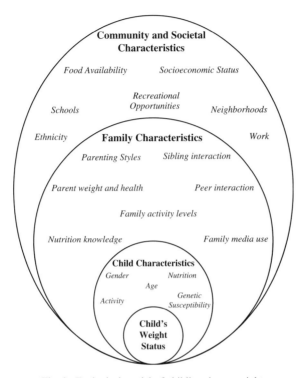

Fig. 2. Ecological model of childhood overweight.

to effective research, but complements the translational medicine approach. This chapter summarizes research efforts aimed at elucidating the complex genetic, behavioral, and social relationships causing overweight and obesity, and highlights targeted efforts to advance treatment and prevention using an integrated approach.

Complex diseases require complex approaches

The completion of the sequence of the human genome has been heralded as the advent of a new era in biomedical research [10]. However, despite all efforts, the impact on clinical medicine and disease management, not only in the area of obesity, has been relatively small. The primary reason for this slow progress is the fact that the genetic factors influencing obesity are complex and multifaceted. The early success stories in medical genetics have shown that mutated genes can be identified in disorders such as cystic fibrosis [11] and sickle cell anemia [12]. However, in all of these cases, a single gene in the human genome is mutated so that it no longer produces a functional protein. In almost all cases, these so-called "monogenic disorders" are recessive—that is, the child needs to inherit one mutated copy of the gene from each parent. Although the clinical consequences of these disorders are usually severe, only a relatively small number of individuals are affected, and the diseases are relatively rare in the general population.

Unfortunately, most common diseases that affect a much larger percentage of children, such as obesity, have a more complicated genetic basis. For these disorders, not just one but several genes are believed to be mutated [13]. However, in contrast to diseases like cystic fibrosis, each of these mutations by itself does not cause the disease, and only the accumulation of a relatively large number of mutations in different genes across the entire genome will ultimately lead to the clinical manifestations of these polygenic disorders. The identification of all these genetic changes is further complicated by the fact that the clinical manifestations of the disorder are also influenced by environmental factors such as nutrition and behavior in the case of obesity. Only the complex interplay of a significant number of genetic mutations and the "wrong" environmental conditions will result in obesity.

This complexity is the primary reason for the slow progress in the identification of genetic causes of obesity. However, despite the adversity of this complex research challenge, significant progress has been made in the last few years, albeit with as-of-yet little impact on clinical disease management in children or adults. The development of high-throughput technologies to examine large numbers of single nucleotide polymorphisms (SNPs) across the human genome has permitted the systematic analysis of the role of these sequence differences in the development of obesity [14]. SNPs are single base pair changes in the DNA sequence. Humans are genetically 99.9% identical on the sequence level [15], which in turn means that an individual's genome sequence differs (on average) from another individual's sequence in three million positions. The majority of these differences consists of single base pair differences in the DNA sequence ("spelling errors"), and includes known mutations responsible for disorders such as cystic fibrosis. However, nothing is known about the effect of the majority of these sequence changes, and it is possible that some of these in combination are responsible for the development of common polygenic disorders such as obesity. In addition to our improved ability to interrogate and examine these SNPs across the entire human genome [16], the clinical ascertainment of large patient cohorts and the accurate diagnosis of obesity-related abnormalities in these individuals allow researchers for the first time to identify sequence changes shared among large numbers of obese individuals [17].

Although it has become easier to identify potential sequence changes that are associated with obesity, the actual verification of the genetic effect and the analysis of its physiologic consequences have been even more challenging. Historically, researchers have examined the effect of mutations on gene function by expressing the mutated gene in cells in vitro and examining the effect of the resulting mutated protein on physiologic responses to external stimuli such as hormones (eg, leptin or insulin). The approach is labor intensive but has yielded significant insights into gene function of individual genes and its mutations. However, such an analysis is no longer feasible when numerous sequence changes in a significant number of different genes have to be examined in parallel. Not only is the sheer number of genes that need to be examined beyond our current capabilities, it is also unclear what kind of effect the different sequence changes will have on the physiology of target organs. The numerous mutations will not have as dramatic an effect as the mutations reported for monogenic disorders. If they did, it is likely that only one or a few mutations would suffice to cause disease, and the onset and severity of the disorder would be much more dramatic than the gradual onset commonly seen in polygenic disorders such as obesity. Thus, research needs to advance from its current state of functional analysis to integrate genomic approaches with extensive clinical analyses to fully understand the complex interplay of genes, nutrition, and behavior that leads to the development and progression of obesity. Genetics can only provide a small yet crucial portion of the answer to this medical challenge, and it cannot do this in the isolation of a basic science research laboratory.

Genetics of feeding behavior

Treatment of obesity has been best conceptualized as an interdisciplinary (ie, physicians, dietitians, psychologists, physical therapists) approach to a chronic disease [18], but there is not a single, effective, standardized treatment approach. Behavioral treatment programs typically result in some short-term weight loss; however, long-term weight maintenance is extremely difficult and successful in a marginal number of patients [19]. In the field of pediatrics, the most successful interventions have been in controlled studies involving behavioral modification [20–23]. In keeping with the ecological model of obesity, translational medicine and research should include investigation of behaviors.

It is challenging to identify which behaviors are genetically related to obesity owing to a variety of research methodologic issues [24]. In their review of the obesity genetic literature, Faith and coauthors [24] recognized that food intake, parenting behavior, physical activity, and eating disorders have genetic influences, whereas personality styles do not. Behavioral genetics studies have identified the genetic preference for specific food types, but the majority of the variance in eating behavior is owing to shared environmental and genetic factors. These can be difficult to clearly separate from genetics [25,26]. Twin studies have found that children with parents who are obese preferred vegetables less, responded greater to cues for food, had a higher desire for drinks, but did not have greater food intake compared with children with parents of normal weight [26]. Animal studies have found links between chromosomes 1 and 4 on weight gain at 8 and 10 weeks, and for 2-week weight gain (ie, difference between weeks 10 and 8), chromosome 6 (which coincides with human 7q) was found to play a role [27]. In review of human studies, the β-2 adrenergic receptor Gln27Gln genotype, and mutations in the *MC4R* gene have been linked with changes in body composition and for the latter in binge eating [25,28]. In addition, dietary restraint has been coupled with chromosomes 3 and 6, and taste sensitivity to 6-*n*-propylthiouracil (PROP) (ie, ability to perceive fat) has been linked to chromosome 7q and relates to food preferences [25].

Children are born with the inherit preference for sweet and salty tastes and reject sour and bitter tastes, and they have the capacity to regulate their amount of food consumption in 24-hour periods. However, parents that do not allow self-control over foods can dominate the child's inborn system that results not only in the disruption of the internal hunger and satiety cues but also in child food preferences [29]. Well-intending parents that seek to control their child's eating practices, especially if the child is at greater risk for obesity [30], set the stage for negativity around food by limiting food choices, a cascade that ultimately leads to weight gain. These findings could influence anticipatory guidance and feeding recommendations in the near future.

Little work has been done to account for the genetic role in physical activity as it relates to obesity. Reviews of animal studies find that "diet, hypothalamic lesions, genetics, age, and sex all affect activity as well as weight gain [31]." One study of adult monozygotic twins found that vigorous exercise can lower the genetic influences on body mass index (BMI), but that it has little influence on blood chemistry results illustrating the strength of genetic vulnerability with regard to medical comorbidities from overweight [32]. A study of adult women found that the β-2 adrenergic receptor Glu27Glu genotype corresponded to lower endurance performance when compared with women with the Gln27Gln and Gln27Glu genotypes [33]. Clearly, more research is needed in this area to ascertain the relationship between diet, physical activity, genetics, and environmental factors and obesity development and weight reduction.

There has been ongoing debate as to whether obesity and psychopathology are connected. Does psychopathology cause obesity, or does obesity cause psychopathology? Although there are no answers to the questions above, studies have found individuals with greater overweight have greater psychosocial problems [34]. Is there a genetic link? Comings and coauthors [35] pioneered one of, if not the most instrumental study that correlated chromosome 7 with obesity and depression. However, not all obese persons are depressed, especially men; yet, evidence has indicated that the BMI–depression relationship is consistent across ethnicities [36]. It appears that researchers are getting closer to uncovering the genetic associations of obesity and its related comorbidities, but sex and socioeconomic status and associated factors may mediate the differences [34,37]. Considering that exercise reduces levels of depression, what might the gene–environment/ behavioral interaction be that also helps lessen body weight? Both obesity and psychopathology are linked with other health problems that make untangling this complex web of interaction extremely difficult.

One of the most exciting areas of research is the use of functional magnetic resonance imaging (fMRI) and positron emission tomography (PET) to pinpoint areas of the brain underlying lifestyle experiences commonly associated with obese individuals. Review of the existing literature identified several studies that examined dopaminergic areas tied to the anticipation, not necessarily the consumption, of food [38]. Differences in the functional architecture between the brains of lean and obese individuals have been identified. However, these investigators note poignantly that in the attempt to uncover the cause of obesity, we are often left with more questions, reaffirming that there is no simple test to recognize those at greatest risk.

Nutrition meets genetics

The underpinnings of nutrition's role in obesity become much more complicated with the tools of genetics and genomics. In particular, the fields of proteomics and metabolomics provide key insight into how the body uses nutrients. For every turn of the Krebs cycle, there are vast arrays of proteins, metabolites, enzymes, and transporters that are controlled by genes. For every one of these genes, there is variation between individuals, all adding up to slight differences in how we use calories. And for every gene, there may be a key vitamin or mineral that influences expression of the gene, which, if not ingested in proper quantities, can lead to abnormal function. This study of food–gene interaction is called *nutritional genomics*, or *nutrigenomics*.

The goal of this research is to elucidate how diet can regulate gene function, why components of a person's diet can increase risk of one disease and lower the risk of another, and how dietary intervention can be tailored to genotype to improve health. Still in its infancy, nutritional genomics has already found applications in cancer, diabetes, and heart disease [39]. In terms of obesity treatment and prevention, this field could unlock the differences in human response to exercise, caloric deprivation, and basal metabolic rate.

Peroxisome proliferator-activated receptors (PPARs) are nuclear receptors that regulate genes involved in the storage and metabolism of fats. A polymorphism in one subtype, PPAR-γ, has been linked to dietary-induced obesity. PPAR-γ affects insulin resistance and blood pressure. Individuals with the Pro12Ala polymorphism appear to be prone to obesity and hyperinsulinism depending on dietary intake of fats. A low polyunsaturated-to-saturated (P/S) fat ratio is associated with an increase in body mass index and fasting insulin levels in individuals who carry the Ala allele, with the reverse occurring with high P/S fat ratios (Ala carriers have lower BMIs and insulin levels) [40]. This relationship is further modified by physical activity [41].

In a mouse model, adiposity has been shown to be altered by maternal diet. When the agouti gene is overexpressed in mice, they develop a yellow coat and early-onset obesity, as well as increased mortality levels [42]. Investigators were able to modify the phenotypes of genetically identical mice by manipulating maternal dietary methyl supplementation, with mice having different color coats depending on the amount of supplementation [43]. Subsequent genomic studies have revealed 28 genes regulated by diet, genotype, or diet–genotype interaction that map to diabetes/obesity quantitative trait loci [44].

Nutrigenomic research is making its way quickly into clinical medicine and could yield relevant findings in the near future. Researchers studying a gene involved in adipocyte fatty acid release (perilipin) found that carriers of the minor allele on a low-calorie diet were resistant to weight loss yet had a lower body weight at baseline (before dietary intervention) [45]. The framework for studies such as this were in animal models, but more such research could soon lead to "personalized" dietary interventions based on genotype.

The neuroendocrine pathway

The discovery of leptin in 1994 was important in many ways. It showed that hunger was more than a craving centered in the brain or a signal from an empty stomach. In a story that continues to evolve, leptin and many other hormones, in conjunction with the nervous system and its signals, regulate short- and long-term control of hunger and weight. Additionally, the adipocyte, previously thought to be a passive reservoir of lipids, is a hormonal organ with multiple actions. The complex pathways delineated to date are all targets for therapy and intervention, both in treating comorbidities resulting from obesity as well as weight issues themselves. Fig. 3 represents some of the major elements of hunger and weight control.

Leptin, produced primarily by adipocytes, acts as the main signal to the brain from fat stores. Therefore, when a person becomes obese, leptin levels should increase, signaling the brain to decrease intake and increase energy expenditure. The gene for leptin was discovered in the *ob/ob* mouse, which was homozygous for a mutation in the gene, resulting in a deficiency in leptin production. As a consequence, mice gained weight at an increased rate [1]. Despite the promise of leptin as a treatment target for obesity, it has found limited clinical use. There have only been a few cases of either leptin deficiency or leptin receptor mutations, with the former being amenable to leptin replacement therapy [46,47]. In obese patients with normal (ie, functional) leptin and leptin receptor genes, treatment with leptin has not resulted in dramatic effects [48], and it appears that obese patients have a form of "leptin resistance." Regardless, leptin is still under investigation as a treatment modality [49].

Ghrelin is one of the many enteric hormones discovered in the wake of leptin. It was originally discovered in the rat, with the human homolog identified shortly thereafter [50]. It is expressed mainly in the fundus of the

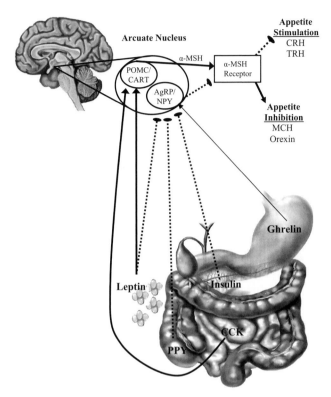

Fig. 3. Neuroendocrine control of appetite. Solid arrows represent stimulation, and dotted lines represent inhibition. AgRP, agouti-related peptide; CART, cocaine-amphetamine–regulated transcript; CCK, cholecystokinin; CRH, corticotrophin-releasing hormone; MCH, melanocortin hormone; α-MSH, alpha-melanocyte–stimulating hormone; NPY, neuropeptide Y; POMC, pro-opiomelancortin; TRH, thyrotropin-releasing hormone.

stomach and acts as an appetite stimulant, primarily in short-term appetite control. Further studies in humans have found that levels are lower in obese patients [51], who also appear to have increased sensitivity to the appetite-stimulating effects of the hormone [52]. The role of ghrelin in appetite and obesity make the development of antagonists likely as potential therapeutic agents.

Alpha-melanocyte–stimulating hormone, found in mice to increase energy expenditure and decrease energy intake, has been studied extensively as an anorexigenic agent in animals [53]. Studies in mice and humans have identified defects in the melanocortin 4 receptor (MC4R, the target of α-melanocyte–stimulating hormone), with null mutations increasing food intake and insulin levels [54]. Nearly 6% of people with long-term, severe obesity were found to have a mutation in the *MC4R* gene [55], making *MC4R* deficiency the most common monogenic form of obesity. Therapies are under development for those with this form of severe obesity [56].

In addition, neuropeptide Y, an orexigenic (appetite stimulating) peptide released from the arcuate nucleus, is another potential target for an intervention. Antagonists of neuropeptide Y could lead to sustained decreases in appetite [53].

Peptide YY (PYY) is an enteric-derived hormone that was identified in studies of rodents [57,58]. Released by enteroendocrine cells of the ileum and colon, PYY acts as an "ileal brake" and delays gastric emptying, thereby decreasing energy intake. It acts centrally as well on the arcuate nucleus to inhibit appetite. Animal studies were translated quickly to human studies, and results on feeding inhibition were promising. Much like leptin, the initial promise of therapies using PYY analogs have not materialized, but interest remains high [59].

Another peptide hormone, glucagon-like peptide-1 (GLP-1), is produced in the central nervous system and the small intestine and acts on satiety by multiple mechanisms. It slows gastric emptying, decreases gastric acid secretion, and stimulates insulin release [60,61]. Much like other appetite-suppressing peptides, it is a rational target for drug investigation. GLP-1 may have positive effects on diabetes and cardiovascular function and may have potential in the treatment of heart disease and diabetes [61].

Finally, amylin is a peptide cosecreted with insulin that has been shown to slow gastric emptying and lower food intake in animals [62,63]. The amylin analog pramlinitide has been studied primarily as adjunctive therapy in diabetes, but has resulted in sustained weight loss [64].

A promising therapy using newly discovered mechanisms of appetite control is rimonabant. Whereas currently available appetite suppressants rely on stimulant properties to reduce appetite, rimonabant selectively blocks the canabinoid-1 receptor, a G protein–coupled receptor found in the central nervous system and in various peripheral tissues. Blocking the action of this receptor prevents overactivation of the endocannabinoid system, centrally and peripherally [65]. In the first large-scale trial in North America, rimonabant produced sustained weight loss above dietary intervention alone [66]. More exciting is the independent effect the drug appeared to have on the amelioration of cardiovascular risk factors (diabetic risk, high-density lipoprotein, triglycerides, waist circumference). Given its lack of stimulant properties, rimonabant may offer the promise of long-term weight control.

Is obesity an infection?

There is mounting evidence of possible infectious contributions to the etiology of obesity. An adenovirus inoculation (and later other viruses) has been identified as a cause of increased adiposity in animals [67,68]. Mice and chickens were then inoculated with human adenovirus, which resulted in increased adipose tissue and lower cholesterol and triglycerides [69]. This was later found to be a transmissible effect in other animal studies [70]. Human studies found that a higher percentage of obese subjects had adenovirus-36 antibodies when compared with nonobese controls [71]. Paradoxically, the patients with adenovirus antibodies had lower serum cholesterol and triglycerides, as was found in human virus inoculation of chickens and mice. These relatively new findings imply that treating infections (using antivirals) at an early age could potentially prevent later onset of obesity.

Adipocytes as an endocrine organ

The further investigation of the role of adenovirus infection may not lead to a focused antiviral treatment for obesity but may find new pathways and mechanisms, similar to the discovery of leptin and subsequent research into weight control that has found the adipocyte to be an active endocrine organ. Increasing adiposity leads to increasing levels of "adipokines," adipocyte-derived inflammatory markers that act in pro- and antiinflammatory pathways [72,73]. Additionally, macrophages found in adipose tissue likely have a role in the obese–inflammatory state and its related disease [74]. Laboratory and animal research has led to the understanding that obesity is a state of chronic inflammation. Infection may be the link among adipocytes, macrophages, and inflammation, or at least a contributor.

Translating clinical knowledge into community action

In 1998, health care providers, public health officials, schools, and communities were asked to start working together to bring attention to the epidemic of childhood obesity. This condition, not defined as a disease, was prioritized with diseases such as diabetes, asthma, and cancer [75]. Rapid increases in obesity rates [76–78], rising health care costs (estimates of $14 billion per year is spent caring for overweight children and their comorbid conditions), [79] and media attention have accelerated interest in this epidemic.

In 2003 the National Institute of Health Obesity Research Task Force was formed and began to develop a strategic focus of research agenda. National collaborative programs such as Action for Kids, VERB, 5 a day, Ways to Enhance Children's Nutrition and Physical Activity (WE CAN), Active Living by Design, and Steps to a Healthier US were launched to help the prevention of overweight and obesity in both children and adults through community action, strategic partnership, and national outreach. These initiatives could be enhanced further by using techniques that were successful in other public health campaigns such as smoking cessation [80]. Clinical intervention, educational programs, regulatory policies, economic approaches, and comprehensive programs that incorporate these facets have synergistically influenced the reduction of smoking [81,82]. Applying the above characteristics within the context of the Ecological Model of Childhood Overweight [9] framework has the potential to reduce modifiable risk factors in genetically susceptible individuals and reverse the obesity epidemic (Table 1).

Table 1
Modifiable risk factors of the ecological model of childhood obesity

	Clinical interventions	Educational programs	Regulatory efforts	Economic factors
Child	Poor nutrition Sedentary activity Activity level	School curriculum Day care curriculum After school programs	School Wellness policy Limited physical education Competitive food Sales Vending machine Food as reward	Pricing of nutrient-poor foods
Family	Parent: • Style • Weight • Health • Media use • Nutrition knowledge Family: • Activity • Eating behaviors • Sedentary behavior	Worksite wellness programs	Work site policy: • Smoking cessation • Support • Breastfeeding • Food environment	Tax breaks for physical activity participation Working bonus for reducing excess weight
Community	Health care providers: • Relay consistent message • Improve self efficacy	Media campaign Health Fairs Public health messages	Built environment: • Urban sprawl • Walkability • Safety • Transportation • Recreational opportunities [100] Food environment • Access to nutrient-dense foods • Reduce marketing for unhealthful foods [101]	Tax on nutrient-poor foods Support for Farmers Markets

Clinical interventions

Health care providers of children have been advised by the American Academy of Pediatrics policy statement to monitor high risk patients, calculate and plot BMI yearly, encourage breastfeeding, and discuss physical activity and snacks as part of each anticipatory guidance opportunity [83]. Many health care providers report decreased self-efficacy when attempting to counsel patients on nutrition and physical activity. Physicians are more likely to counsel regarding exercise if they are currently active themselves [84]. With education, health care providers can become more confident. As Crawford and coworkers [85] report, staff wellness training improved the perceptions of their own health beliefs and counseling self-efficacy.

One of the most modifiable risk factors for childhood obesity is reducing the amount of television screen time [86]. Proposed mechanisms for pediatric weight gain owing to television consumption include displacement of physical activity, lowering of metabolic rate during viewing, and negative effects on nutritional intake [87]. Consistent evidence supports the direct correlation between television exposure time and increased weight [88,89]. Although associated with obesity and poor school performance [90], 30% of children younger than 3 years, 43% of children aged 4 to 6 years, and 68% of those aged 8 to 18 years have televisions in their bedrooms [91,92]. Helping families understand that excessive television viewing can have a negative impact on their child's long-term health is a necessary part of every well child visit.

Family environment risk factors

Whereas the effect of guidance from health care providers can be influential on health behaviors [93], family environment is paramount. Children are exposed to both the genes and the environment of their parents. Davison and Birch [94] report that overweight parents tend to exercise less, derive less enjoyment from physical activity, and consume an increased percentage of calories from fat. Although modeling poor dietary and physical activity habits increases the risk of pediatric overweight, parental support and modeling physical activity have been shown to increase girls' physical activity [95]. Parental health behavior change predicts the initial and the maintained decrease in a child's BMI in family-based weight management programs [96]. Discussions with families regarding the weight status of their children should therefore include an assessment of the parental health practices to facilitate long-lasting healthy habits.

Community-based change

Children are currently exposed to an "obeseogenic" environment in the larger community. Children spend the majority of their time away from home at school. Changes to their environment at school can be successful, acceptable, and efficacious to decrease screen time, increase fruit and vegetable intake, and increase moderate to vigorous activity in middle school children [97,98]. Children also spend on average 2 to 5 hours per day in the media environment [99] in which they will see between 12 and 30 food commercials. Ludwig and Gortmaker [87] describe children viewing food advertisements as increasing their energy intake significantly, increasing consumption of fast food and sweetened beverages, and decreasing consumption of fruits and vegetables. Health care providers must advocate for regulatory efforts to decrease such advertising policies. Sweden and the Netherlands have passed legislation that prevents direct food advertising toward children.

Summary

Obesity is becoming a major health problem in children. The number of overweight individuals is rapidly increasing, and the impact of basic research into the genetic and physiologic basis of obesity has not been successfully translated into clinical management and prevention of this new epidemic. The factors influencing the development and progression of obesity are complex, and comprehensive, integrated efforts are required to unravel the causes of the disorder and develop novel options for prevention and treatment. Using the Ecological Systems Theory as a model, a thorough understanding of the physiologic, behavioral, and environmental components and the systems in which they are embedded and interact will lead to a holistic approach, maximizing the impact of translational medicine in the approach to childhood obesity.

Acknowledgment

The authors would like to thank Nancy Pejsa for her assistance in preparing the figures.

References

[1] Zhang Y, Proenca R, Maffei M, et al. Positional cloning of the mouse obese gene and its human homologue. Nature 1994;372(6505):425–32.
[2] Perusse L, Rankinen T, Zuberi A, et al. The human obesity gene map: The 2004 update. Obes Res 2005;13(3):381–481.
[3] Kirk S, Scott BJ, Daniels SR. Pediatric obesity epidemic: treatment options. J Am Diet Assoc 2005;105(5, Suppl 1):S44–51.
[4] Stewart L, Houghton J, Hughes AR, et al. Dietetic management of pediatric overweight: development and description of a practical and evidence-based behavioral approach. J Am Diet Assoc 2005;105(11):1810–5.
[5] Bautista-Castano I, Doreste J, Serra-Majem L. Effectiveness of interventions in the prevention of childhood obesity. Eur J Epidemiol 2004;19(7):617–22.

[6] Kiess W, Reich A, Muller G, et al. Obesity in childhood and adolescence: clinical diagnosis and management. J Pediatr Endocrinol 2001;14(Suppl 6):1431–40.

[7] Yanovski JA. Intensive therapies for pediatric obesity. Pediatr Clin North Am 2001;48(4): 1041–53.

[8] Yanovski SZ, Yanovski JA. Obesity. N Engl J Med 2002;346(8):591–602.

[9] Davison KK, Birch LL. Childhood overweight: a contextual model and recommendations for future research. Obes Rev 2001;2(3):159–71.

[10] Lander ES, Linton LM, Birren B, et al. Initial sequencing and analysis of the human genome. Nature 2001;409(6822):860–921.

[11] Riordan JR, Rommens JM, Kerem B, et al. Identification of the cystic fibrosis gene: cloning and characterization of complementary DNA. Science 1989;245(4922):1066–73.

[12] Cao A, Galanello R, Rosatelli MC. Prenatal diagnosis and screening of the haemoglobinopathies. Baillieres Clin Haematol 1998;11(1):215–38.

[13] Clement K. Genetics of human obesity. Proc Nutr Soc 2005;64(2):133–42.

[14] Zak NB, Shifman S, Shalom A, et al. Genetic dissection of common diseases. Isr Med Assoc J 2002;4(6):438–43.

[15] Sachidanandam R, Weissman D, Schmidt SC, et al. A map of human genome sequence variation containing 1.42 million single nucleotide polymorphisms. Nature 2001;409(6822): 928–33.

[16] Kwok PY. Methods for genotyping single nucleotide polymorphisms. Annu Rev Genomics Hum Genet 2001;2:235–58.

[17] Hirschhorn JN. Genetic approaches to studying common diseases and complex traits. Pediatr Res 2005;57(5 Pt 2):74R–7R.

[18] Rippe JM, Crossley S, Ringer R. Obesity as a chronic disease: modern medical and lifestyle management. J Am Diet Assoc 1998;98(10, Suppl 2):S9–15.

[19] Wilson GT, Brownell KD. Behavioral Treatment for Obesity. 2nd edition. New York: The Guilford Press; 2002.

[20] Epstein LH. Family-based behavioural intervention for obese children. Int J Obes Relat Metab Disord 1996;20(Suppl 1):S14–21.

[21] Epstein LH, McCurley J, Wing RR, et al. Five-year follow-up of family-based behavioral treatments for childhood obesity. J Consult Clin Psychol 1990;58(5):661–4.

[22] Epstein LH, Roemmich JN, Raynor HA. Behavioral therapy in the treatment of pediatric obesity. Pediatr Clin North Am 2001;48(4):981–93.

[23] Epstein LH, Valoski A, Wing RR, et al. Ten-year outcomes of behavioral family-based treatment for childhood obesity. Health Psychol 1994;13(5):373–83.

[24] Faith MS, Johnson SL, Allison DB. Putting the behavior into the behavior genetics of obesity. Behav Genet 1997;27(4):423–39.

[25] Faith MS, Keller KL, Johnson SL, et al. Familial aggregation of energy intake in children. Am J Clin Nutr 2004;79(5):844–50.

[26] Faith MS. Development and modification of child food preferences and eating patterns: behavior genetics strategies. Int J Obes 2005;29(6):549–56.

[27] Zhang S, Gershenfeld HK. Genetic contributions to body weight in mice: relationship of exploratory behavior to weight. Obes Res 2003;11(7):828–38.

[28] Potoczna N, Branson R, Kral JG, et al. Gene variants and binge eating as predictors of comorbidity and outcome of treatment in severe obesity. J Gastrointest Surg 2004;8(8): 971–81.

[29] Birch LL, Fisher JO. Development of eating behaviors among children and adolescents. Pediatrics 1998;101(3 Pt 2):539–49.

[30] Faith MS, Berkowitz RI, Stallings VA, et al. Parental feeding attitudes and styles and child body mass index: prospective analysis of a gene-environment interaction. Pediatrics 2004; 114(4):e429–36.

[31] Tou JC, Wade CE. Determinants affecting physical activity levels in animal models. Exp Biol Med 2002;227(8):587–600.

[32] Williams PT, Blanche PJ, Krauss RM. Behavioral versus genetic correlates of lipoproteins and adiposity in identical twins discordant for exercise. Circulation 2005;112(3):350–6.

[33] Moore GE, Shuldiner AR, Zmuda JM, et al. Obesity gene variant and elite endurance performance. Metabolism 2001;50(12):1391–2.

[34] Stunkard AJ, Faith MS, Allison KC. Depression and obesity. Biol Psychiatry 2003;54(3): 330–7.

[35] Comings DE, Gade R, MacMurray JP, et al. Genetic variants of the human obesity (OB) gene: association with body mass index in young women, psychiatric symptoms, and interaction with the dopamine D2 receptor (DRD2) gene. Mol Psychiatry 1996;1(4): 325–35.

[36] Faith MS, Matz PE, Jorge MA. Obesity-depression associations in the population. J Psychosom Res 2002;53(4):935–42.

[37] Butler MG, Hedges L, Hovis CL, et al. Genetic variants of the human obesity (OB) gene in subjects with and without Prader-Willi syndrome: comparison with body mass index and weight. Clin Genet 1998;54(5):385–93.

[38] Tataranni PA, DelParigi A. Functional neuroimaging: a new generation of human brain studies in obesity research. Obes Rev 2003;4(4):229–38.

[39] Kaput J, Rodriguez RL. Nutritional genomics: the next frontier in the postgenomic era. Physiol Genomics 2004;16(2):166–77.

[40] Luan J, Browne PO, Harding AH, et al. Evidence for gene-nutrient interaction at the PPARgamma locus. Diabetes 2001;50(3):686–9.

[41] Franks PW, Luan J, Browne PO, et al. Does peroxisome proliferator-activated receptor gamma genotype (Pro12ala) modify the association of physical activity and dietary fat with fasting insulin level? Metabolism 2004;53(1):11–6.

[42] Wolff GL, Roberts DW, Mountjoy KG. Physiological consequences of ectopic agouti gene expression: the yellow obese mouse syndrome. Physiol Genomics 1999;1(3):151–63.

[43] Cooney CA, Dave AA, Wolff GL. Maternal methyl supplements in mice affect epigenetic variation and DNA methylation of offspring. J Nutr 2002;132(8 Suppl):2393S–400S.

[44] Kaput J, Klein KG, Reyes EJ, et al. Identification of genes contributing to the obese yellow Avy phenotype: caloric restriction, genotype, diet x genotype interactions. Physiol Genomics 2004;18(3):316–24.

[45] Corella D, Qi L, Sorli JV, et al. Obese subjects carrying the 11482G > A polymorphism at the perilipin locus are resistant to weight loss after dietary energy restriction. J Clin Endocrinol Metab 2005;90(9):5121–6.

[46] Montague CT, Farooqi IS, Whitehead JP, et al. Congenital leptin deficiency is associated with severe early-onset obesity in humans. Nature 1997;387(6636):903–8.

[47] Farooqi IS, Matarese G, Lord GM, et al. Beneficial effects of leptin on obesity, T cell hyporesponsiveness, and neuroendocrine/metabolic dysfunction of human congenital leptin deficiency. J Clin Invest 2002;110(8):1093–103.

[48] Bell-Anderson KS, Bryson JM. Leptin as a potential treatment for obesity: progress to date. Treat Endocrinol 2004;3(1):11–8.

[49] Lo KM, Zhang J, Sun Y, et al. Engineering a pharmacologically superior form of leptin for the treatment of obesity. Protein Eng Des Sel 2005;18(1):1–10.

[50] Kojima M, Hosoda H, Date Y, et al. Ghrelin is a growth-hormone-releasing acylated peptide from stomach. Nature 1999;402(6762):656–60.

[51] Tschop M, Weyer C, Tataranni PA, et al. Circulating ghrelin levels are decreased in human obesity. Diabetes 2001;50(4):707–9.

[52] Druce MR, Wren AM, Park AJ, et al. Ghrelin increases food intake in obese as well as lean subjects. Int J Obes 2005;29(9):1130–6.

[53] Ramos EJ, Meguid MM, Campos AC, et al. Neuropeptide Y, alpha-melanocyte-stimulating hormone, and monoamines in food intake regulation. Nutrition 2005;21(2):269–79.

[54] Vaisse C, Clement K, Guy-Grand B, et al. A frameshift mutation in human MC4R is associated with a dominant form of obesity. Nat Genet 1998;20(2):113–4.

[55] Farooqi IS, Keogh JM, Yeo GS, et al. Clinical spectrum of obesity and mutations in the melanocortin 4 receptor gene. N Engl J Med 2003;348(12):1085–95.

[56] Boyce RS, Duhl DM. Melanocortin-4 receptor agonists for the treatment of obesity. Curr Opin Investig Drugs 2004;5(10):1063–71.

[57] Batterham RL, Cohen MA, Ellis SM, et al. Inhibition of food intake in obese subjects by peptide YY3–36. N Engl J Med 2003;349(10):941–8.

[58] Batterham RL, Cowley MA, Small CJ, et al. Gut hormone PYY(3–36) physiologically inhibits food intake. Nature 2002;418(6898):650–4.

[59] Boggiano MM, Chandler PC, Oswald KD, et al. PYY3–36 as an anti-obesity drug target. Obes Rev 2005;6(4):307–22.

[60] Dhillo WS, Bloom SR. Gastrointestinal hormones and regulation of food intake. Horm Metab Res 2004;36(11–12):846–51.

[61] Edwards CM. The GLP-1 system as a therapeutic target. Ann Med 2005;37(5):314–22.

[62] Reidelberger RD, Kelsey L, Heimann D. Effects of amylin-related peptides on food intake, meal patterns, and gastric emptying in rats. Am J Physiol Regul Integr Comp Physiol 2002; 282(5):R1395–404.

[63] Reidelberger RD, Haver AC, Arnelo U, et al. Amylin receptor blockade stimulates food intake in rats. Am J Physiol Regul Integr Comp Physiol 2004;287(3):R568–74.

[64] Schmitz O, Brock B, Rungby J. Amylin agonists: a novel approach in the treatment of diabetes. Diabetes 2004;53(Suppl 3):S233–8.

[65] Cota D, Marsicano G, Tschop M, et al. The endogenous cannabinoid system affects energy balance via central orexigenic drive and peripheral lipogenesis. J Clin Invest 2003;112(3): 423–31.

[66] Pi-Sunyer FX, Aronne LJ, Heshmati HM, et al. Group RI-NAS. Effect of rimonabant, a canna-binoid-1 receptor blocker, on weight and cardiometabolic risk factors in overweight or obese patients: RIO-North America: a randomized controlled trial. JAMA 2006;295(7):761–75.

[67] Dhurandhar NV, Kulkarni P, Ajinkya SM, et al. Effect of adenovirus infection on adiposity in chicken. Vet Microbiol 1992;31(2–3):101–7.

[68] Dhurandhar NV, Whigham LD, Abbott DH, et al. Human adenovirus Ad-36 promotes weight gain in male rhesus and marmoset monkeys. J Nutr 2002;132(10):3155–60.

[69] Dhurandhar NV, Israel BA, Kolesar JM, et al. Increased adiposity in animals due to a human virus [see comment]. Internat J Obes Relat Metab Disord 2000;24(8):989–96.

[70] Dhurandhar NV, Israel BA, Kolesar JM, et al. Transmissibility of adenovirus-induced adiposity in a chicken model. Int J Obes Relat Metab Disord 2001;25(7):990–6.

[71] Atkinson RL, Dhurandhar NV, Allison DB, et al. Human adenovirus-36 is associated with increased body weight and paradoxical reduction of serum lipids. Int J Obes 2005;29(3): 281–6.

[72] Fantuzzi G. Adipose tissue, adipokines, and inflammation. J Allergy Clin Immunol 2005; 115(5):911–9 quiz 920.

[73] Hutley L, Prins JB. Fat as an endocrine organ: relationship to the metabolic syndrome. Am J Med Sci 2005;330(6):280–9.

[74] Bouloumie A, Curat CA, Sengenes C, et al. Role of macrophage tissue infiltration in met-abolic diseases. Curr Opin Clin Nutr Metab Care 2005;8(4):347–54.

[75] Hill JO, Trowbridge FL. Childhood obesity: future directions and research priorities. Pedi-atrics 1998;101(3 Pt 2):570–4.

[76] Hedley AA, Ogden CL, Johnson CL, et al. Prevalence of overweight and obesity among US children, adolescents, and adults, 1999–2002. JAMA 2004;291(23):2847–50.

[77] Popkin BM, Udry JR. Adolescent obesity increases significantly in second and third gener-ation US immigrants: the National Longitudinal Study of Adolescent Health. J Nutr 1998; 128(4):701–6.

[78] Freedman DS, Srinivasan SR, Valdez RA, et al. Secular increases in relative weight and adiposity among children over two decades: the Bogalusa Heart Study. Pediatrics 1997; 99(3):420–6.

[79] Marder W. Childhood Obesity: costs, treatment patterns, disparities in care, and prevalent medical conditions. Thomson Medstat Research Brief. Ann Arbor (MI): Thompson Medstat; 2006.

[80] Mercer SL, Green LW, Rosenthal AC, et al. Possible lessons from the tobacco experience for obesity control. Am J Clin Nutr 2003;77(4 Suppl):1073S–82S.

[81] Reducing Tobacco use: a report of the Surgeon General. Department of Health and Human Services, Centers for Disease Control and Prevention, National Center for Chronic Disease and Health Promotion, Office of Smoking and Health. 2000;2–16.

[82] Population-based smoking cessation: proceedings of a conference on what works to influence cessation in the general population. Department of Health and Human Services, National Institutes of Health, National Cancer Institute, Monograph Number 12; 2000.

[83] Krebs NF, Jacobson MS. American Academy of Pediatrics Committee on Nutrition. Prevention of pediatric overweight and obesity. Pediatrics 2003;112(2):424–30.

[84] Abramson S, Stein J, Schaufele M, et al. Personal exercise habits and counseling practices of primary care physicians: a national survey. Clin J Sport Med 2000;10(1):40–8.

[85] Crawford PB, Gosliner W, Strode P, et al. Walking the talk: Fit WIC wellness programs improve self-efficacy in pediatric obesity prevention counseling. Am J Public Health 2004;94(9):1480–5.

[86] Robinson TN. Reducing children's television viewing to prevent obesity: a randomized controlled trial. JAMA 1999;282(16):1561–7.

[87] Ludwig DS, Gortmaker SL. Programming obesity in childhood. Lancet 2004;364(9430): 226–7.

[88] Berkey CS, Rockett HR, Field AE, et al. Activity, dietary intake, and weight changes in a longitudinal study of preadolescent and adolescent boys and girls. Pediatrics 2000;105(4):E56.

[89] Gordon-Larsen P, Adair LS, Popkin BM. Ethnic differences in physical activity and inactivity patterns and overweight status. Obes Res 2002;10(3):141–9.

[90] Borzekowski DL, Robinson TN. The remote, the mouse, and the no. 2 pencil: the household media environment and academic achievement among third grade students. Arch Pediatr Adolesc Med 2005;159(7):607–13.

[91] Center on Media and Child Health, Henry J. Kaiser Family Foundation. The effects of electronic media on children ages zero to six: a history of research:1–16, Issue brief #7239; 2005.

[92] Roberts DF, Foehr UG, Rideout V. Generation M: Media in the lives of 8–18 Year-olds. Henry J. Kaiser Family Foundation. 1–145, Issue brief #7251; 2005.

[93] Galuska DA, Will JC, Serdula MK, et al. Are health care professionals advising obese patients to lose weight? JAMA 1999;282(16):1576–8.

[94] Davison KK, Birch LL. Child and parent characteristics as predictors of change in girls' body mass index. Int J Obesity Relat Metab Disord 2001;25(12):1834–42.

[95] Davison KK, Cutting TM, Birch LL. Parents' activity-related parenting practices predict girls' physical activity. Med Sci Sports Exerc 2003;35(9):1589–95.

[96] Wrotniak BH, Epstein LH, Paluch RA, et al. Parent weight change as a predictor of child weight change in family-based behavioral obesity treatment. Arch Pediatr Adolesc Med 2004;158(4):342–7.

[97] Gortmaker SL, Peterson K, Wiecha J, et al. Reducing obesity via a school-based interdisciplinary intervention among youth: Planet Health. Arch Pediatr Adolesc Med 1999;153(4): 409–18.

[98] Wiecha JL, El Ayadi AM, Fuemmeler BF, et al. Diffusion of an integrated health education program in an urban school system: planet health. J Pediatr Psychol 2004;29(6):467–74.

[99] Coon KA, Tucker KL. Television and children's consumption patterns. A review of the literature. Minerva Pediatr 2002;54(5):423–36.

[100] Brisbon N, Plumb J, Brawer R, et al. The asthma and obesity epidemics: the role played by the built environment–a public health perspective. J Allergy Clin Immunol 2005;115(5):1024–8.

[101] Sloane DC, Diamant AL, Lewis LB, et al. Improving the nutritional resource environment for healthy living through community-based participatory research. J Gen Intern Med 2003;18(7):568–75.

PEDIATRIC CLINICS

OF NORTH AMERICA

ELSEVIER
SAUNDERS

Pediatr Clin N Am 53 (2006) 795–806

Index

Note: Page numbers of article titles are in **boldface** type.